Seward's Bedside Diagnosis

D0873144

Seward's Bedside Diagnosis

David Mattingly MB FRCP (London) FRCGP

Emeritus Professor of Postgraduate Medical Studies and formerly Director, Postgraduate Medical School, University of Exeter; Honorary Consultant Physician, Royal Devon and Exeter Hospital, Exeter

The late Charles Seward MD FRCP (Ed)

Honorary Consultant Physician, Royal Devon and Exeter Hospital, Exeter; Honyman Gillespie Lecturer

THIRTEENTH EDITION

CHURCHILL LIVINGSTONE
EDINBURGH LONDON MELBOURNE AND NEW YORK 1989

CHURCHILL LIVINGSTONE
Medical Division of Longman Group UK Limited

Distributed in the United States of America by
Churchill Livingstone Inc., 1560 Broadway, New York,
N.Y. 10036, and by associated companies, branches and
representatives throughout the world.

First Edition 1949   Eighth Edition 1969
Second Edition 1952   Ninth Edition 1971
Third Edition 1955   Tenth Edition 1974
Fourth Edition 1957   Eleventh Edition 1979
Fifth Edition 1960   Twelfth Edition 1985
Sixth Edition 1962   Thirteenth Edition 1989
Seventh Edition 1965

ISBN 0-443-04077-X

British Library Cataloguing in Publication Data
Mattingly, David
   Seward's bedside diagnosis.
   1. Medicine. Diagnosis
   I. Title   II. Seward, Charles
   616.07′5

Library of Congress Cataloging in Publication Data
Mattingly, David.
   Seward's bedside diagnosis/David Mattingly, Charles
   Seward. — 13th ed.   p.   cm.
   Includes index.
   1. Diagnosis.   2. Symptomatology.   3. Physical
   diagnosis.
I. Seward, Charles.   II. Title.
RC71.3.S43 1989   88–19220
616.07′5 — dc19   CIP

Produced by Longman Singapore Publishers (Pte) Ltd.
Printed in Singapore.

Preface

This present edition marks the fortieth year since the original publication of *Bedside Diagnosis* in 1949. It was written by Charles Seward during the closing stages of the Second World War when he was serving in the Royal Army Medical Corps in India. In it he classified the causes of a disease according to the symptoms and signs it produces rather than its aetiology and pathology, this being the way in which it presents in clinical practice. This novel approach was encouraged by the late Lord Cohen of Birkenhead, Professor of Medicine at the University of Liverpool and later President of the General Medical Council. In a foreword to the first edition he said that the student who masters the principles on which this handbook is based will have an intelligent and rewarding approach to the diagnosis of disease, and will have laid a foundation which will remain whatever stress the superstructure of later knowledge may impose upon it. And even the experienced practitioner will learn much from its text.

The almost unparalleled demand for *Bedside Diagnosis* over the past 40 years has resulted in thirteen English editions and its translation into Czechoslovakian, German, Greek, Portuguese and Spanish. Its continuing success is a tribute to the wisdom and vision of Charles Seward who died in November 1987 at the age of 89.

The ever-increasing advances in clinical medicine and diagnostic techniques by the seventh edition called for the help of a younger colleague in active hospital practice, and in 1964 he enlisted my help in the task of updating successive editions. Many of the chapters have been completely rewritten and none have gone unaltered. In the present edition there are new sections on such topics as the acquired immunodeficiency syndrome (AIDS), Alport's syndrome, the adult respiratory distress syndrome, anorexia nervosa, Cryptosporidia infection, diabetes mellitus, epiglottitis, the haemolytic-uraemic syndrome, hypertrophic cardiomyopathy, hypothyroidism, IgA nephropathy, the neuroleptic malignant syndrome, parvovirus infection and Reye's syndrome.

I am grateful to Mr Patrick Beasley and Mr Wilfred Selley for their advice on dysphagia and facial pain, and to Dr Harry Hall for his chapter on Coma. Dr Ian Cruikshank and Dr Dilwyn Morgan kindly supplied up-to-date statistics on the prevalence of infectious diseases and mortality rates in Britain. Thanks are also due to Dr John Barraclough, Dr Tom Hargreaves and Dr Miles Joyner for their help in compiling the tables of 'Normal Values' which complete the book.

I am particularly indebted to Mrs Mary Wood, secretary to the Postgraduate Medical School of the University of Exeter, who has spent many hours typing the manuscripts for this and previous editions of the book. Finally I remain obliged as always to Churchill Livingstone for the help and support that I have received from them.

Exeter, 1989   D. M.

Contents

Introduction

This book has been written to meet what is believed to be a need both of the medical student and the qualified practitioner. Its aim is to provide a link between the clinician's findings at the bedside or in the consulting room and the systematic description of diseases in the more orthodox textbooks of medicine.

The first concern of any doctor when confronted with an ill patient is to reach a diagnosis as soon as possible, for on this depends the management of the case. The means to this end are his or her clinical knowledge and skill in eliciting the history and physical signs, supplemented where necessary by laboratory and radiological investigations.

Some disorders may be recognized at the first encounter but if not recourse to textbooks may be of little immediate help — they tend to group and describe diseases under physiological systems. This presumes, of course, that a tentative diagnosis has already been made. A more rational approach is to determine the most significant symptoms or signs and to consider their most likely causes in the light of the age, sex and other circumstances of the individual patient. This is the approach adopted in this book. There are not many major symptoms and signs, and the most important are considered in separate chapters.

The starting point is to obtain a full and, if possible, accurate history. The student is sometimes instructed to let the patient tell his own story but one may be baffled by a garrulous, confused, nervous, forgetful or untruthful patient. In these circumstances it is necessary to guide him towards eliciting the primary symptom, rather than those arising from it. A few examples may clarify the principles involved.

A patient complains of dyspnoea, palpitations and retrosternal pain on exertion and presents an appearance of pallor. Anaemia is a possibility and the blood picture must therefore be ascertained. If anaemia is found it is likely to be the significant physical sign, and its causes should be considered rather than those of the other symptoms mentioned, which proceed from and are secondary to it.

However, the anaemia may in turn be due to a more fundamental cause, such as haemorrhage. Thus a patient may consult the doctor because of giddiness or faintness. On being interrogated he describes what has evidently been a loss of blood in his stools. Clearly this is the significant condition which calls for investigation. Another patient may complain of debility and loss of weight but if abdominal pain, vomiting, diarrhoea, pyrexia or anaemia are present the causes of these should be considered first.

No consultation is complete without an enquiry as to the taking of drugs prescribed or bought over the counter. Drug-induced symptoms have been reported in as many as 20% of hospital patients, and in one general practice in Britain it was found that 87% of patients over the age of 75 were on medication. In old people then, in whom there may be a slowing of metabolism and impaired renal excretion, the possibility of side-effects should always be borne in mind.

Arrangement of chapters

Most chapters are concerned with a symptom or sign and begin with a synopsis of its more important causes. The pathophysiology is then considered. The diagnostic approach which follows is intended to show how the clinician, with the synopsis of causes in mind, should analyse it. This analysis will narrow down the field of possible causes and allow the doctor to select the most likely.

Diseases are important not on account of their rarity or scientific interest but in the degree to which they affect the life and health of the population. The student should cultivate a preference for the probable; a small bird on a chimney top may certainly be a canary, but it is much more likely to be a sparrow.

In the text the aetiology and clinical features of each cause or disease are discussed, followed by the relevant investigations. Many disorders present with more than one symptom or sign and a given entry may be brief to avoid unnecessary repetition. Where a fuller description is given in another chapter this is indicated by a reference to the appropriate page.

The alternative to some such diagnostic approach as is given in this book is a haphazard consideration of the most likely causes that come to mind. This is no way to undertake that most fascinating, responsible and rewarding of all forms of detection — the diagnosis of disease.

The index

At the bedside or in the consulting room the clinician is confronted not with diseases but with symptoms and signs. In this book a score of these is considered and the synopsis of each chapter analyses each symptom or sign under discussion into its causes or the diseases giving rise to it.

The index, which is chiefly one of diseases, is the reverse of the structure of the book in that it refers back from a disease to the chapters where each symptom or sign to which it may give rise is discussed. It has the additional purpose of listing the more important ways by which a disease may manifest itself. Bold type is used to indicate the fullest description of the condition.

CHAPTER 1
The physiology of pain

We all experience pain at some time or another — it is the commonest and therefore the most important symptom of disease. The term encompasses a wide variety of unpleasant sensations associated with tissue damage caused by trauma, inflammation, neoplasia, ischaemia or extremes of temperature. Pain may be described as dull, aching, colicky, stabbing, constant, burning or agonising depending upon the site and nature of the injury. Moreover, the response to pain varies greatly in different individuals and is modified by temperament and psychological factors. This adds to the diagnostic difficulties because, in addition to the objective analysis of pain in the various parts of the body which is the subject of this book, the clinician will have to assess the patient's psychological make-up.

Peripheral receptors

Peripheral pain receptors in most tissues consist of three-dimensional plexuses of unmyelinated fibres passing between the cells in all directions. Similar plexuses are present in the walls of arteries, arterioles, veins and venules and encircle each blood vessel embedded in the adventitial sheath. Free nerve endings appear to be largely confined to the cornea, teeth, tendons and ligaments.

Pain impulses arise from the depolarization of these sensory nerve endings which occurs in response to mechanical deformation or to a change in the composition of the surrounding fluid. The latter may be caused by an alteration in the hydrogen ion concentration or by the release of compounds such as histamine, bradykinin, serotonin (5-hydroxytryptamine) and prostaglandins from damaged cells. Prostaglandins are particularly important in this context as they appear to enhance and prolong the effect of other pain-producing substances. Prostaglandins are long-chain fatty acids derived from arachidonic acid which is liberated from membrane-bound phospholipids. The analgesic properties of aspirin and other non-steroidal anti-inflammatory drugs stem from their ability to act as prostaglandin synthetase inhibitors.

Peripheral pathways

'Somatic' pain originates in the skin, adjacent mucous membranes, subcutaneous tissues, musculoskeletal system and the parietal serous membranes.

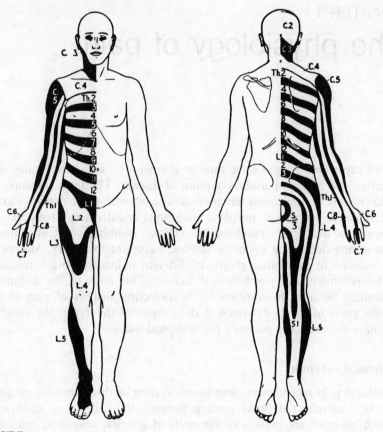

FIGURE 1

The impulses that give rise to somatic pain are carried by fine myelinated and unmyelinated sensory nerves to the spinal cord via the posterior root and trigeminal ganglia. The parietal serous membranes lying within the body cavity include the outer coverings of the dura, pleural spaces, pericardium and peritoneum, and pain arising from these structures is interpreted as coming from the corresponding dermatome. Similarly, when a sensory nerve is damaged anywhere along its course, the pain produced is felt in the peripheral tissue from which it comes. Examples of such 'referred' pain are the pain felt in the ring and little finger when the ulnar nerve is compressed at the elbow, or the sciatic pain that arises from pressure on posterior nerve roots in the lumbar spine.

Pain impulses generated in the viscera and the membranes associated with them follow a different route to the posterior root ganglia. They travel in afferent sympathetic nerves to the corresponding ganglia of the sympathetic trunk before joining nerves from the rest of the body. Visceral and deep somatic pain are more diffuse and less well-localized than pain arising from more superficial structures. This is possibly because there are fewer sensory receptors in the deeper tissues. Nearly all the sensory nerves enter the spinal cord via the posterior roots and terminate in the grey matter of the dorsal columns.

Spinal pathways

On entering the cord the pain fibres divide into many branches and form synapses in the superficial layers of the dorsal horns. Most of the noxious impulses which eventually reach consciousness in the cerebral cortex enter the central nervous system via the substantia gelatinosa. Here an intricate network of interconnecting neurones begins the task of filtering and modulating the signals before transmitting them to the brain.

The nature of the neurotransmitters in the spinal cord is still uncertain. However they may include excitatory aminoacids such as L-glutamate and L-aspartate, or one of the many polypeptides that have been isolated from nervous tissue. Substance P is the most promising of these polypeptides. Opioid peptides such as enkephalins are present in the dorsal horns and probably play a major role in weakening pain signals at this level by binding to the opiate receptors there. Epidural injections of small doses of morphine in man have been shown to produce complete analgesia for many hours.

According to the 'gate control' theory of Melzack and Wall the perception of pain is regulated by some kind of neurological gate in the substantia gelatinosa which can be opened or shut by appropriate stimuli. Incoming signals from large tactile sensory fibres and descending spinal pathways 'close the gate' by presynaptic inhibition of the neurones carrying the pain traffic, thereby reducing it to acceptable levels.

Whether this mechanism involves the release of enkephalins is still debatable but the theory would explain why vigorous massage relieves pain by 'rubbing it better' and provides a physiological basis for pain relief by transcutaneous electrical nerve stimulation. It has been suggested that the apparent analgesic effect of acupuncture works in a similar way. The afferent impulses from the acupuncture point may inhibit the pain traffic either locally in the spinal cord or — more likely — by activating the descending inhibitory pathways from the brain-stem nuclei. It may be relevant that the Chinese have claimed that acupuncture is more successful the higher up the body one goes, being particularly effective when applied to the neck.

From the dorsal horns the pain impulses ascend by two main routes, a multisynaptic short fibre system which communicates with other segments of the cord before reaching the reticular formation in the brainstem, and oligosynaptic long-fibre tracts in which the axons cross the midline and ascend directly to the reticular formation or the thalamus itself. The lateral spinothalamic tract is largely concerned with carrying discriminative somatic sensations which will help to locate the source of the pain. The spinoreticulothalamic tract conveys the messages which determine the quality and intensity of the pain.

Pathways in the brain

The reticular formation in the brain stem contains a number of nuclei which serve as relay stations on the spinoreticulothalamic pathways. From here the painful messages are passed on to the thalamus to be further processed before reaching consciousness in the cerebral cortex. The autonomic manifestations of sweating, peripheral vasoconstriction, tachycardia, nausea and vomiting which may accompany any severe pain are probably mediated by the fibres which radiate from the reticular formation to other centres in the brain stem and the hypothalamus.

In addition to these ascending pathways fibres descend from the grey matter adjacent to the aqueduct and floor of the third ventricle to the raphe nucleus in the reticular formation. This nucleus is the origin of the descending dorsolateral tract which terminates in the substantia gelatinosa of the spinal cord. All these neural junctions contain opiate receptors and high concentrations of endogenous opioid peptides. Morphine and other opiate drugs probably exert their main analgesic effect by binding to these receptors, thus reducing synaptic transmission in the ascending pathways and at the same time activating descending inhibitory impulses which close the 'gates' to incoming noxious signals in the dorsal horns.

The influence of the psyche on an individual's response to a particular painful situation may be exerted at any level in the central nervous system. Whilst it may not be possible to 'wish a pain away' there is no doubt that mechanisms do exist which allow some control by the mind over the physical discomforts of the body.

Neuroendocrine interactions

This brief and inevitably simplified account of the physiology of pain would be incomplete without some reference to the presence of endogenous opioid peptides in the pituitary gland. Soon after the discovery of the enkephalins in brain tissue and the gut it was realised that the met-enkephalin sequence of groups within the molecule was present in beta-lipotrophin, a polypeptide secreted by the anterior lobe of the pituitary. It was also present in three distinct fragments of this hormone which have been found in the peripheral blood; these are now known as endorphins. All these substances have opiate-like activity but differ from the enkephalins in having a longer-lasting action. Beta-lipotrophin and its related endorphins are derived from the same precursor molecule as corticotrophin and their plasma concentrations also rise in response to stress. The role of these opiate hormones in modulating pain perception has still to be determined, but their increased secretion during stressful situations might explain the transient freedom from pain which has been reported immediately after a severe injury. That they are potentially capable of achieving this is shown by the recent demonstration that the intrathecal injection of a few milligrams of a synthetic endorphin produced total analgesia for more than 24 hours in some patients with intractable cancer pain.

DIAGNOSTIC APPROACH

The distinctive features of any pain are of great diagnostic importance and it is recommended that they should be analysed in the following order.

Position, radiation and character

The site of the pain must be ascertained as precisely as possible. Somatic pain is usually well localised to the affected area but referred pain from the deeper tissues may be misleading. This particularly applies to pain arising from the spine and parietal serous membranes. For example, the dome of the diaphragm is supplied by the phrenic nerve (C4) and inflammatory lesions above or below the diaphragm may cause pain in the shoulder.

Visceral pain, on the other hand, is usually dull, diffuse and poorly localised, being felt mainly in the midline of the body. It too may radiate to involve other structures; thus the pain of renal calculi may pass from loin to groin whilst pain from an ischaemic heart or inflamed pericardium may be referred to arms, jaw or back.

The terms in which a patient describes his pain reflect both the character of the pain and the patient's temperament. A pain may be described as stabbing or colicky in nature but it may be disabling to one patient and merely inconvenient to another. Colicky or griping pain is caused by spasm of smooth muscle in the gut or genito-urinary system whilst one which pulsates in time with the heart beat is usually vascular in origin.

Duration and incidence

The time a pain has lasted from its first appearance should be ascertained. Acute pain is relatively short-lived but there may have been previous attacks of a similar kind. The frequency of these should be determined and it should be noted whether they are increasing or decreasing in severity and duration. Examples of recurrent pain include trigeminal neuralgia, migraine, angina pectoris and attacks of gallstone or renal colic. Pain which recurs daily but does not last all day is termed 'diurnal'. The patient should be asked for an account of its occurrence from the time of waking onwards. An example is the pain of peptic ulceration which may recur daily for weeks with intervals of freedom from pain between the bouts.

Chronic pain persisting for weeks or months is often only partially relieved by the milder analgesics. It may be constant, as in cranial arteritis and the later stages of invasive carcinoma, or it may fluctuate in intensity without disappearing completely. In severe rheumatoid arthritis, for example, the pain and stiffness in the joints are usually at their worst on waking but may ease off during the day.

Aggravating and relieving factors

These will be referred to where they are relevant to the disorder under discussion. They include the emotional state of the patient, the menses, taking of meals or any particular food, evacuation of the bowels or bladder, coughing and breathing, posture and movements of the body. The effect of any drugs, particularly analgesics, upon the symptoms should be noted.

Accompanying symptoms

These may not be volunteered and should be sought. Thus migraine may begin with scotomata and end with vomiting. Chest pain accompanied by some shortness of breath is likely to arise from the heart or pleura, and in patients with oesophageal disease there may be a history of dysphagia. In the abdomen renal pain is often accompanied by dysuria, haematuria and vomiting. Finally it should not be forgotten that any severe pain, particularly if it arises from the viscera, may be associated with extreme anxiety, sweating, tachycardia and nausea from stimulation of the autonomic nervous system.

CHAPTER 2
Head pain

The term head pain is used to cover the causes of facial pain as well as the more familiar headache.

SYNOPSIS OF CAUSES*

INTRACRANIAL

INFLAMMATORY

Meningism; **Meningitis**; Encephalitis; Poliomyelitis; Malaria; Cerebral abscess; Cranial arteritis.

NON-INFLAMMATORY

Migraine; Cluster headache; Concussion; Extradural haemorrhage; Subdural haemorrhage; **Subarachnoid haemorrhage; Stroke**; Neoplasm; Benign intracranial hypertension.

CRANIAL

Dental disease; Otitis and mastoiditis; Sinusitis; Disease of skull.

EXTRACRANIAL

Trauma; Cervical spondylosis; **Glaucoma; Corneal ulcer; Iritis**; Scleritis; Trigeminal neuralgia; Temporo-mandibular neuralgia.

GENERAL

Fever; Hypertension; Drugs; Psychogenic causes.

* Bold type is used for causes more commonly found in Europe and North America.

PHYSIOLOGY

Most people suffer from headache from time to time. Pain in the head, like pain elsewhere, is conveyed to the cerebral cortex by sensory nerves; it may be localised in their surface distribution or felt diffusely in the head as a whole. The nerves mainly concerned are:

1. The fifth or trigeminal nerve which supplies the face and underlying structures, the anterior two thirds of the scalp and the underlying perios-

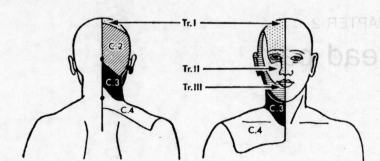

FIGURE 2

teum outside the skull. Within the skull it supplies the dura and vessels of the anterior and middle fossae in front of the tentorium cerebelli.

2. The first three cervical nerves which supply the posterior third of the scalp and periosteum and the trapezius muscle outside the skull. Within the skull they supply the dura posterior to the tentorium and the vessels of the posterior fossa.

CRANIAL PAIN

The skull itself is insensitive to pain; bony lesions such as metastases or Paget's disease seldom give rise to any discomfort. Pain may be due to dental disease, acute sinusitis, otitis or mastoiditis.

INTRACRANIAL PAIN

The brain itself is insensitive to pain. The pain-sensitive tissues are the cerebral and dural arteries, the large veins and the venous sinuses. Pain may arise from:

1. Inflammation of cerebral arteries, as in cranial arteritis
2. Dilatation of arteries as in migraine, fever or due to the effects of drugs, including alcohol
3. Traction or displacement of cerebral blood vessels, such as may occur in tumour, abscess or haemorrhage
4. Inflammation of the dura, as in meningitis

EXTRACRANIAL PAIN

Sustained spasm of the scalp or neck muscles is a common cause of pain in tension headache or cervical spondylosis. It is often accompanied by local tenderness felt mainly in the frontal and trapezius muscles. Pain may arise from inflammation, dissection or dilatation of extracranial arteries. For example, the superficial temporal artery is frequently involved in cranial arteritis. Ocular disease such as acute glaucoma or iritis causes varying degrees of extracranial pain.

Finally it may be said that the great majority of headaches are due to vascular disturbance or to sustained muscular contraction in the extracranial muscles.

DIAGNOSTIC APPROACH

The complaint of headache calls for four preliminary enquiries:

1. *Is the headache a 'casual' one?* By 'casual' is meant the occasional headache which many people get for no apparent reason. It is discussed at the end of this chapter under Psychogenic causes, but the possibility of an underlying biochemical disturbance cannot be excluded.
2. *Did head injury precede the onset of the headache immediately or by weeks or even months?* Such a headache may be a sequel to concussion or subdural haemorrhage.
3. *Is fever present?* If so, its causes must be considered. In certain infections, notably typhoid and infections caused by arboviruses, headache may be of such severity as to overshadow the presence of fever.
4. *Are drugs being taken which might account for the headache?* Women should be specifically asked whether they are taking the contraceptive pill.

Position, radiation and character

Descriptions of the character of pain vary so much with the personality of the patient that it is more useful to try to determine the degree of severity. Is this such as to render physical or mental work impossible? The pain of such catastrophes as acute meningitis or subarachnoid haemorrhage is so intense as to be outside the patient's previous experience. Vascular headaches are throbbing in character and are made worse by coughing, jolting and straining.

The position of the pain may be of considerable value in determining the likely pathology. Frontal headaches are by far the commonest and most are casual in type and respond to mild analgesics. Unilateral pain, on the other hand, occurs in migraine, cluster headache, cranial arteritis, trigeminal neuralgia, sinusitis, dental disease and inflammation of the ear. Vertex headache, especially if resistant to mild analgesics, suggests a psychogenic cause.

Duration and incidence

The time the headache first appeared should be established. The tendency to have casual headaches may be lifelong. Migraine often appears first in childhood while cranial arteritis and trigeminal neuralgia occur in the elderly. The incidence may be:

1. *Sudden*, as in subarachnoid haemorrhage or trigeminal neuralgia
2. *Diurnal*, that is occurring about the same time each day. The morning headache in hypertension and the headache of the insulin-dependent diabetic with nocturnal hypoglycaemia fall into this category
3. *Episodic*, seen typically in migraine and cluster headaches
4. *Constant*, as in meningitis and cranial arteritis

Aggravating and relieving factors

Headaches of vascular origin are frequently increased by stooping, coughing or sneezing. Some dislike of bright light is common in many forms of headache, but photophobia should make one think of meningitis. Eating may precipitate both trigeminal and temporomandibular neuralgia.

Many head pains are relieved by rest, the application of cold or the use of mild analgesics. This is not the case, however, in headaches associated with meningitis, subarachnoid haemorrhage or cerebral tumour.

Associated symptoms

Nausea and vomiting accompany many severe headaches, especially migraine, which is frequently preceded by disturbances of vision. In acute glaucoma nausea and vomiting may suggest an intra-abdominal cause. Vomiting occurs in cerebral tumours and in organic disease of the brain headache may be accompanied by confusion and personality changes. Finally, the likelihood of a psychogenic cause may become apparent as the interview proceeds.

Investigations

These will be determined by the history and severity of the symptoms. However, in persistent headache they should include measurement of the blood pressure and examination of the optic fundi. In the differential diagnosis a polymorph leukocytosis and a raised ESR point to an inflammatory cause; a positive blood culture will confirm the presence of sepsis.

Whilst examination of the cerebrospinal fluid (CSF) is invaluable in the diagnosis of meningitis and subarachnoid haemorrhage, lumbar puncture can be extremely hazardous and is contraindicated in the presence of papilloedema. Plain X-rays of the skull are seldom helpful but may reveal a fracture, enlarged pituitary fossa or Paget's disease. Although the invasive techniques of cerebral angiography and air encephalography have been widely used in the past in the search for space-occupying lesions, they have been largely replaced by the non-invasive and much safer procedure of computed tomography (CT scanning).

INTRACRANIAL CAUSES

Intracranial causes of head pain have been divided into inflammatory and non-inflammatory groups. With the obvious exceptions of migraine and cluster headache most of these are potentially life-threatening conditions.

INFLAMMATORY CAUSES

Meningism

Increased intracranial pressure without meningeal inflammation sometimes accompanies the onset of any acute infection, particularly in childhood. The patient is feverish with severe headache and neck stiffness; photophobia and Kernig's sign are often present. Only a lumbar puncture will enable meningitis to be excluded; in meningism the cerebrospinal fluid is normal but under increased pressure.

Meningitis

Aetiology
Inflammation of the meninges is due to a wide variety of microorganisms ranging in size from viruses to amoebae. The infection may spread from an adjacent source such as an infected skull fracture, or be blood-borne from a distant focus in the upper respiratory tract, lungs or middle ear. *Meningococcal meningitis* due to *Neisseria meningitidis* is still the commonest bacterial form in Britain, affecting mainly children and young adults. The organism is normally conveyed in the bloodstream from the nasopharynx. Two thirds of cases occur before the age of 5. Despite antibiotic therapy it continues to have a mortality rate of about 20%.

Fulminant meningococcal septicaemia, the Waterhouse–Friderichsen syndrome, is occasionally seen. Circulatory failure and widespread haemorrhage due to disseminated intravascular coagulation often lead rapidly to death despite antibiotic and corticosteroid therapy; the belief that death in this condition is due to adrenal failure is no longer tenable.

The next most common bacterial form of meningitis in young children is that due to *Haemophilus influenzae* and usually follows a respiratory or ear infection. In the neonate meningitis is commoner in low birthweight infants and may be due to a wide variety of organisms of which the most important are haemolytic streptococci and *Esch. coli*. *Streptococcus pneumoniae* is the commonest pathogen to be involved in meningitis following head injury, and alcoholics and diabetics are particularly susceptible. *Tuberculous meningitis* has become increasingly rare in Britain but remains a serious health hazard in developing countries.

Non-bacterial meningitis is now the commonest of all forms in the British Isles and is usually due to an enterovirus of the echo or coxsackie group, being seen most often in children and young adults. It is usually benign and short-lived but may complicate such diseases as infectious mononucleosis or leptospirosis. *Syphilitic meningitis* is now rare but if it is suspected the appropriate serological tests must be carried out. Amoebae are a very rare cause but isolated cases have appeared in Europe after swimming in contaminated water.

Meningitis is sometimes the first indication of infection by the *human immunodeficiency virus* (HIV-1) before seroconversion has taken place. Meningo-encephalitis occurring in a patient with the acquired immuno-deficiency syndrome (AIDS) is more likely to be due to an opportunistic organism such as cytomegalovirus, the herpes simplex virus, *Toxoplasma gondii* or *Cryptococcus neoformans*.

Clinical features
Common to all acute forms of meningitis are malaise, fever, severe head-ache, photophobia and vomiting. In infants the onset may be insidious with drowsiness, irritability and sometimes brief convulsions following a respir-atory or ear infection. Tuberculous meningitis in older children and adults is also of more gradual onset. It presents with malaise, irritability and slight fever; if untreated the patient becomes comatose and dies within a few weeks.

In all forms of meningitis, with the possible exception of meningitis in the infant, there will be signs of meningeal irritation such as neck stiffness and a positive Kernig's sign. Papilloedema is rare and is associated with grave complications such as cortical thrombophlebitis, cerebral abscess and subdural empyema. A purpuric rash is common in meningococcal menin-gitis and this may appear before the cerebral symptoms. A viral cause should be suspected if there is a maculopapular rash.

Investigations
Examination of the cerebrospinal fluid (CSF) is invaluable since its compo-sition may provide a clue to the cause and bacteria may be seen on mi-croscopy or cultured on appropriate media. The presence of papilloedema, however, makes this procedure extremely hazardous and on these rare occasions it may be wiser to forego a lumbar puncture. The presence of a polymorph leukocytosis suggests a bacterial cause and treatment with several antibiotics may then be started whilst awaiting the results of blood cultures. These should in any case be taken in every patient with suspected bacterial meningitis — the meningeal inflammation is nearly always part of a septicaemia.

The differences in appearance and composition of the CSF between bacterial and non-bacterial meningitis are shown in Table 2.1.

Tubercle bacilli may be seen in the CSF but are grown on culture only after a delay of several weeks. Earlier confirmation of the diagnosis of tuberculous meningitis may be provided by the finding of miliary mottling on a chest X-ray or choroid tubercles in the retina. In likely cases antitu-berculous drugs should be started immediately without waiting for positive identification of this organism.

In suspected viral meningitis specimens of CSF and stool should be sent

TABLE 2.1 Characteristics of the CSF in bacterial and non-bacterial meningitis

	Bacterial[1]	Non-bacterial
Appearance	Turbid	Clear
Pressure[2]	Raised	Raised
Cell content[3]	Polymorphs+++	Lymphocytes+
Protein	Raised	Normal or raised
Glucose	Reduced	Normal

1. In tuberculous meningitis the fluid is often clear and contains an excess of lymphocytes
2. The normal CSF pressure is less than 180 mmH$_2$O
3. The white cell count is normally less than 5 cells per mm^3

for viral studies and the advice of the microbiologist sought. Echo- and coxsackieviruses are sometimes grown from the CSF but poliovirus can only be isolated from stools. A rising titre of antibodies to a particular virus in blood samples taken at least 10 days apart is evidence of recent infection.

Encephalitis

This term is used to describe diffuse non-suppurative inflammation of the brain. It is usually associated with viral infections, particularly that due to the Herpes simplex virus. In recent years it has been recognised as a complication of infection by the human immunodeficiency virus (HIV-1) which causes AIDS. Encephalitis may occur during the initial viral infection when seroconversion is taking place, or as a sinister manifestation of the relentless destruction of brain cells by the HIV virus during the latter stages of the disease.

Encephalitis is a potentially fatal disorder and appears chiefly in children and young adults; permanent brain damage is not uncommon in survivors. It commences abruptly as a rule with headache, restlessness, fever and vomiting; stupor, delirium, convulsions and finally coma often follow. There is no increase in the white cell content of the CSF unless there is an accompanying meningitis, but the protein concentration may be raised. If AIDS is suspected blood should be taken for HIV antibodies. The causative organism may only be identified by brain biopsy.

The type of encephalitis which occasionally complicates recovery from measles or mumps or follows vaccination is more insidious in onset. It appears within 1–3 weeks of the initial illness or vaccination and is probably due to an abnormal immunological response to virus protein.

Poliomyelitis

Aetiology

The poliovirus is excreted in great numbers in the pharyngeal secretions and faeces of infected individuals, especially in the early stages of the illness. Less commonly it is spread by contaminated food or water. The incubation period is about 1 week. Active immunization has reduced this disease to the point of rarity in Britain but poliomyelitis is still a serious problem in developing countries.

Clinical features
In the absence of overt involvement of the central nervous system polio is indistinguishable from other viral infections. Tiredness, mild headache, catarrh or sore throat may be its only manifestations. In less than 1% of cases this minor illness is followed within a few days by meningitis. Most of these patients will recover without paralysis, but when paralysis does occur any muscle group may be affected. Within 2–3 days its final extent can be assessed. The onset of dysphagia or respiratory distress from brain-stem involvement are clearly grave manifestations; respiratory arrest was the commonest cause of death in past epidemics.

Investigations
The CSF will show the characteristic features of a non-bacterial meningitis. In the first week of the illness the virus may be isolated from faeces, pharyngeal swab or throat washings. The diagnosis is usually made, however, from the fourfold rise in the level of polio antibodies in sera taken at the onset and about 10 days later.

Malaria (see also Fever, p. 312)

In acute *plasmodium falciparum* infections occlusion of cerebral blood vessels by clumps of parasitized erythrocytes leads to widespread hypoxia, cell necrosis and gross cerebral oedema. Malaria should always be considered in the differential diagnosis of severe headache in travellers who have recently returned from the tropics. Enquiry may reveal that prophylactic treatment was inadequate or discontinued too soon. The headache is usually accompanied by fever and mental confusion, and there may be vomiting or diarrhoea. Cerebral malaria is often fatal within a few days in the absence of prompt treatment. The diagnosis can be rapidly confirmed by finding the parasite in thick blood films.

Cerebral abscess

Aetiology
Pyogenic infection of the brain localizing as an abscess may, like meningitis, arise from an adjacent source such as otitis media or sinusitis. Alternatively, it may be blood-borne from a distant site as in bronchiectasis, lung abscess or endocarditis.

Clinical features
The onset is insidious as a rule and may be without fever, particularly if antibiotics have been given. Headache, drowsiness and personality changes may be the only evidence of the presence of cerebral abscess. Focal symptoms such as fits and palsies may not appear for a long time; papilloedema is rare.

Investigations
Leukocytosis and a raised ESR may be found. Lumbar puncture is rarely helpful and is certainly contraindicated in the presence of papilloedema. The CSF is often normal but may contain a few pus cells and sometimes shows a slight increase in the protein content. A skull X-ray is seldom informative and an electroencephalogram (EEG) is of limited value but will probably show a focus in one or other hemisphere. Where computed tomography is available this is the investigation of choice. It will enable the lesion to be located and its probable nature to be determined. In the absence of this sophisticated technique more limited information may be obtained from an isotope scan or cerebral angiography. The precise diagnosis in life can, however, be made only by the neurosurgeon aspirating pus and by identification of the causal organism.

Cranial arteritis

Aetiology
It is now well recognised that temporal or cranial arteritis is only one manifestation of a widespread inflammation of blood vessels throughout the body. It is clearly related to polymyalgia rheumatica and many such cases have cranial artery involvement. The deposition of immune complexes in the vessel wall is thought to be responsible both for this and for other vascular diseases such as polyarteritis nodosa.

Clinical features
Cranial arteritis is seen almost entirely in the elderly of both sexes. Severe, dull, throbbing and persistent pain is felt most commonly at one temple. Whilst constant it may exacerbate sharply at times. Pain is often felt in the masseter muscles in the act of chewing.
   Intracranial vasculitis may cause mental symptoms and lead to a mistaken diagnosis of senility. Retinal artery involvement is of serious import as it may result in sudden loss of vision in one or both eyes; this was the first complaint in half of one series of reported cases. Because of the value of steroid therapy in averting or mitigating loss of vision prompt treatment is imperative. With or without eye symptoms the disorder should be regarded as a medical emergency. Pain elsewhere in limbs and joints is common, whilst cerebral and myocardial infarction occur occasionally. There is a general disturbance of health which may manifest itself as malaise, anorexia, weight loss, fever or night sweats.
   On examination the temporal and sometimes the occipital arteries may be found to be hard, thickened, tender and pulseless; the overlying skin may be reddened. Retinal haemorrhages and papilloedema are not infrequent but fundal changes may be slight even when the sight has been lost. The blood pressure is usually normal.

Investigations
Leukocytosis is sometimes present and the ESR is usually greater than

50 mm/h (Westergren). A normocytic, normochromic anaemia is often found. Serum electrophoresis may show a non-specific increase in gamma-globulin. Biopsy of the affected temporal artery will usually confirm the presence of a giant-cell arteritis.

NON-INFLAMMATORY CAUSES

Migraine

Aetiology

Migraine was described by the Sumerians 5000 years ago and later by Hippocrates. It is the most frequent cause of severe headache and is said to affect about 5% of the population. There is a family history of migraine in about two-thirds of cases, the mother being usually the relative affected. Attacks often begin at puberty and are apt to occur in women before the onset of a period; they may remit during pregnancy. An initial constriction of branches of the common carotid artery gives rise to the prodromal symptoms. This is followed by vasodilatation and distension of the vessels with throbbing pain. In many patients platelet aggregation is persistently increased during an attack and it has been suggested that the initial vaso-constriction is due to the release of serotonin from the platelets. As the levels of this substance decline the vessels dilate and the release of neuro-kinins and prostaglandins from the aggregated platelets sensitise the pain receptors in the vessel walls.

Clinical features

Attacks are episodic. Precipitating factors include psychological stress, tyramine-containing food such as cheese and chocolate, red wine and the oestrogen-containing contraceptive pill. The pain often appears on waking but when it arises during the day prodromal symptoms are common and characteristic. These include changes in mood, fortification spectra, visual field defects and occasionally transient hemiparesis or paraesthesia. Vertigo may occur, especially in later life.

These phenomena are usually followed within the hour by a severe unilateral headache which may spread to involve the whole forehead. The pain may last several hours and is often accompanied by photophobia, nausea and vomiting. Examination rarely reveals any abnormality but attacks are likely to be more frequent if hypertension is present. The head-ache is sometimes accompanied by redness of the eye and swelling of the nasal mucosa on the affected side.

Investigations

These are seldom indicated unless the blood pressure is raised or neuro-logical signs persist after the attack.

Cluster headache

Migrainous neuralgia, as it is also termed, is seen mainly in men between the third and sixth decades. Sudden attacks of severe throbbing pain begin in one nostril and spread to the adjacent orbit and temple. They may occur during the day but are commoner at night. The pain rarely persists for more than 2 hours but it can recur daily, often at the same time of day. After a cluster of attacks lasting several weeks there may be a pain-free interval of several months before the next cluster begins. Alcohol and vasodilator drugs appear to be precipitating factors, suggesting a vascular origin for these headaches. Cluster headache differs from migraine, however, in the absence of prodromal symptoms, vomiting and a positive family history.

Concussion

Concussion is the name given to the sudden loss of consciousness caused by a blow to the head. This may be momentary or persist for many hours. It is often followed by headache and amnesia. In Britain traffic accidents, industrial injuries and miscellaneous falls cause over 500 000 head injuries each year. Of these some 15% of cases have continuing symptoms. The incidence of headache following concussion was recorded in one series of 200 consecutive admissions to hospital of males over the age of 13 years. Excluding cases who died, were transferred elsewhere or became demented, headache was absent in nearly 60%, admitted on questioning in 30% and complained of spontaneously in only 11%.

Apart from a skull X-ray there is no need for further investigations unless coma persists or focal neurological signs develop. It should not be forgotten, however, that head pain following accidents may be due to extracranial causes such as injury to the cervical spine.

Extradural haemorrhage

This results from fracture of the parietal bone or the thin temporal bone with laceration of the middle meningeal artery. A haematoma forms and steadily increases in size, pressing the dura upon the adjacent brain. There may be initial loss of consciousness followed by a lucid interval. Within hours or sometimes days more severe headache develops with hemiparesis, vomiting, drowsiness and confusion merging into coma. A skull X-ray may disclose the fracture line, whilst computed tomography should confirm the diagnosis. If this condition is suspected immediate referral to a neurosurgeon is essential since the degree of recovery is proportional to the speed with which surgery is undertaken.

Subdural haemorrhage

Aetiology

This results from tearing of the sagittal veins. Haemorrhage occurs in the subdural space and slowly increases. It may be seen in infants, in whom the possibility of 'battering' must be borne in mind, or in the elderly following a trivial fall. In nearly 40% of one series of 389 cases of subdural haematoma there was no initial history of trauma though such an event, thought at the time to be trivial, was often recalled after recovery.

Clinical features
The initial complaint is of headache which is worse on waking and is increased by exertion. Relatives may have noticed some mental deterioration with failing memory and confusion. Focal signs such as hemiparesis may develop and be mistakenly attributed to cerebral thrombosis. In the infant evidence of injury such as bruising or fracture should be sought; retinal haemorrhages are nearly always present in the 'battered child'.

Investigations
The EEG is usually abnormal. The CSF may be clear, blood-stained or xanthochromic. The only certain way of establishing this diagnosis is by computed tomography, which will reveal both the site and nature of the lesion. When suspected, such a case should be referred to a neurosurgeon without delay.

Subarachnoid haemorrhage
Aetiology
This is due as a rule to the rupture of a congenital aneurysm, situated in most cases in the anterior part of the circle of Willis. It occurs chiefly in middle age and is responsible for about 2% of sudden deaths. In one series of 312 patients, of whom nearly half succumbed, headache persisted in one-third of the survivors. The contraceptive pill, multiple pregnancies, hypertension and cigarette smoking have all been implicated as risk factors. The pain is probably due to distention or traction upon the vessels.

Clinical features
When loss of consciousness is not immediate the subject is stricken with intense head pain and vomiting is common. This may soon be followed by loss of consciousness, and even after recovery there is often protracted stupor and confusion. On examination neck stiffness and a positive Kernig's sign are nearly always present. In a minority of cases subhyaloid haemorrhage and papilloedema may be found. Paralysis of cranial nerves, usually the third, and transient limb palsies are sometimes seen. The knee and ankle reflexes are often absent and the plantar responses may be extensor. Hydrocephalus is a rare but surgically-treatable complication of subarachnoid haemorrhage. It should be strongly suspected if dementia, excessive drowsiness, urinary incontinence or ataxia appear in the weeks following the initial bleed.

Investigations
A cautious lumbar puncture will reveal blood evenly mixed in the specimen. If over 12 hours have elapsed the fluid after centrifuging will have a yellow tint. Cerebral angiography will locate the site of the aneurysm in about 80%

of cases but this investigation is only justified if surgery is contemplated. If hydrocephalus is present computed tomography will show the dilated ventricles.

Stroke (see also Coma, p. 339)

Severe headache may accompany cerebral haemorrhage, embolism or thrombosis but paralysis or coma are the presenting features of a stroke. Vomiting may occur at the onset. The presence of atrial fibrillation would favour embolism as the most likely cause. Investigations are rarely helpful in establishing the precise aetiology but computed tomography can be used to exclude other causes of paralysis or coma, and may enable a distinction to be made between infarct and haemorrhage.

Transient ischaemic attacks are due to detachment of small thrombi from atheromatous carotid or vertebral arteries and occur mainly in hypertensive subjects. These 'little strokes' may precede a major embolism and are characterised by their sudden onset, brevity and repetitive nature. Headache is reported to be prominent during and after an attack in about 30% of cases, and may be unilateral. Accompanying these headaches there may be transient hemiparesis or monocular blindness. Horner's syndrome has been noticed in a few cases. Aortic angiography is sometimes of value in demonstrating surgically remedial stenosis, but is not without the risk of detaching further thrombi. Non-invasive tests which may be of value in establishing the diagnosis include ultrasound scanning of the carotid bifurcation and digital subtraction angiography.

Neoplasm

Cerebral tumours are an uncommon cause of head pain but headache is rarely the only presenting symptom. It arises from distortion of intracranial structures or increased intracranial pressure. The headache is usually of recent origin and often accompanied by vertigo or vomiting. It is frequently worst on waking and is aggravated by anything which may raise the intracranial pressure such as stooping, coughing, lifting a weight or straining at stool.

Relatives may have noticed a change in personality or intellectual impairment, while focal fits or transient hemiparesis are evidence of a progressive neurological disorder. Cerebral metastases should be suspected if there is a history of cancer surgery or heavy cigarette smoking.

No abnormality may be found on examination but the presence of papilloedema or an extensor plantar response will obviously make the diagnosis more likely. Skull X-rays are seldom helpful and the most cost-effective investigation is computed tomography. Cerebral angiography will help to delineate the extent of the abnormality and may provide some clues to its probable pathology. These patients should be referred to a neurosurgical unit without delay.

Pituitary tumours rarely give rise to head pain unless they are very large and have encroached upon the surrounding bone. In acromegaly headache is usually associated with a large, often cystic, tumour and the expanded pituitary fossa is clearly visible on a lateral skull X-ray.

Benign intracranial hypertension

Aetiology

This rare cause of severe headache is seen typically in obese young women. It may occur in association with pregnancy, oral contraceptives or the treatment of acne with tetracycline and vitamin A; it may also be seen during corticosteroid therapy. On rare occasions other drugs such as indomethacin, nalidixic acid and nitrofurantoin have been implicated. It has also been reported occasionally in Addison's disease, Cushing's syndrome and hypoparathyroidism. The cause of the raised intracranial pressure is thought to be either some disturbance in the function of the choroid plexus leading to an accumulation of cerebrospinal fluid or to intracellular hyper-hydration within the brain.

Clinical features

The condition usually presents acutely with severe throbbing headache which may be accompanied by nausea, vomiting, ataxia, blurring of vision or diplopia. In those cases associated with drugs there may be a delay of weeks or months between starting treatment and the onset of symptoms. Recurrences can occur many months after apparent recovery but the ultimate prognosis is good. On examination there will be papilloedema of varying degree with some concentric constriction of the visual fields and an occasional sixth nerve palsy.

Investigations

The CSF is normal in appearance and constitution but the pressure is usually raised. An EEG may show a mild excess of non-specific theta activity without focal or diagnostic features. Computed tomography of the brain, by excluding other causes of raised intracranial pressure, has greatly simplified the diagnosis of this condition.

CRANIAL CAUSES

Dental disease

This is the commonest cause of facial pain and the pain impulses are conveyed by the alveolar branches of the second and third divisions of the trigeminal nerve. Caries leads to pulpitis and abscess formation at the root of the tooth, but this may not be obvious on X-rays. Gingivitis may spread to the supporting tissues around the tooth and result in periodontitis and abscess formation. Sharp pain is induced by chewing or percussion and by hot, cold, sweet or salt fluids in the mouth. It may be referred to the adjacent ear or maxillary sinus.

Otitis and mastoiditis

Inflammation of the middle ear and mastoid bone can give rise to severe pain and fever is likely to be present; in a young child the pain of otitis media may not be localised. Examination of the ears, which is best carried out last in young children, should include the external auditory meatus as well as the drumhead in any case of earache or pyrexia. The mastoid area should be examined for swelling or tenderness.

Sinusitis

Aetiology
The maxillary, frontal, sphenoid and ethmoid sinuses all communicate with the nasal passages through small and easily blocked ostia. They are vulnerable to infection following colds, influenza and infectious fevers. The sinus most commonly infected in this way is the maxillary antrum. Root abscesses in the upper jaw may cause maxillary sinusitis. The upper respiratory tract is also open to attack by a variety of allergens such as pollen, house dust and industrial chemicals.

Clinical features
In acute suppuration of the sinuses pain is felt in the forehead or face. It may be throbbing in character and tends to recur daily at the same time. Nasal and postnasal discharge and fever are likely to be present, with tenderness over the affected sinus. Examination of the nose may show oedematous mucosa bathed in mucopus. Similar symptoms without fever result from nasal obstruction and rhinorrhoea of allergic origin. In chronic sinusitis pain is not a prominent feature and is often absent.

Investigations
X-rays of the skull may show total opacity of the infected sinus, a fluid level or apical abscess. Antral lavage is sometimes carried out to relieve the symptoms and to identify the offending organism.

Disease of the skull
Conditions affecting the cranium are all rare causes of headache; pain arises from involvement of the periosteum. Myeloma deposits never give rise to head pain but extensive Paget's disease of the skull may do so.

EXTRACRANIAL CAUSES

Headaches are often attributed to uncorrected errors of refraction, but there is little evidence to support this view. Discomfort may be due to screwing up the eyes in concentrated reading or bright light. There are, however, some eye disorders which do give rise to severe head pain and these are discussed below. Many studies of computer operators have reported head-ache as a common complaint. The cause of this is unknown but it could be due to the inaudible acoustic component of the non-ionizing electromagnetic radiation which is emitted from visual display units.

Trauma

In concussion loss of consciousness and the history of injury dominate the clinical picture. Most individuals who have an injury to their head have local pain or tenderness at the site of impact for a few hours or even a few days after the event. This post-traumatic headache is often due to extra-cranial local tissue injury and sustained contraction of the muscles of the scalp and neck. It may arise from torsion of the cervical spine and the muscles attached to it and is common after 'whiplash injury'. This last frequently occurs in road traffic accidents when the forward lurch and recoil of the body may result in strain of cervical intervertebral joints or ligaments, bruising of the greater occipital branch of the second cervical nerve, actual fracture of a vertebra or a disc protrusion. Severe headache starting within hours or days of concussion is, however, an important symptom of extradural haemorrhage.

Cervical spondylosis

Aetiology
This term is used to include arthritis, disc degeneration and the late effects of trauma just referred to. Pain is felt in the occipital region from a lesion of muscle, ligaments or joints in the cervical spine. In the upper two cervical vertebrae, which are not separated by an intervertebral disc, trauma or increasing age may result in osteoarthritis with resulting headache and limitation of head movements. In the lower cervical vertebrae there may be pressure upon the thecal dura by a protruding disc or fragment of a disc. Such degeneration and consequent osteophyte formation in the intervertebral foramina is common with advancing age. Radiological evidence of cervical disc degeneration has been found in 80% of adults over the age of 55 years. The non-segmental reference of pain has been attributed to pressure upon the pain-sensitive dura.

Clinical features
Occipital headache is apt to be felt on waking and lasts a few hours. The scalp may be tender, particularly at the occiput, with tender nodules in the neck muscles. Movements of the head are limited and painful.

Investigations
X-rays of the cervical spine usually reveal narrowing of the intervertebral spaces and osteophyte formation.

Glaucoma

Aetiology

This term is used to describe a number of disorders which cause the intra-ocular pressure to rise with consequent ischaemia of the optic nerve head. The increased pressure is due to obstruction to the flow of aqueous humour into the canal of Schlemm. It may be due to injury, inflammation or more commonly to structural abnormalities. Glaucoma is rare before middle-age, after which its incidence increases with each decade. It is estimated that between 1% and 2% of those over 40 will eventually suffer from it. The family incidence is high.

Clinical features

The commonest form is open-angle glaucoma which affects both sexes equally, is insidious in onset, rarely causes headache and presents with blurring of vision and field loss. Narrow-angle glaucoma, on the other hand, occurs more frequently in women with hypermetropia and often presents with head pain. One eye is usually affected more severely than the other.

Subacute attacks of narrow-angle glaucoma are heralded by unilateral headache and blurring of vision which may be mistaken for migraine. This usually occurs in the evening and resolves by morning and is characteristically accompanied by the appearance of 'halos' around lights. On examination there may be cupping of the discs and some field loss. Mild attacks often recur for several months before the onset of an acute episode which presents with severe headache, nausea and vomiting. Delay in recognising the ocular origin of these symptoms may result in permanent loss of vision.

In acute glaucoma the eye is reddened, the cornea steamy and the pupil enlarged and sluggish in its reaction to light. The intra-ocular pressure is markedly raised and the affected eye may feel stony hard to gentle digital pressure compared with the eye on the other side. This is an emergency, calling for immediate reference to an ophthalmologist.

Corneal ulcer

Certain types of corneal ulcer cause intense neuralgic headache. The dentritic ulcers of herpes simplex can seriously damage the eye. Involvement of the cornea is very common in herpes zoster of the first branch of the trigeminal nerve and is often followed by postherpetic neuralgia, especially in the elderly.

Iritis

Inflammatory conditions of the eye are sometimes found in chronic bowel and joint disorders and give rise to pain. Iritis is seen occasionally in Crohn's disease and ulcerative colitis and is not infrequent in ankylosing spondylitis and Reiter's syndrome. The eye is red and painful and vision is blurred. The pupil is small in contrast to the dilated oval, fixed pupil of glaucoma.

Scleritis

Scleritis is of unknown aetiology but is sometimes associated with connective-tissue disease. There is neuralgic pain in the areas supplied by the first and second divisions of the trigeminal nerve. It is often distressing and seemingly out of proportion to the bluish discoloration visible beneath the conjunctiva, which may be raised.

Trigeminal neuralgia

This is fortunately rare. It is seen chiefly in the elderly; when seen in the young multiple sclerosis should be considered. It is thought to result from ischaemia of unknown cause affecting a branch of the trigeminal nerve on one side of the face, usually the second division.

The onset is sudden and violent. The pain may last seconds only to recur from such stimuli as eating, speaking, brushing the teeth or shaving which act like a trigger firing off the attack. Spasmodic twitching of the face sometimes occurs on the affected side giving rise to the term 'tic douloureux'. Attacks come at first at rare intervals but these tend to shorten and the pain lasts longer. Eventually they may recur several times a day and increase in severity. Accompanying symptoms include salivation, watering eyes and running nose. No abnormality is found on examination or in X-rays of the skull.

Temporomandibular neuralgia

Dysfunction of the temporomandibular joint can give rise to pain in the face, teeth, ear or temple. It is likely to be seen by dental surgeons in tense young women suffering perhaps from domestic stress. The pain is usually unilateral and is brought on by involuntary clenching of the teeth. Osteoarthritis of the joint is common in the old, particularly in the endentulous or those with ill-fitting dentures. Pressure on the joint evokes pain and clicking upon opening or closing the jaws may be felt.

GENERAL CAUSES

These include fever, hypertension, disturbances of the psyche and many drugs. Iatrogenic headache is not uncommon but frequently unrecognised.

Fever

Headache is one of the symptoms which accompany fever and it is usually overshadowed by it. It appears to be due, as is that induced by histamine, to distension of the cerebral arteries. Headache is severe and striking, however, and so of some diagnostic value in meningitis, encephalitis, typhoid, typhus, malaria, influenza and leptospirosis.

Hypertension

The systemic blood pressure is a continuous variable and the 'normal' range is therefore an arbitrary one. The World Health Organization defines hypertension as a systolic pressure of more than 160 mmHg or a diastolic pressure greater than 95 mmHg. Mild hypertension is usually symptomless except in pregnancy, being found as a rule on routine examination. As the blood pressure rises still further headache is often the first symptom to appear. It may long precede any evidence of heart failure, renal impairment or vascular damage to the eyes or brain. It is usually intermittent to begin with and it may be many months before the patient seeks advice. The headache is usually dull or throbbing in nature and is often present on waking in the morning, easing off as the day progresses. Apart from the raised blood pressure there may be nothing else to find on examination.

Most patients with a persistently elevated blood pressure have 'essential' hypertension which, as its name implies, is of unknown aetiology. Less than 10% of cases have a recognisable cause such as Conn's syndrome, Cushing's syndrome, diabetes or renal diseases like glomerulonephritis or an ischaemic kidney. Coarctation of the aorta and phaeochromocytoma are rare conditions which are likely to be seen only once in a lifetime. In pregnancy a blood pressure of 140/90 is abnormal and is likely to be accompanied by other signs of pre-eclampsia such as ankle oedema, hydramnios or proteinuria. Diabetes and Cushing's syndrome are usually readily recognised but Conn's syndrome (primary aldosteronism) can be missed for years if hypokalaemia is not present or is wrongly attributed to diuretic therapy.

In 'malignant' or 'accelerated' hypertension the blood pressure is markedly elevated and the patient presents with severe prostrating headache, vertigo, blurring of vision, vomiting, confusion and focal neurological signs. Papilloedema is often present and there will be retinal haemorrhages and fluffy white exudates. The urine will contain protein, red cells and granular casts. This is a medical emergency requiring immediate admission to hospital. These grave symptoms and signs will gradually subside as the blood pressure is lowered by hypotensive drugs, but overenthusiastic treatment may lead to permanent blindness or hemiplegia.

Drugs

The mechanisms involved in drug-induced headache are not fully understood but in some cases such headache is associated with a rise in blood pressure. Severe headache may appear abruptly in patients taking isocarboxazid, phenelzine or tranylcypromine for depression. These drugs are monoamine-oxidase inhibitors and interfere with the metabolism of tricyclic antidepressants and sympathomimetics contained in proprietary cough medicines and decongestant nasal drops. This interaction can lead to a dangerous accumulation of pressor amines with consequent hypertension and even subarachnoid haemorrhage. Similarly, the pressor effect of tyramine present in cheese, pickled herring, broad beans, Bovril, Oxo, Marmite and red wine is greatly potentiated by these drugs.

Headache is not uncommon in women taking oral contraceptives and pre-existing migraine may be made much worse by the pill; it does not appear to be associated with hypertension in the majority. Other hormonal preparations which may cause headache are bromocryptine and stanozolol. Headache is also a side-effect of many drugs which act on the central nervous system, such as the benzodiazepines, chlormethiazole edisylate, meprobamate and the barbiturates.

In patients with heart disease the commonest drugs to cause headache are glyceryl trinitrate and isosorbide mononitrate or dinitrate used in the treatment of angina. These vasodilators presumably cause headache by producing dilatation of cerebral vessels. Headache is also a well-recognised side-effect of treatment with amiodorone hydrochloride, nifedipine, enalapril maleate and phenindione. Bronchodilators such as salbutamol and other selective beta-adrenoceptor stimulants can also cause headache, particularly when taken by mouth. In insulin-dependant diabetics headache on waking is almost always due to unsuspected hypoglycaemia during the night. It can be prevented by a suitable reduction in the evening insulin dose.

PSYCHOGENIC CAUSES

Most people experience casual headaches at one time or another and some react more readily to minor stresses and feel them more acutely than their tougher brethren. To label such people as neurotic is neither kind nor justified but a certain number of their complaints may be written off, not as to their genuineness but as to their significance. A history of such headaches is likely to be found.

That the head is conceived as taking the impact of emotional stress is recognised in the popular use of such expressions as of someone being a 'regular headache' or a 'pain in the neck', whilst 'holding one's head up' is symbolic of responding well to life's difficulties.

The 'furrowed brow of care' points to the mechanism of production of such tension headaches in which a sustained contraction of the scalp and shoulder muscles is mediated through the trigeminal, second cervical and trapezius nerves (C3–C4). The pain is felt at the vertex as a tight cap, or in the frontal and occipital regions, and tenderness is often present at the occiput and along the upper border of the trapezius muscle.

CHAPTER 3
Thoracic pain

SYNOPSIS OF CAUSES*

INTRATHORACIC

RESPIRATORY
Tracheitis; **Pleurisy; Pulmonary embolism; Pneumothorax**; Neoplasm.

CARDIOVASCULAR
Angina pectoris; Myocardial infarction; Pericarditis; Cardiomyopathy; Aortic aneurysm.

OESOPHAGEAL
Oesophagitis; Achalasia; Oesophageal spasm; Rupture.

THORACIC WALL

NON-INFLAMMATORY
Trauma; Tietze's syndrome; Osteoarthritis; **Osteoporosis**; Osteomalacia; Paget's disease; Neoplasm.

INFLAMMATORY
Herpes zoster; Bornholm disease; Tuberculosis; Ankylosing spondylitis.

EXTRATHORACIC

Cervical spondylosis; Gallstones; Hepatic abscess; Subphrenic abscess; Splenic disease; **Psychogenic causes**.

---

* Bold type is used for causes more commonly found in Europe and North America.

PHYSIOLOGY

The *thorax* extends from the supraclavicular fossae to the rib margins in front and to the level of the twelfth thoracic vertebra and ribs behind. In the thoracic wall the *shoulder area* extends from the root of the neck to the level of the axillae in front and behind. It is supplied by the third and fourth cervical nerves. The trapezius muscle, which arises from the occiput and cervical and thoracic spine, shares this innervation.

The fifth cervical to the first thoracic nerves comprise the *brachial plexus* and supply the upper limb and pectoralis muscles on each side. Lesions of

27

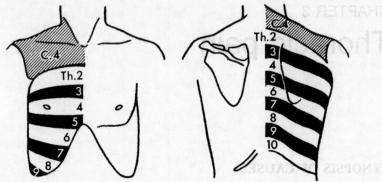

FIGURE 3

the lower cervical spine can therefore cause pain referred to the upper chest as well as to the shoulder. The dome of the diaphragm is supplied by the *phrenic nerve* (C3–C5) and when this is inflamed pain is referred to the shoulder. The chest wall from the axillae to the costal margins, comprising skin and underlying muscle, ribs and parietal pleura, is supplied by the second to the eighth thoracic nerves.

Within the thorax the viscera are supplied by afferent fibres of the sympathetic nervous system and stimulation of their nerve endings gives rise to deep-seated visceral pain. Inflammation of the visceral pleura may, however, spread to the overlying parietal pleura where it will give rise to more localised pain referred to the corresponding somatic segment. This accounts for the sharply localised pain of pleurisy and the pain referred to the shoulder when the diaphragm is involved.

The *heart and pericardium* are innervated by the first to the fifth thoracic sympathetic nerves. In ischaemic heart disease and pericarditis visceral pain is felt behind the sternum and sometimes in the epigastrum. It may be referred to the arm, jaw or interscapular area. The thoracic aorta is supplied by the first to eighth thoracic sympathetic nerves but seldom gives rise to pain.

The *oesophagus* is also supplied by the third to the eighth thoracic sympathetic nerves and thus shares in part the innervation of the heart and great vessels. Pain arises from inflammation or spasm and is felt behind the sternum or in the epigastrium. It may be mistaken for pain of cardiac origin especially if it is referred to the jaw or to the back.

DIAGNOSTIC APPROACH

In the introduction to this book it was said that the nature of some disorders may be obvious at the first encounter, or at least a tentative diagnosis can be made. Thus in practice by far the commonest cause of severe thoracic pain in the middle-aged or elderly is ischaemic heart disease. Pain which is made worse by breathing is almost always pleuritic in origin, and in a woman on the Pill or in a postoperative patient should suggest a pulmonary embolus. Trauma is a likely cause in the young whilst extrathoracic causes increase in frequency with advancing age. There remain a minority of cases where the diagnosis is obscure and in these a more methodical approach is necessary.

Position, radiation and character
The position of the pain and its possible radiation into the neck, face, back or arms should be determined. Its character may range from a dull ache to the severe constricting pain characteristic of myocardial ischaemia.

Duration and incidence
The time and circumstances of the first appearance of the pain should be ascertained and whether the incidence is sudden, diurnal, episodic or constant. A sudden onset is seen in such major disorders as myocardial infarction, pulmonary embolism, pneumothorax and vertebral collapse.

Aggravating or relieving factors
In cardiac disease pain is often aggravated by exertion or emotional stress. It is relieved by rest and, in the case of angina, dramatically eased by the administration of trinitroglycerin. Pleuritic pain is increased by coughing and deep inspiration whilst pain arising from the spine is often increased by sneezing, blowing the nose and movement. Changes of posture such as lying down or bending encourage oesophageal reflux, and the pain of reflux oesophagitis is usually relieved by milk or antacids.

Associated symptoms
Cardiac disorders are often associated with dyspnoea, palpitations and oedema of the lower limbs. Cough, especially if there is purulent or bloody sputum, points to a pulmonary cause, whilst dysphagia is almost always of oesophageal origin. Anorexia and rapid weight-loss are ominous symptoms which may suggest an underlying carcinoma of the oesophagus or bronchus; both are commoner in smokers.

INTRATHORACIC CAUSES

Thoracic pain has been classified under intrathoracic, thoracic-wall and extrathoracic causes. Of these the most frequent are causes originating within the chest. They are discussed under respiratory, cardiovascular and oesophageal sections.

RESPIRATORY CAUSES

Tracheitis
Upper respiratory tract infection, such as the common cold or influenza,

frequently involves the trachea. There is a painful cough and a feeling of rawness beneath the upper sternum. A little purulent sputum may be coughed up as the condition resolves.

Pleurisy

Aetiology
This is a surface manifestation of some underlying disease. The commonest causes in practice in the UK are pneumonia and pulmonary embolism. Less commonly, pleurisy is a complication of tuberculosis, bronchiectasis, lung abscess, bronchial carcinoma and connective-tissue disease.

Clinical features
The pain of pleurisy is characteristically stabbing in nature and exacerbated by coughing and inspiration. Deep breathing is prevented by pain and there is reduced movement on the affected side. When the diaphragm is involved pain may be referred to the shoulder. Local tenderness is often present and a friction rub is usually audible, disappearing with the onset of effusion. Pulmonary embolism is very likely if there is evidence of deep vein thrombosis in the lower limbs or frank blood in the sputum; the absence of such symptoms, however, does not exclude pulmonary embolism.

Investigations
Any sputum should be sent for culture and, if malignancy is suspected, for cytology. AP and lateral chest X-rays may reveal an underlying lesion but it should be remembered that many pulmonary emboli cast no shadow. A polymorph leukocytosis will suggest an inflammatory cause but the ESR is raised in many of these disorders and is therefore of little help in the differential diagnosis.

Pulmonary embolism

Aetiology
Embolism with infarction of the lung is increasingly recognised as being a major cause of chest pain, dyspnoea and sudden death. In a minority of cases the clot arises in a failing heart but in some 90% the emboli have their source in the leg or pelvic veins. Thrombosis in the veins is made more likely by immobilization, damage to the vessel wall and increased coagulability of the blood. Embolism is therefore a complication of surgery, pregnancy, cardiac failure and injury of the lower limbs. It also occurs in malignant disease such as carcinoma of the bronchus or pancreas, though the reason for this is not clear.

Deep vein thrombosis, with the ever-present risk of pulmonary embolism, frequently follows myocardial infarction in the elderly, particularly if there is a history of angina or if congestive cardiac failure is present. There is an increased risk of embolism in women on oral contraceptives, probably due to some effect of the oestrogen content on clotting mechanisms.

Clinical features

The picture varies widely but three presentations can be recognised:

1. A massive embolus blocking a pulmonary artery or one of its main branches presents with sudden collapse, dyspnoea, cyanosis, hypotension and chest pain suggestive of myocardial infarction. It is likely to be rapidly fatal.

2. Smaller emboli entering peripheral pulmonary arteries give rise to the more classical picture of sudden pleuritic pain with varying degrees of dyspnoea, cough and sometimes bloody sputum. The temperature and pulse rate are usually raised and there may be a pleural rub at the site of the pain. Small emboli do not necessarily give rise to pain and when this is absent the only indication of their presence may be increasing shortness of breath. Bronchospasm, appearing in congestive cardiac failure or following surgery, may be induced by emboli.

3. Recurrent micro-emboli may shower into the pulmonary arterioles silently over a period of many months. Gradual obliteration of the vascular bed leads to pulmonary hypertension, dyspnoea and finally cor pulmonale.

All these presentations may be preceded or accompanied by thrombophlebitis of the lower limbs which can be symptomless or accompanied by swelling, oedema, increased skin temperature and tenderness of the affected calf. Thickened tender veins may be palpable in the popliteal fossa or thigh.

Investigations

A normal chest X-ray is compatible even with massive embolism, but commonly there is significant absence of lung markings with translucency in the affected area. The pulmonary artery may be prominent and the heart dilated. If infarction has occurred a rounded or wedge-shaped shadow may be seen at the periphery of the lung; the diaphragm may be elevated and an effusion may develop. An isotope lung scan may show areas of reduced or absent perfusion due to infarcts, despite a normal chest X-ray.

In massive embolism the ECG may show signs of acute cor pulmonale with right bundle-branch block, large P waves and right axis deviation. The serum enzymes will be elevated if there is extensive tissue damage. Pulmonary angiography is the definitive investigation if operative removal of the clot from the pulmonary artery is thought feasible. This procedure is surprisingly well-tolerated even when the patient is desperately ill.

Pulmonary infarction is usually accompanied by a rise in the ESR and a polymorph leukocytosis. Secondary infection may occur in the infarcted areas of lung, with production of purulent blood-stained sputum. In the absence of objective signs of thrombophlebitis in the limbs the presence of thrombosis may be confirmed by venography, the use of radioactive labelled fibrinogen or ultrasound; none of these techniques, however, is infallible.

Pneumothorax

Aetiology

Total or partial collapse of the lung from entry of air into the pleural cavity results from penetrating wounds of the thorax or a fractured rib. In the absence of injury this sometimes occurs spontaneously in bronchitis and emphysema and rarely complicates tuberculosis or lung cancer. However, the great majority of cases of spontaneous pneumothorax are due to rupture of a congenital bulla on the surface of the pleura. This condition is seen most frequently in otherwise healthy young men and is apt to recur.

Clinical features

As a rule sudden severe pain is experienced on one side of the chest without any obvious precipitating cause. The pain is continuous in nature and is usually followed by increasing dyspnoea. It may be referred to the shoulder on the same side, the epigastrium or behind the sternum. In this last situation it may be mistaken for myocardial infarction in older patients.

On examination, movement of the affected side is diminished with hyperresonance on percussion and faint or absent breath sounds. When the tear in the pleura acts as a one-way valve tension pneumothorax develops. The patient becomes increasingly dyspnoeic, distressed and cyanosed. This is a medical emergency requiring immediate reduction of the raised intra-thoracic pressure by prompt insertion of a wide-bore needle or intercostal catheter connected to an underwater drain.

Investigations

Normally the edge of the partially collapsed lung is clearly visible on a chest X-ray as a line beyond which there are no lung markings. A small pneumo-thorax, however, may only be detected on expiration. An otherwise clear film, particularly one taken after re-expansion of the lung, will exclude tuberculosis or neoplasm.

Neoplasm (see also Cough, p. 232)

Thoracic pain is said to appear late in bronchial cancer. It was, however, the presenting symptom in one-third of one series of 4000 cases. The pain may be pleuritic in character from an unresolved pneumonia beyond a blocked bronchus or from direct invasion of the pleura.

CARDIOVASCULAR CAUSES

Ischaemic heart disease is one of the major health hazards in the world today. In Britain it is responsible for one-third of all deaths over the age of 45. This ischaemia, unless it results from severe anaemia or advanced aortic valvular disease, is due to *atherosclerosis* of the coronary arteries.

Atherosclerosis is multifactorial in origin and risk factors include cigarette smoking, diabetes mellitus, hypertension, hypothyroidism and hyperlipi-daemia. The incidence of deaths from ischaemic heart disease in Australia and the United States has been falling during the past 20 years. It has not been possible to identify any specific reduction of one or other risk factor to account for this decline but a similar trend is now becoming appparent in Britain.

The first manifestations of this disease are uncommon in men and rare in women before the age of 40. Widespread atheroma may, however, be present in early adult life. This was demonstrated by the finding of gross changes in the coronary arteries of young soldiers who died unexpectedly after sport or vigorous exercise. In premenopausal women atheroma is almost always associated with diabetes, hypertension, hypothyroidism or the oestrogen-containing contraceptive pill. After the age of 40 it becomes increasingly common in both sexes, the mortality in postmenopausal women approaching but never quite catching up with that of men of a similar age.

Atherosclerosis of the coronary arteries progresses silently over many years, as was shown by the Framingham survey in the United States. 30 000 people were studied over a long period, being examined at regular intervals. In one group with no complaint of chest pain or other symptoms and with previously normal electrocardiograms, the survey disclosed the development of abnormal ECG findings in 20%. Eventually the disease becomes clinically apparent with the onset of cardiac failure, angina pectoris or myocardial infarction.

Angina pectoris

Aetiology
In the majority of cases anginal pain is due to narrowing of the major coronary arteries by atherosclerosis. However, any condition which obstructs coronary flow or increases cardiac work may result in inadequate oxygenation of the myocardium, leading to the accumulation of pain-producing substances in the ischaemic muscle. Thus angina may occur as a complication of syphilitic aortitis, aortic valve disease, hypertrophic cardiomyopathy, hypothyroidism and severe anaemia. In addition, coronary angiography has shown that arterial spasm alone can cause angina at rest in some individuals and, if prolonged, may even result in myocardial infarction.

Clinical features
Anginal pain is typically episodic, being provoked by physical activity or emotional stress and relieved by rest and trinitroglycerin. It is sometimes accompanied by some shortness of breath. Occasionally the pain occurs at night and wakens the patient from sleep. The first attack often appears unexpectedly in the course of a customary effort such as climbing stairs or walking up an incline, particularly after a meal or in cold weather. The pain varies from a mild ache to a boring or vice-like pain felt behind the sternum; attacks rarely last more than a few minutes but may recur frequently. Sometimes the pain is felt in the epigastrium where it may be attributed by the patient to 'indigestion' since it is often accompanied by abdominal bloating and belching. It may radiate to the jaws, neck,

shoulders and arms and pain and paraesthesiae may be felt in the fingers; the left side is more frequently affected than the right.

Attacks often recur unchanged in character for years but are likely to increase in severity and frequency and culminate in acute myocardial infarction or sudden death. On examination, nothing abnormal may be found but during an attack the patient will be anxious and sweating with a rapid pulse; the blood pressure may be elevated and a fourth heart sound is often present.

Investigations

The ECG is normal as often as not, but transient evidence of myocardial ischaemia in the form of elevation or depression of ST segments or inversion of T waves may be evoked by exercise. Bundle-branch block or pathological Q waves point to previous myocardial infarction. Anaemia, diabetes mellitus, hyperthyroidism, hypothyroidism and syphilis are possible accompanying or causal conditions which must be excluded.

Myocardial infarction

Aetiology

As has already been said, acute myocardial infarction is due in the great majority of cases to atherosclerosis of the coronary arteries. It is predominantly a disease of the left ventricle and interventricular septum. Obstruction to the coronary blood flow from thrombosis or subintimal haemorrhage leads to acute necrosis of the cardiac muscle. Rare causes include coronary embolism complicating bacterial endocarditis or left atrial thrombosis, Marfan's syndrome, with cystic necrosis of the media of the coronary arteries, and polyarteritis nodosa. Myocardial infarction without coronary obstruction occasionally occurs in patients with severe aortic stenosis if the perfusion pressure suddenly drops during sustained effort.

Clinical features

The main presenting symptom is the sudden onset of severe prolonged pain in the chest or epigastrium where it may be mistaken for 'indigestion'. It is similar to the pain of angina but more intense and often persists for hours unless relieved by opiates. The pain is usually described as crushing or constricting in character and may radiate to the neck, jaw or upper limbs. It is frequently accompanied by some dyspnoea from pulmonary oedema. In a minority of cases, especially in diabetics and the elderly, pain is absent and dyspnoea and syncope are the presenting features. Most deaths occur in the first few hours after infarction but arrythmias are common for several days afterwards and are the major cause of cardiac arrest in hospital. Premonitory symptoms such as an increase in the frequency of pre-existing anginal attacks or abnormal tiredness for weeks beforehand may be elicited from relatives or survivors.

On examination the patient will be apprehensive and in pain unless opiates have already been given. There may be pallor, sweating, cyanosis and a poor peripheral circulation, depending on the degree of cardiogenic shock. Auscultation of the lung bases may reveal the crepitations of pulmonary oedema. The heart sounds will be faint and distant but a fourth heart sound is usually present and there may be a soft systolic murmur at the apex suggesting mitral regurgitation. A pericardial friction rub is occasionally heard. Bradycardia is evidence of heart block and a systolic blood pressure below 100 mmHg is an ominous sign. The temperature is often elevated for a few days after an infarct and recovery may be complicated by pulmonary embolism or the postmyocardial infarction syndrome. The latter occurs a week or more after the attack and presents with pericarditis and pleurisy. It responds dramatically to corticosteroids or nonsteroidal anti-inflammatory drugs.

Investigations
A chest X-ray may show cardiac enlargement or pulmonary oedema but can safely be deferred until the patient is ambulant. A polymorph leukocytosis is often present initially and a raised ESR can persist for several weeks.

The diagnosis is largely confirmed by changes in the ECG though this may be normal in the first day or two after an attack. Elevation of the ST segment in one or more leads indicates myocardial damage and is usually the first abnormality to appear. As a rule this returns within a few days to the baseline and the T wave becomes inverted. If there is necrosis of the greater part of the ventricular wall a deep Q wave appears and may persist indefinitely. Because of this changing pattern serial ECGs are often necessary to establish the diagnosis. Anterior infarcts produce changes in AVL and the anterior chest leads whilst inferior or posterior infarcts are shown up in standard leads III and AVF. Persistent elevation of the ST segment is sometimes seen in aneurysmal dilatation of the ventricular wall; angiography will be necessary to confirm this complication.

The ECG is usually enough to confirm the diagnosis but the changes may be equivocal or difficult to interpret, particularly if there has been a previous infarct. In such cases additional help is gained from enzyme estimations. Tissue necrosis releases enzymes into the circulation and a rise in the levels of these will occur if infarction has taken place. The time at which the serum level begins to rise, the peaks and the intervals before return to normal vary with each enzyme. It is therefore desirable to obtain a specimen of blood as near to the peak time as possible.

1. *Creatine kinase (CK)*. The rise occurs earlier than with the other enzymes and usually within 4–8 hours of onset, reaching a peak in 16–24 hours. It declines rapidly in 2–4 days. The normal levels are less than 130 IU/l in women and 182 IU/l in men.

2. *Aspartate aminotransferase (ASAT)*. The level begins to rise some 6 hours after onset, reaches a peak within 48 hours and falls to normal within 4–5 days. The normal levels are 0–25 IU/l.

3. *Lactate dehydrogenase (LDH)*. This reaches its peak between 48 and 72 hours after onset, falling to normal levels with 7–10 days. The normal levels are 160–480 IU/l.

With regard to the enzyme tests it should be noted that the normal ranges for a particular laboratory may differ from those given above and should be ascertained before attempting to interpret the results. The hour and day of onset and the time and date of the sampling must be known. Ideally the specimen should not be taken earlier than 8–12 hours after the onset. When blood is taken more than 3 days afterwards the lactate dehydrogenase estimation is likely to be the most informative.

Pericarditis

Aetiology
Acute pericarditis is most frequently viral in origin and often due to coxsackie- or echoviruses. It is usually accompanied by inflammation of the underlying myocardium. It may occur in rheumatic fever and is common in myocardial infarction. It is part of the postmyocardial infarction syndrome and sometimes results from trauma and operations on the heart. Rare causes include malignant infiltration, Q fever and connective-tissue disorders such as systemic lupus erythematosus. As a chronic condition, pericarditis is usually painless and may be due to tuberculosis or be present in uraemia.

Clinical features
The pain of acute pericarditis is often sharp or aching in character in contrast to the deep visceral pain of cardiac ischaemia. It is felt in the precordium and may radiate to the neck, back or left shoulder. It is exacerbated by inspiration, movements of the trunk and lying down and is relieved by sitting up and learning forward. Fever is usually present and there may be dyspnoea. A pericardial rub confirms the diagnosis but is not invariably found. The presence of other features such as polyarthritis or a rash should make one think of systemic lupus erythematosus. In most cases of viral pericarditis recovery is complete within a few weeks, but relapses do occur.

Investigations
The initial ECG may be normal, but repeated tracings will usually show ST segment elevation or inversion of the T waves in one or more of the chest leads. These abnormalities often persist for some weeks after apparent recovery. On X-ray the heart shadow is usually normal unless there is underlying heart disease. The ESR and serum enzymes may be elevated depending on the amount of tissue damage. Viral studies may reveal the causative agent in retrospect and Q fever should not be forgotten as an occasional cause. If systemic lupus erythematosus is suspected LE cells and DNA antibodies should be looked for in the blood.

Cardiomyopathy

Hypertrophic cardiomyopathy is a rare inherited disorder which results in massive patchy hypertrophy of the ventricular muscle. The myocardium fails to relax normally in diastole and this leads to a rise in left ventricular end-diastolic pressure. Outflow tract obstruction due to bulging of the septum or a mid-cavity muscular obstruction may be present. Dyspnoea, palpitations, syncope and severe and prolonged angina on effort are the presenting features.

Although this condition can appear at any age it should always be considered in the differential diagnosis of angina in a young adult, particularly if there are none of the usual risk factors for ischaemic heart disease or there is a family history of sudden death. On examination the heart will be clinically enlarged and a double apical impulse may be felt. A third heart sound and late systolic murmur may be heard at the apex. The ECG will show left ventricular hypertrophy and left bundle-branch block. The diagnosis is usually confirmed by echocardiography and cardiac catheterization.

Aortic aneurysm

Aetiology
Atherosclerosis is now a much commoner cause of aortic aneurysm than syphilis. The most usual site is in the descending aorta where it may give rise to thoracic or abdominal pain. It is seen as a rule in elderly males but occurs at an earlier age in such rare conditions as coarctation of the aorta and Marfan's syndrome.

Clinical features
An aneurysm is ordinarily silent until rupture or dissection occurs. In a typical case of dissecting aneurysm the onset consists of sudden severe substernal pain which may radiate to the back, abdomen and limbs; it is accompanied by shock. This may at first be mistaken for myocardial infarction or pulmonary embolism. Death commonly follows within hours from rupture into the pericardium or lungs. On examination transmitted pulsation may be seen in the upper chest. The apex is likely to be displaced laterally and an aortic diastolic murmur may be audible. The radial and femoral pulses may differ in force and timing on the two sides of the body. A syphilitic aneurysm of the arch or descending aorta may give rise to severe pain in the back from erosion of ribs or vertebrae.

Investigations
A chest X-ray will usually show enlargement of the aortic shadow and, if time permits, aortography will confirm the diagnosis. However the prognosis is very poor and even if surgery is undertaken the operative mortality is high. Serological tests for syphilis should not be forgotten.

OESOPHAGEAL CAUSES

Oesophagitis

Aetiology
Acute oesophagitis sometimes follows an upper respiratory infection,

prolonged gastric intubation or a *Candida* infection in a debilitated subject, particularly if on immunosuppressive therapy. The swallowing of corrosives is another important cause, seen mainly in children.

Chronic oesophagitis is nearly always due to oesophageal reflux, which may exist alone or occur with an hiatal hernia. It is seen commonly in the middle-aged and elderly, particularly in the obese and more often in women; it may appear for the first time during pregnancy. Ulceration leads to occult bleeding and fibrous stricture; haematemesis is rare. Another cause of chronic oesophagitis which is being increasingly recognised in the elderly is the retention of swallowed tablets at the lower end of the gullet. Drugs which have so far been implicated include emepronium bromide, Slow-K tablets, ferrous sulphate, antibiotics and non-steroidal anti-inflammatory drugs. In elderly patients the risk is increased by taking such tablets without adequate fluid and at bedtime.

Clinical features
In acute oesophagitis there is a temporary substernal discomfort on swallowing sufficient to deter the patient from taking nourishment. In chronic oesophagitis painful dysphagia is common. The pain has a similar distribution to that of cardiac ischaemia for which it is sometimes mistaken. It is dull and boring in character and felt behind the xiphisternum or in the epigastrium, spreading upwards into the neck. If reflux is present the discomfort will be increased by recumbency or stooping; it may then be accompanied by acid regurgitation into the mouth. Milk or antacids will provide temporary relief.

Investigations
A barium swallow may show a hiatus hernia or merely reflux through the patulous sphincter. Irregularity of the inflamed oesophageal mucosa is sometimes seen. The presence of oesophagitis can only be confirmed with certainty by endoscopy. A full blood count frequently discloses an iron-deficiency anaemia from chronic blood loss; the stools should therefore be tested on more than one occasion for occult blood.

Achalasia (see also Dysphagia, p. 109)

In this rare disorder of adult life there is impairment of the normal relaxation of the lower oesophageal sphincter leading eventually to obstruction. Intermittent retrosternal pain, similar to that seen in reflux oesophagitis, is an early complaint. It varies in intensity and may last for hours but is rapidly relieved by drinking cold water. The diagnosis is made on a barium swallow which shows the dilated and elongated oesophagus.

Oesophageal spasm (see also Dysphagia, p. 110)

Diffuse spasm of the lower half of the oesophagus is an obscure and uncommon cause of dysphagia and substernal pain. The latter may be so severe as to be mistaken for myocardial infarction. Oesophageal spasm is seen mainly in the middle-aged and elderly of both sexes. Attacks may be triggered off by emotional stresses, hasty meals or food which is too hot or too cold. When the pain comes on during eating the patient may abandon the meal — further mouthfuls only exacerbate the discomfort. Antacids may provide relief if there is an associated oesophagitis. A barium swallow is often normal but beads of contrast media may be seen trapped in the spastic lower oesophagus. Oesophagoscopy will show no abnormality unless there is an accompanying oesophagitis, but manometry will reveal abnormal contractions.

Rupture of the oesophagus

Aetiology
The commonest cause is traumatic perforation of the oesophagus during endoscopy, dilatation of a stricture or oesophageal surgery. Less commonly it may result from a traffic accident with injuries to the chest. Spontaneous rupture is rare but can follow a prolonged bout of vomiting.

Clinical features
The patient will complain of retrosternal pain which may mimic that of myocardial infarction. Since most perforations involve the mediastinal pleura the signs of a pleural effusion on one or both sides soon develop. Surgical emphysema may be palpable in the neck and audible on ausculation. When mediastinitis appears the patient will be very ill with high fever and rigors.

Investigations
A chest X-ray will show widening of the mediastinum and air in the soft tissues; there may be a pleural effusion. A marked polymorph leukocytosis is usual. This is a surgical emergency and even a delay of a few hours may be fatal.

THORACIC WALL CAUSES

For convenience, these have been divided into non-inflammatory and inflammatory sections. One cannot, however, exclude an inflammatory basis for such disorders of unknown aetiology as osteoarthritis or Paget's disease.

NON-INFLAMMATORY CAUSES

Trauma

Aetiology
Aching tender muscles occur in many situations, particularly after unaccustomed exercise. In the thorax such pain is felt chiefly in the back. Pain of varying degrees of severity follows damage to the soft tissues of the

thoracic cage; this may be sustained in sport, traffic accidents or assault. Such a cause is usually self-evident but a rib may be fractured in a bout of coughing in the chronic bronchitic or result from minimal trauma in the elderly, especially in the presence of osteoporosis. Fracture of a vertebra may be frankly traumatic but as with the ribs can follow trivial injury if the bones are already softened by osteoporosis, osteomalacia or metastases.

Clinical features

There may be tenderness, bruising or abrasions at the site of injury. The pain of rib fracture is increased by a deep breath, coughing, sneezing or movements of the trunk. 'Springing' the rib cage by pressure upon the sternum and release will cause pain at the fracture site. The pain of vertebral collapse may be localised to the damaged vertebra or may radiate around the chest wall; it is also exacerbated by coughing, sneezing and movement.

Investigations

A chest X-ray will disclose such complications as pneumothorax or haemothorax but oblique views are usually necessary to show rib fractures. A lateral picture of the thoracic spine will disclose the characteristic wedge-shaped appearance of a compression fracture. If the bones appear to be abnormally translucent the appropriate tests to exclude osteomalacia and myeloma should be done. Only a bone biopsy will provide substantive evidence of osteoporosis or osteomalacia, though these diagnoses are often inferred from radiological appearances alone.

Tietze's syndrome

Aetiology

Painful swelling of one or more costochondral junctions was first described by Alexander Tietze of Breslau in 1921. The cause is unknown, but it may be due to minor trauma since it has been reported after persistent coughing or sneezing. It is sometimes preceded by a respiratory infection and is seen both in children and adults.

Clinical features

Pain over the affected cartilages is the first symptom and may be sharp, aching or dull in character. It sometimes spreads over the anterior chest wall and into the arms; in an adult this may be mistaken for angina pectoris, particularly in patients who have already suffered a myocardial infarction. The pain may be aggravated by coughing or deep inspiration and usually follows a fluctuating course for weeks or even months before subsiding. The patient is otherwise well.

On examination a firm tender swelling of the affected cartilage will be found. The commonest sites are the second and third costochondral junctions but more than one may be involved, usually on the same side. The overlying skin moves freely and is not inflamed. The swelling slowly regresses but rarely disappears completely.

Investigations

A normal blood count, ESR and chest X-ray should exclude other rarer causes of swelling of the costochondral junction such as neoplasia, infection or rheumatoid arthritis.

Osteoarthritis

This becomes increasingly common as age advances. It has been estimated that some 60% of the population of Britain over the age of 65 suffer from this condition. In the thorax pain may be referred to the chest wall from involvement of the apophyseal and costovertebral joints or from prolapse of an intervertebral disc. Such pain tends to appear following gardening or prolonged sitting in an awkward position; it is usually relieved by mild analgesics. Occurring in the praecordium it may be severe enough to suggest myocardial infarction but it is not accompanied by dyspnoea and can be reproduced by movements of the spine. X-rays of the thoracic vertebrae in such subjects may disclose narrowing of the intervertebral spaces and the presence of osteophytes.

Osteoporosis

Aetiology

Osteoporosis is defined as a reduction in bone mass per unit volume and is due to increased bone resorption relative to bone formation. Some loss of bone substance is part of the normal process of ageing and is probably caused by the decline in sex hormone production in later life. In women it begins around the menopause and in men about a decade later. Osteoporosis occurs at an earlier age in Turner's syndrome and other hypogonadal states. It is occasionally seen as a familial disorder. Excessive bone resorption is also seen in Cushing's syndrome, prolonged corticosteroid therapy, hyperthyroidism, hyperparathyroidism, alcoholism with or without liver disease, renal failure and myelomatosis.

Clinical features

In the thoracic spine the weight of the torso results in a wedge-shaped compression of the softened vertebral bodies and the consequent characteristic stoop and loss of height. Thoracic pain of a segmental nature is often severe and increased by movement.

Investigations

Lateral X-rays of the thoracic spine will show the collapsed vertebrae and general loss of bone density. In hyperparathyroidism rarefaction of the skull and subperiosteal erosions of the phalanges may be seen on X-ray. The serum chemistry is usually normal in osteoporosis but the calcium will be elevated in primary hyperparathyroidism and may be raised in hyperthyroidism and myelomatosis. A full blood count, ESR, renal and liver function tests, sex-hormone estimations and tests of thyroid or adrenal function may be indicated in appropriate cases.

Osteomalacia

Aetiology

Osteomalacia is the adult counterpart of rickets and is due to the defective mineralization of bone from lack of vitamin D. The two sources of this fat-soluble vitamin are: 1) the irradiation of 7-dehydrocholesterol in the skin by sunlight; and 2) the dietary intake of fortified foods and fish oil. Milk and other dairy products contain only trivial quantities, although they are important sources of calcium and phosphate. It is now recognised that vitamin D itself is inactive and first undergoes hydroxylation in the liver to 25,hydroxycholecalciferol.

A second hydroxylation then occurs in the renal tubular cells to produce 1,25dihydroxycholecalciferol, which is the active metabolite. It is the concentration of this substance in the blood which regulates the intestinal absorption of calcium and phosphate and their deposition in bone and other tissues. Deficiency of this essential compound may result from reduced exposure to sunlight, inadequate dietary intake of vitamin D, steatorrhoea, defective hydroxylation in the liver or kidneys or a combination of these factors. In Britain osteomalacia is seen mainly in the housebound elderly, in Asian immigrants and in chronic renal failure. Its occasional occurrence in epileptics on anticonvulsant therapy is thought to be due to hepatic enzyme induction leading to accelerated metabolism of vitamin D metabolites in the liver.

Clinical features

Pain in the thoracic or lumbar vertebrae is aching in character and is made worse by prolonged sitting or standing. It may radiate to the chest wall. The typical waddling gait of the more severe forms of this disorder is due to a proximal myopathy but even in the milder cases there may be difficulty in getting out of a chair. Tetany is uncommon — the tendency to develop hypocalcaemia is usually corrected by a compensatory increase in para-thormone secretion. There may be evidence of intestinal malabsorption in the form of loose and fatty stools. A history of liver or renal disease, partial gastrectomy or anticonvulsant therapy may point to the most likely cause.

Investigations

X-rays of the spine will show a non-specific decrease in bone density and may reveal biconcave or 'codfish' vertebrae and compression fractures. A full skeletal survey is necessary to demonstrate the characteristic ribbon-like zones of rarefaction which occur in the more severe cases. These are known as Looser's zones or Milkman fractures and are found in the shafts of the long bones, the pubic rami and the lateral borders of the scapulae.

In most cases of osteomalacia, with the exception of those due to chronic renal failure, the serum calcium or phosphate will be at or below the normal range. The serum alkaline phosphatase is elevated except in the early stages of the disease and in vitamin-D-resistant rickets (which is rare); it is the best screening test if other causes, such as Paget's disease, can be excluded.

The serum 25,hydroxycholecalciferol levels are usually low in osteomalacia secondary to dietary deficiency, malabsorption or hepatic causes but may be normal in the elderly and those with renal disease. Whenever possible the diagnosis should be confirmed by bone biopsy; this will show excess osteoid combined with a disrupted calcification front.

Paget's disease

The thoracic vertebrae are not commonly affected in Paget's disease but when they are, severe incapacitating pain may result from vertebral collapse or pressure on adjacent nerve roots. X-rays of the spine will show replacement of the normal trabecular pattern by a coarser disorganised one. The serum alkaline phosphatase will be very high, the level depending to some extent on the amount of bone involved.

Neoplasm

Myeloma and metastases from breast, bronchus, kidney or prostate are the commonest neoplasms to affect the spine. Pain results from vertebral collapse and pressure on or infiltration of the posterior nerve roots. If X-rays show no abnormality but suspicion persists an isotope bone scan or computed tomography may disclose the lesion. Metastases in the ribs may remain painless and radiologically invisible for a long time until the periosteum is involved or fracture occurs.

INFLAMMATORY CAUSES

Herpes zoster

This is due to a virus identical with that of varicella, to which it may give rise in contacts — there are therefore two diseases caused by the one organism. A history of recent contact with varicella is, however, exceptional and it may well be that herpes zoster is due to activation of a latent virus from a previous attack of chickenpox. It affects the posterior horn, ganglion and peripheral nerve of one and occasionally two adjacent spinal segments and the rash is usually unilateral. Thoracic dermatomes, most commonly the third to the fifth, are affected in half the cases. Constitutional symptoms are uncommon.

The first complaint is of pain, burning and neuralgic in character and of segmental distribution. Within 3–4 days macules appear, developing into vesicles on an erythematous base. These become crusts which separate and may leave small, eventually paper-white scars. The pain may last for weeks and sometimes persists indefinitely or recurs spasmodically as a distressing postherpetic neuralgia. The character of the pain, its situation, the history and the typical scars when present will establish the diagnosis.

Bornholm disease

Aetiology

Bornholm disease, or epidemic myalgia as it is also known, is due to an acute infection by viruses of the coxsackie B group. These organisms also cause meningitis, gastroenteritis, myocarditis, pericarditis and orchitis, which have all been reported as occasional complications of this disease. Its name is taken from the Danish island of Bornholm, in the Baltic Sea, where a large outbreak was described in 1930. Epidemics usually occur in summer or early autumn and have been reported from most parts of the globe. All age groups are affected but the highest incidence is in children and young adults. The incubation period ranges from 2–5 days.

Clinical features
A small number of cases experience prodromal symptoms such as a feverish cold, headache and anorexia for some days beforehand but severe spasmodic pain in the chest or abdomen is the presenting symptom in the majority. In the thorax the pain is usually localised to the lower ribs but may spread up the chest wall and even involve the muscles of the shoulder girdle and neck. It is aggravated by respiration and movement and is often accompanied by a high fever, headache, cough and anorexia. On examination, visible splinting of the chest may be seen during paroxysms of pain and local tenderness may be elicited in those areas where pain is present; a pleural rub confined to the lower half of the chest may also be found. The illness usually subsides in a week or two but relapses can occur as long as a month after apparent recovery.

Investigations
The virus may be isolated from throat washings or stools at the onset of the illness, but the diagnosis is usually confirmed retrospectively from the rise in viral antibody levels in paired acute and convalescent sera.

Tuberculosis

In tuberculosis of the spine pain, sometimes of segmental distribution, results from an abscess involving two adjacent vertebrae and the intervening disc. The resulting collapse may subsequently cause neurological symptoms in the lower limbs from pressure on the spinal cord. The mid- and lower thoracic vertebrae are the ones usually involved and referred abdominal pain may suggest an intra-abdominal condition; local tenderness, rigidity of the spine and lateral X-rays will, however, disclose the real cause.

Ankylosing spondylitis (see also Fever, p. 326)

Although this disorder mainly affects the sacroiliac joints and lumbar spine it can involve the costovertebral joints of the thoracic spine and give rise to pain and limited chest expansion. At this stage of the disease the diagnosis is usually obvious from the history, examination and characteristic X-ray changes in the spine and pelvis. These consist of sclerosis, erosion and fusion of the sacroiliac joints, with 'squaring' of the vertebral bodies and calcification of the anulus fibrosus to form the classical 'bamboo spine'.

EXTRATHORACIC CAUSES

Except for psychogenic conditions, extrathoracic causes of pain in the chest are uncommon.

Cervical spondylosis

Pressure upon a lower cervical nerve root may be due to osteophyte formation or to a displaced intervertebral disc. The pain is normally referred to the neck, shoulder and arm but may also be felt in the pectoral muscles, which share the same innervation (C5–C7). Exacerbation of the pain on movement of the neck points to a cervical origin.

Gallstones (see also Lateral abdominal pain p. 92)

Impaction of a gallstone results in severe epigastric or right hypochondriac pain which is commonly referred to the right shoulder and scapular area.

Hepatic abscess (see also Lateral abdominal pain p. 91)

Abscess of the liver is usually amoebic; it may remain symptomless for some time until the onset of secondary infection. Along with malaise, fever and sweating the liver becomes tender. The abscess may reach the surface in an intervertebral space with pain and tenderness; there may be right shoulder tip pain. Fluid appears in the pleural cavity and rupture may take place into the pleural space or peritoneum.

Subphrenic abscess (see also Fever, p. 332)

In this elusive disorder pleuritic pain and effusion are frequent. Pain is occasionally referred to the shoulder from the inflamed dome of the diaphragm.

Splenic disease

Splenic enlargement from whatever cause is ordinarily painless, but rupture, abscess or infarct can cause pain of pleuritic character in the left lower chest.

PSYCHOGENIC CAUSES

Praecordial pain is a common somatic expression of anxiety, though some unremembered tear of a few fibres of thoracic muscle may be its source. In the psychoneurotic subject its situation readily gives rise to fear of heart disease. In the effort syndrome, described in the chapter on Tachycardia, it has been discussed as occurring along with palpitation and dyspnoea. A careful history and examination should be followed by explanation and reassurance.

CHAPTER 4
Abdominal pain

Pain felt in the abdominal area may have its origin within the abdomen, in the abdominal wall or be referred from an extra-abdominal source in the spine or thorax. Abdominal pain is most often due to causes within the abdominal cavity. It may be somatic or visceral in type and the distinction between these is of some diagnostic value.

SOMATIC PAIN

Pain originating in the abdominal wall or referred from the spine or thorax is localised to one or two adjacent dermatomes and is usually felt to one side or the other. It is typically described as burning, aching or stabbing in character and may be exacerbated by movement and coughing. When the parietal peritoneum is involved the pain may be agonizing in intensity and is less well-localised. At times it may be indistinguishable from visceral pain; it arises in three ways:

1. when the inflamed surface of a solid or hollow viscus comes into contact with the pain-sensitive parietal peritoneum
2. when gastric or intestinal contents, pancreatic secretions or blood leak into the abdominal cavity and similarly irritate the parietal peritoneum
3. from traction upon the parietal peritoneum of the posterior abdominal wall where it is prolonged on to the mesentery and mesocolon and shares their nerve supply

VISCERAL PAIN

It has been established that the abdominal organs, with their visceral peritoneal covering, are insensitive to such stimuli as pricking, cutting, squeezing or burning which would cause pain if applied to the skin. This is not surprising, for pain is an aid to survival and occurs in a structure or viscus when its vitality is threatened. In the natural order of things, however, these internal organs are not exposed to such attacks and health and survival would not be preserved by the possession of such sensibility. Experiments have shown that this lack of sensibility extends also to the healthy mucosa of gastric and colonic fistulae. If, however, there is congestion or inflammation of the mucous membrane the application of mechanical or chemical stimuli such as mustard will evoke pain of considerable intensity. In these experiments on the healthy mucosa of fistulae it was found, moreover, that the deliberate induction in the subject of feelings of anger or frustration resulted in an increase of mucus and lysozyme secretion, reddening of the gut and spontaneous bleeding; hypermotility was shown by strong muscular contractions following touching of the gut — bowels of wrath indeed!

Visceral pain is described as colicky, gripping, dull or aching in character depending on its source. It may be accompanied by secondary autonomic manifestations such as sweating, pallor, restlessness, nausea and vomiting. Unlike somatic pain it is poorly localised and this may be due to the fact that there are few pain receptors in the viscera compared to the skin. These visceral receptors are sensitive to stretching and chemical irritation.

Organs such as the stomach, pancreas, biliary tract, intestines, uterus and bladder, which are derived from midline structures in the embryo, have a bilateral nerve supply, and pain from them will tend to be felt centrally. The diaphragm, gall-bladder, liver, spleen, kidney, ureter, fallopian tube and ovary on the other hand have a predominantly unilateral nerve supply and pain from these structures tends to be felt laterally.

Visceral pain, then, arises from:

1. stimulation of an inflamed mucosa, as in peptic ulcer
2. bacterial or chemical inflammation, as in cholecystitis, salpingitis or infarction of bowel
3. muscular spasm, as in biliary, renal or intestinal obstruction
4. psychogenic causes

PSYCHOGENIC CAUSES

The whole alimentary tract, from the oesophagus to the rectum, is readily played upon by emotional disturbances. This reaction takes the form of spasm or hypermotility with resulting vomiting, diarrhoea or pain; these symptoms will be discussed in the following chapters. There may be oesophageal spasm, pylorospasm and the intestinal hurry of nervous diarrhoea or irritable colon. Proctalgia fugax is considered by many to have a psychological basis and recent studies have shown it to have a high incidence in patients with the irritable bowel syndrome.

Whilst a psychological cause for a symptom has to be one of exclusion positive features which may be confirmatory should be sought in the history, for these may not conform to any recognizable pattern of disease. Thus there may be other evidence of nervous disorder such as longstanding fatigue, headache, insomnia, palpitations or the hyperventilation syndrome. An anxiety state or symptoms of depression may be evident.

TOPOGRAPHY

For the purposes of diagnosis it is necessary to divide the abdomen into regions. The customary division into nine such regions by the horizontal subcostal and intertubercular lines and the vertical midclavicular lines is undesirable, for it encourages us to continue to think in watertight compartments. In practice, moreover, neither memory of the pain nor its actual location when present is precise.

A division into upper and lower abdominal areas would deprive us of the distinction between epigastric pain in gastric disorders, umbilical pain in small bowel disease and hypogastric pain in colonic conditions. It would rob us, moreover, of the distinction between lateral pain, which is frequently somatic, and central pain, which is usually visceral. Finally, whilst the customary transverse lines give three areas of similar depth in the young, in the elderly stooped subject the ribs may reach or even overlap the pelvic brim so that there is no umbilical zone at all!

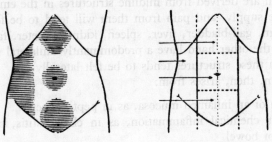

FIGURE 4

In the authors' topography, as shown in the diagrams, the linea alba is divided, as recommended by Glisson in 1676, into equal thirds giving epigastric, umbilical and hypogastric regions. There are thus three central and two lateral regions in the abdomen. In practice the pain is usually localised by the patient as being around, above or below the umbilicus or distinctly to one side of the abdomen. The most important question is therefore 'At, above or below the navel?'

CHAPTER 5
Epigastric pain

SYNOPSIS OF CAUSES*

INTRA-ABDOMINAL

OESOPHAGUS, STOMACH AND DUODENUM
Oesophageal disease; Gastritis; Peptic ulcer; Perforation of peptic ulcer; Dumping syndrome; Gastric cancer.

INTESTINE
Irritable bowel; Diverticulitis; Neoplasm; Lead poisoning.

LIVER, BILIARY TRACT AND PANCREAS
Hepatic disease; **Gallstones; Pancreatitis; Cancer of the pancreas**

VASCULAR
Aortic aneurysm; Upper mesenteric ischaemia.

EXTRA-ABDOMINAL

Muscular strain; **Heart disease**; Bornholm disease; **Psychogenic causes**.

---

* Bold type is used for causes more commonly found in Europe and North America.

PHYSIOLOGY

The epigastrium is the uppermost of the three central regions of the abdomen. It is bounded above by the rib margins sloping downwards and outwards from the xiphisternum and laterally by the mid-clavicular lines. Its vertical extent is that of the upper third of the linea alba. In practice, epigastric pain is central and definitely above the umbilicus.

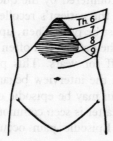

FIGURE 5

The sixth to the ninth intercostal nerves supply the skin, muscles, parietal pleura and peritoneum of the area. Within the abdomen they are joined by the corresponding sympathetic fibres from the viscera and blood vessels and enter the sixth to the ninth thoracic segments of the spinal cord.

DIAGNOSTIC APPROACH

Epigastric discomfort or pain is a common symptom and most frequently of intra-abdominal origin. Such causes are therefore considered first but the possibility of the source being outside the abdomen or of being psychogenic in origin must not be overlooked.

As is the case elsewhere in the abdomen epigastric pain may present as a single acute episode or as a chronic complaint of 'indigestion' or 'dyspepsia'. An acute onset with diarrhoea and vomiting is frequently seen in gastroenteritis but is usually short-lived and is rarely confused with more serious disorders. In adults a single episode of intense and even prostrating pain with signs of shock occurs in perforation of a peptic ulcer, gallstone colic and acute pancreatitis. In all of these radiation to the back may occur. Rarer causes are rupture of an aortic aneurysm in the elderly or of the oesophagus following endoscopy. It should not be forgotten that the pain of myocardial infarction may be felt in the epigastrium as well as in the thorax. All these conditions present so abruptly that the patient can often give the precise time of onset. Vomiting is common to all of them.

In practice the distinction between an abdominal crisis which may require urgent surgical intervention and a heart attack is rarely difficult, provided that due attention is paid to the history and physical signs.

Much more common is the chronic or intermittent discomfort of 'indigestion'. This requires a different approach. The age of the patient may be an important guide; duodenal ulcer, for example, is seen most often in middle-aged men, though women are not exempt. Gallstones, pancreatitis and neoplasms occur later in life, while vascular lesions are seen only in the elderly unless there is pre-existing rheumatic heart disease with atrial fibrillation.

The duration and incidence of the pain are the most important factors to be established and it may require patience to discover the time of the first appearance of the symptom. The frustrating answer of 'some time ago' and its variations may be countered by the question 'Days, weeks, months or years?'. Having pushed the patient's recollection back to say, 6 months ago, a further question must be put: 'Then, up to then you had no discomfort, no wind, nothing?' The patient will often reply that he has 'of course' had indigestion on and off for years. This proves on enquiry to be the epigastric pain with which the interview began.

The incidence of the pain may be episodic or diurnal, that is, occurring daily but not all day. The latter is seen commonly in peptic ulcer and rarely in mesenteric ischaemia. Episodic pain occurs in cholecystitis, while a constant nagging pain is sometimes a feature of the late stages of a gastric or pancreatic neoplasm.

Aggravating and relieving factors should be discovered. The pain of peptic ulceration appears an hour or more after meals and, with duodenal ulcer, may wake the patient from sleep; it is often temporarily relieved by more food or antacids. In reflux oesophagitis pain is brought on by stooping or recumbency and is again relieved by antacids or milk.

Associated symptoms include nausea, vomiting, anorexia, heartburn, flatulence, abdominal distension and diarrhoea. The presence of any of these symptoms helps to exclude an extra-abdominal cause. Significant loss of weight is an ominous sign; in the adolescent female it is likely to be due to anorexia nervosa while in the elderly it suggests neoplasia. With the asking of these questions, which take longer to describe than to carry out, the pain has been fully analysed and a tentative diagnosis can often be made before the patient is even examined.

INTRA-ABDOMINAL CAUSES

The great majority of cases of epigastric pain are due to causes arising in the stomach or duodenum. The gastro-oesophageal junction is here regarded as lying within the abdomen.

OESOPHAGUS, STOMACH AND DUODENUM

Oesophageal disease (see also Thoracic pain, p. 37)

The commonest condition is reflux oesophagitis, which gives rise to burning lower sternal or epigastric pain provoked by recumbency and accompanied by 'heartburn'. In rupture of the oesophagus the intense pain and shock may be indistinguishable from the much more frequently occurring perforation of a peptic ulcer. Although dysphagia is the commonest presenting symptom of oesophageal cancer, it can give rise to epigastric pain.

Acute gastritis

Aetiology

The stomach is open to insult to a degree and in a variety of ways suffered by no other organ. Though its tolerance of abuse is high, acute gastritis, with or without enteritis, is very common. Acute infections and the ingestion of bacterial toxins in food are frequent causes, whilst allergy to certain food such as milk, eggs or fish may produce it in susceptible individuals. Acute inflammation of the gastric mucosa is an undesirable side-effect of many drugs, including alcohol. Of those most commonly prescribed aspirin and other non-steroidal anti-inflammatory drugs are the most frequent offenders. Metabolic causes include uraemia and diabetic ketoacidosis.

Clinical features
The sudden onset of epigastric discomfort or pain, often accompanied by nausea and vomiting, occurs during the course of a febrile illness or following the ingestion of food or drugs. The vomited material may contain only mucus, but gastric erosions produced by drugs may bleed freely and result in haematemesis. The attack usually subsides in a day or two provided that the insult is not repeated. In diabetic ketoacidosis the onset is more gradual, being preceded by thirst, polyuria, lassitude and the smell of acetone on the breath. In such cases the severity of the pain, the presence of abdominal rigidity and the vomiting of copious brown ill-smelling fluid can be mistaken for a surgical emergency.

Investigations
Because of its transient nature investigations are rarely necessary. If haematemesis has occurred endoscopy may show gastric erosions and a blood count performed some hours after the event will disclose the degree of blood loss. In diabetic ketoacidosis the urine will be loaded with sugar and ketones and the blood glucose level will be grossly elevated.

Chronic gastritis

This is an ill-defined entity which usually develops after repeated bouts of acute gastritis and can only be diagnosed from biopsies of the stomach wall. There will be a long history of epigastric pain or discomfort which is unrelated to meals. Gastroscopy will show no ulceration but chronic inflammatory changes will be present in the gastric mucosa. The role of *Campylobacter pylori* in the aetiology of this condition is still uncertain, but this organism has been frequently found in biopsy specimens.

Chronic atrophic gastritis, on the other hand, is an autoimmune phenomenon which occurs in most patients with pernicious anaemia. It appears to be due to circulating antibodies to parietal cells and intrinsic factor, and may be accompanied by metaplasia of the gastric mucosa. There is a high risk of gastric cancer developing in these patients. A barium meal will often show an absence of rugal markings on the greater curve and fundus of the stomach.

Peptic ulcer

Aetiology
The term peptic ulcer is used to describe both acute and chronic inflammatory lesions in the stomach and duodenum. Acute ulcers are largely confined to the stomach and, with the rare exception of those accompanying extensive burns, are usually associated with alcohol excess or aspirin and other non-steroidal anti-inflammatory drugs. They are frequently multiple and may bleed, especially in the elderly. Perforation is extremely uncommon for they rarely penetrate deeper than the muscularis mucosae; spontaneous healing is the rule within a week or two.

Chronic ulcers probably begin as small breaks in the mucosal surface which expose the underlying tissues to proteolytic digestion by the gastric juices. Why the normal mucosal defences break down remains a mystery. During their active phase they penetrate the muscular layer and damage the underlying blood vessels so that haemorrhage or perforation may result. When healing occurs the ulcer crater is reduced in size by the contraction of fibrous tissue at its base and the growth of granulation tissue. Recurrent ulceration at the same site leads to extensive scarring with consequent deformity; in the case of pyloric and duodenal ulcers this may be severe enough to cause pyloric obstruction.

Chronic gastric ulcers are commoner in the lower social classes, in heavy cigarette smokers and in patients with chronic bronchitis; the peak incidence is in middle age. Ulceration usually occurs in an area of abnormal mucosa and is therefore a complication of chronic gastritis. The reflux of bile from the duodenum is thought to damage the gastric mucosa in some individuals and to encourage ulcer formation.

Duodenal ulcers occur mainly in the first part of the duodenum. In Britain and many other countries they are much commoner than gastric ulcers and men are far more often affected than women. The peak incidence is in middle age and stress, alcohol and cigarette smoking have all been implicated as causal factors. They are usually associated with hypersecretion of both acid and pepsin by the parietal cells of the stomach. Hypercalcaemia stimulates acid secretion, which probably accounts for the known occurrence of duodenal ulcers in primary hyperparathyroidism. In the Zollinger–Ellison syndrome duodenal ulceration accompanies gastrin-secreting tumours of the pancreas or duodenum. This rare disorder should be suspected if a duodenal ulcer does not respond to medical treatment or recurs after gastric surgery, particularly if there is unexplained diarrhoea.

Although chronic gastric and duodenal ulcers appear to arise from different pathological processes they occasionally co-exist in the same patient. Whether corticosteroid therapy actually initiates peptic ulceration is still controversial but there is little doubt that steroids are a common cause of indigestion, may delay healing of existing ulcers and increase the risk of haemorrhage and perforation. One striking and so far unexplained feature of peptic ulceration is the wide variation in its incidence in different parts of the world and even within the British Isles; in Scotland the prevalence of duodenal ulcer is much higher than it is south of the border.

Clinical features

The commonest symptom is upper abdominal pain related to meals. It is usually localised to the epigastrium and varies in intensity from a vague discomfort to a dull gnawing pain which may be temporarily relieved by food, milk, antacids or histamine H_2-antagonists. When the pain radiates through to the back it is likely that the ulcer has penetrated the wall of the stomach or duodenum to involve the pancreas and other retroperitoneal tissues.

Classically the pain of gastric ulceration is maximal in the first hour after a meal, while that of a duodenal ulcer is temporarily relieved by eating and at its worst some 2–3 hours after food. Hunger pain, waking the patient from sleep and relieved by milk or antacids is very characteristic of a duodenal ulcer and the patient should always be asked if he suffers from it. However this pattern is not invariable and the history cannot always be relied upon to differentiate between the two types of ulcer.

Peptic ulcer pain is episodic in nature, occurring in bouts lasting a few weeks and followed by long symptom-free intervals when the ulcers heal. The duration of the present attack must be ascertained and enquiries should be made about previous episodes. The familial incidence of peptic ulcers should not be forgotten and enquiries should be made about other members of the family. Persistent indigestion in a previously symptom-free middle-aged or elderly patient should arouse suspicion of possible malignancy and its relief by antacids or histamine H_2-antagonists is no guarantee of its benign nature.

Nausea, 'heartburn', flatulence and a feeling of abdominal distention or 'bloating' after meals may accompany the pain. Vomiting is unusual and suggests the presence of gastritis or pyloric obstruction; the vomit usually consists of recently ingested food unless bleeding has occurred, when it will contain frank blood or 'coffee grounds'. Anorexia and weight-loss are seen more commonly with gastric ulcers, when the patient may avoid eating for fear of provoking the pain which follows a meal.

On examination there is usually little to find apart from some epigastric tenderness. The major complications of peptic ulceration are acute haemorrhage, anaemia secondary to chronic blood loss in the stools, pyloric obstruction and perforation.

Investigations

The majority of chronic peptic ulcers can be demonstrated by a barium meal, especially if double-contrast techniques are used. Deformity of the duodenal cap is evidence of past or present ulceration even if no actual crater is seen. Barium meals are also helpful in determining whether there is any pyloric obstruction, oesophageal reflux or evidence of gastric atrophy or hypertrophy. What they will not do is to enable a firm distinction to be made between benign and malignant gastric ulcers. Fibreoptic endoscopy has the great advantage that multiple biopsies can be taken when the nature of a gastric ulcer is in doubt, and it will often reveal the presence of small ulcers and superficial gastric erosions which have been missed on barium meal examination.

A routine blood count will reveal anaemia, and occult blood tests on the stools will be positive if there has been recent bleeding. Measurements of gastric acid secretion in the basal state and after maximal stimulation with histamine or pentagastrin are of limited value and have been abandoned in routine clinical practice. In the rare Zollinger–Ellison syndrome the fasting serum gastrin level, determined by radioimmunoassay, is usually greater than 300 pmol/l (600 ng/l).

Perforation of peptic ulcer

Aetiology

This serious and common occurrence is seen more frequently in men than in women. Most of the ulcers involved are situated at the pylorus or in the duodenum. Several thousand cases occur annually in Britain and some 10% are fatal, survival depending upon prompt diagnosis and treatment. Mortality is particularly high in the elderly, in whom the symptoms may be obscured by intercurrent disease. At perforation the gastric contents may pass down the right paracolic gutter to the right iliac fossa and simulate acute appendicitis. Peritonitis may be localised at first but soon spreads over the whole abdominal cavity.

Clinical features

Severe upper abdominal pain is the commonest presenting symptom and the precise time of onset can often be given by the patient. A history of dyspepsia or of known peptic ulcer is likely and should be sought. The pain is felt initially in the epigastrium or to the right of the midline but soon spreads to involve the whole abdomen. It is aggravated by coughing and deep breathing and, in contrast to the restlessness associated with gall-bladder pain and renal colic, the patient is reluctant to move. Enquiry should be made for shoulder-tip pain, because this information is frequently not volunteered and its presence makes perforation more likely. Vomiting is not uncommon at the onset but repeated vomiting is unusual. The pain may deceptively diminish some hours after the event.

On examination there will be marked tenderness and guarding, particularly in the upper abdomen; rebound tenderness may be elicited as low as the right iliac fossa. The abdomen becomes distended and does not move with respiration; bowel sounds disappear with the onset of ileus. The rigidity, like the pain, may diminish in a few hours and give rise to the dangerous impression that improvement is taking place. This is followed, however, by a rise in the pulse rate and the patient's condition becomes more grave with each hour that passes.

What has been said refers of course to acute perforation; we must not overlook the occasional case of chronic posterior perforation of the duodenum with abscess formation behind the cap. A review of the history may then disclose hunger pain in the past and an episode of intense epigastric pain and retching which subsided and has been forgotten.

Investigations

X-rays of the chest and abdomen, taken soon after the event and in the erect position, often show gas under the right diaphragm; this sign may not be present if some hours have elapsed for small quantities of gas may have been absorbed by then. A moderate rise in the serum amylase level is compatible with perforation and only if the level is greater than 1000 units should acute pancreatitis be considered as an alternative diagnosis. Further investigations are largely superfluous for prompt laparotomy will confirm the diagnosis and enable the damage to be repaired.

Dumping syndrome

The too precipitate passage of food into the duodenum following gastric operations may cause epigastric discomfort and fullness, nausea, vomiting and diarrhoea. With this there is a feeling of faintness accompanied by pallor and sweating. This diagnosis should not be accepted until recurrent ulceration at the anastomotic site has been excluded as far as possible by endoscopy.

Gastric cancer

Aetiology

This is one of the commonest malignancies of the gastrointestinal tract and is responsible for about 10 000 deaths a year in England and Wales. There is a logarithmic increase in incidence from middle age onwards but no age is exempt and persistent indigestion in a younger person may be ignored with tragic results. As with peptic ulceration, males are more vulnerable than females. In the aged the condition may long remain silent. Although the cause is unknown it is commonly preceded by gastric atrophy, and it is therefore hardly surprising that cancer develops in a significant proportion of patients with pernicious anaemia. Benign gastric ulcers rarely undergo malignant change. The growth may be infiltrating, ulcerating or hypertrophic in character and occasionally neoplastic changes are confined to the mucosa; about 95% are adenocarcinomas.

Clinical features

The early diagnosis of this condition is extremely difficult — symptoms referable to the stomach are late in appearing and may be indistinguishable from chronic gastritis or peptic ulceration. The growth may reach a considerable size before the patient feels unwell. Vague epigastric discomfort with fullness after meals and waning appetite may respond temporarily to some modification of the diet or antacid therapy. Although some cases present with haematemesis and melaena, an iron-deficiency anaemia from chronic blood loss in the stools is a more common presentation; such patients should always be thoroughly investigated to exclude cancer of the stomach. Dyspepsia arising for the first time in a patient with pernicious anaemia should also arouse suspicion, particularly if it is associated with loss of weight. There may be dysphagia with growths involving the fundus of the stomach, or repeated vomiting from pyloric obstruction.

In the early stages the appearance of the patient is normal and nothing may be found on examination. As the disease advances a cachectic sallow complexion appears and there may be epigastric tenderness and a palpable mass. Hepatic enlargement, ascites and oedema of the legs from thrombosis of the pelvic veins are late manifestations; pelvic metastases may be felt on rectal examination.

Investigations
These are identical to those described under peptic ulceration but endoscopy is essential if an early diagnosis is to be made. This procedure takes precedence over barium meal examinations for even extensive growths in the cardia may be missed on X-ray. Hepatic metastases are detectable by ultrasound scanning or computed tomography.

INTESTINAL CAUSES

Irritable bowel (see also Lateral abdominal pain, p. 90)

Epigastric pain occurred in 42% of a series of 67 cases of this common disorder. This should be remembered when endoscopy and barium studies are negative.

Diverticulitis

Duodenal and jejunal diverticula are uncommon causes of epigastric pain and may long remain silent. When pain does occur it is increased by meals and may be accompanied by nausea and vomiting, borborygmi and bloating of the abdomen. Haemorrhage occurs occasionally and diarrhoea and malabsorption sometimes develop in the 'blind loop' syndrome. The much more common colonic diverticula do not give rise to epigastric pain.

Neoplasm (see also Lateral abdominal pain, p. 88)

An adenocarcinoma of the proximal colon sometimes presents with epigastric pain provoked by meals. It should be thought of in an elderly subject with persistent dyspepsia and a normal barium meal and cholecystogram.

Lead poisoning (see also Umbilical pain, p. 72)

Acute lead poisoning is now rare in Britain though it was once quite common in workers in metal and foundry trades and is still an occupational hazard amongst potters and artists using lead paints. In severe cases there is agonising upper abdominal pain, copious vomiting and stubborn constipation. Blood and urinary lead levels will be elevated.

LIVER, BILIARY TRACT AND PANCREAS

Hepatic disease (see also Lateral abdominal pain, p. 91)

The liver may be the seat of acute or chronic inflammation, abscess, neoplasia or the congestion of cardiac failure. The pain in liver disease is usually felt in the right hypochondrium but in acute conditions may initially be epigastric and so gains mention here. In the prodromal stage of acute viral hepatitis epigastric pain is accompanied by pyrexia, anorexia, nausea and vomiting. Jaundice commonly appears about the fifth day of the illness but is often absent in mild cases.

Gallstones (see also Lateral abdominal pain, p. 92)

Impaction of a gallstone is a common abdominal emergency and sometimes presents with severe epigastric pain and vomiting. Sooner or later, however, the pain shifts to the right hypochondrium. Cholecystitis may follow and the tenderness and guarding become generalised. The condition may then be mistaken for a ruptured viscus or acute pancreatitis.

Pancreatitis

Aetiology

Acute pancreatitis is uncommon in Britain, occurring in some 3000 cases yearly. Although its exact cause is unknown it is frequently associated with biliary tract disease and chronic alcoholism. It is a rare complication of Behçet's syndrome, mumps, viral hepatitis, penetrating duodenal ulcers and primary hyperparathyroidism. In addition it is sometimes seen following treatment with drugs such as corticosteroids, diuretics, azathioprine, phenformin, rifampicin, tetracyclines and oral contraceptives.

Clinical features

The onset is occasionally mild but typically it presents suddenly with severe epigastric pain which radiates through to the back. The patient is reluctant to move and the pain may be eased by leaning forward. It is accompanied by persistent vomiting and there may be signs of peripheral circulatory failure such as tachycardia, hypotension, pallor, cyanosis and cold sweating extremities. Tenderness in the upper abdomen is usual but rigidity and other signs of peritonitis are late in appearing. The patient is febrile and jaundice sometimes results from pressure upon the bile ducts by the swollen gland or from exacerbation of associated biliary tract disease. In the haemorrhagic form bruising may appear in the flanks or around the umbilicus.

Initially the condition may mimic myocardial infarction, cholecystitis, gallstone colic, intestinal obstruction, perforation of a peptic ulcer, mesenteric artery thrombosis or rupture of an aortic aneurysm. It is very important to establish the diagnosis as soon as possible, because surgery in acute pancreatitis is very hazardous and is seldom indicated. The release of large quantities of proteolytic enzymes leads to widespread tissue damage and erosion of major blood vessels, and death in the early stages may result from retroperitoneal haemorrhage or disseminated intravascular coagulation. Infection, particularly by coliform organisms, is a serious and potentially lethal complication leading to abscess formation in the pancreas, lesser sac and left subphrenic space. Recurring attacks of acute pancreatitis are not uncommon in the presence of biliary tract disease or chronic alcoholism.

Investigations

A raised serum amylase level of more than 1000 units is rarely found in any other condition; more modest elevations are however seen in perforation of a duodenal ulcer or following the administration of opiates. Impaired glucose tolerance from damage to the beta cells will result in elevated blood glucose levels. The possibility of myocardial infarction means that an ECG will be required. This may indeed show equivocal changes such as depressed ST segments or inverted T waves in some leads. X-rays of the abdomen occasionally reveal pancreatic calcification or opaque gallstones, while the absence of gas under the diaphragm or of multiple fluid levels make perforated peptic ulcer or intestinal obstruction less likely. A moderate polymorph leukocytosis is usually present. Hypocalcaemia, occurring between the third and fifteenth day, is an ominous sign. A normal serum calcium level during an attack does not exclude hyperparathyroidism; if this is suspected further calcium studies should be done when the patient has recovered. The serum bilirubin may rise during the attack and elevation of the liver enzymes is due either to biliary tract obstruction or associated liver disease.

Cancer of the pancreas

Aetiology
Adenocarcinoma of the pancreas accounts for some 6000 deaths annually in England and Wales. It is commoner in men and occurs chiefly in later life. The incidence is rising in all Western societies and, while no cause has been found, cigarette smoking has been firmly implicated as a risk factor. The growth may commence in the head, body or tail of the organ and symptoms and signs vary accordingly; the head is the commonest site.

Clinical features
More than half the cases present with epigastric pain. It is dull, boring, steadily worsening and often radiating through to the back; a minority present with back pain only. The pain is made worse by food and recumbency, and, traditionally, is eased by sitting forward. Weight loss may be the predominant feature, and obstructive jaundice from occlusion of the common bile duct develops sooner or later. Pruritus is common as in other forms of obstructive jaundice. Anorexia, diarrhoea and steatorrhoea largely account for the progressive loss of weight.

On examination the tumour is seldom palpable but as with any other posthepatic biliary obstruction an enlarged gall-bladder may be felt. In a minority of cases thrombophlebitis of the leg or pelvic veins may herald the onset of this disease.

Investigations
Establishing the diagnosis is often difficult and depends largely upon indirect evidence of pancreatic involvement. Diabetes develops in some patients and a glucose tolerance test will confirm this. A barium meal may show deformity and widening of the duodenal loop. Endoscopic retrograde pancreatography, done by cannulation of the ampulla of Vater through a fibreoptic endoscope, can in skilled hands reveal an otherwise undiagnosable growth. Jaundice, if present, arises from biliary obstruction and the urine will then contain bilirubin and the stools will be pale from excess fat. In some cases only exploratory laparotomy will provide the answer.

VASCULAR CAUSES

These are uncommon causes of epigastric pain and are seen mainly in the elderly of both sexes.

Aortic aneurysm

The usual site of this vascular lesion is below the renal arteries. In Britain the majority are due to atherosclerosis, but inflammatory abdominal aortic aneurysms are recognised as a separate entity and account for about 10% of cases. This latter condition mainly affects men and is probably due to an endarteritis of the vasa vasorum which supply the aortic wall. Both varieties are encountered in elderly hypertensive patients and may exist without symptoms until the occurrence of dissection or rupture. This catastrophe presents acutely with intense epigastric or umbilical pain and shock. Pain in the back is common if the aneurysm is leaking posteriorly and may be mistaken for 'lumbago'. The inflammatory variety differs from the atherosclerotic type in producing pain in the abdomen or back before dissection has occurred, and is associated with a raised ESR.

On examination a pulsatile epigastric mass is felt in the majority and there may be a vascular bruit over it. A plain abdominal X-ray will often show the characteristic curvilinear calcification in the aortic wall, and ultrasonography or computed tomography may be useful in confirming the dilatation of the aorta. Surgical resection and replacement with a prosthetic graft is usually necessary, but low-dose steroid therapy may abolish symptoms and shrink the fibrotic mass in the inflammatory variety.

Upper mesenteric ischaemia

Aetiology
The small intestine is supplied by the coeliac and upper mesenteric arteries which may become stenosed or occluded by atherosclerosis or rarely by embolism. Thus this disorder is found in association with hypertension, ischaemic heart disease and intermittent claudication.

Clinical features
Although this condition is characteristically seen in the elderly, cases still occur in younger patients with rheumatic heart disease and atrial fibrillation. Chronic arterial insufficiency of the small bowel gives rise to epigastric or umbilical pain which appears soon after a meal; this has been described as 'abdominal angina'. It may be so severe as to induce fear of eating, with consequent weight loss; the ischaemia may cause diarrhoea and malabsorption. The condition can continue in this way for a year or two before the onset of acute infarction of the bowel or death from other causes.

Investigations
Selective angiography of the superior mesenteric artery and its branches may enable a firm pre-operative diagnosis to be made.

EXTRA-ABDOMINAL CAUSES

The nerve supply of the epigastrium is shared with the lower thorax and consequently the same conditions can give rise to pain in either region. Spinal lesions of the lower thoracic vertebrae usually cause pain referred to the lateral abdominal area but reference can occur to the epigastrium, particularly in children.

Muscular strain

Unaccustomed exercise involving the abdominal muscles or prolonged coughing may cause pain in the epigastrium and elsewhere in the abdominal wall. It can be reproduced when lying down by lifting the head.

Heart disease (see also Thoracic pain, p. 32)

In ischaemic heart disease and acute pericarditis pain is sometimes referred to the epigastrium where it may be attributed by the patient to 'indigestion'. It is seldom associated with any abdominal rigidity or tenderness and a careful history and electrocardiogram will usually suffice to establish its cardiac origin. In congestive cardiac failure a distended liver may give rise to pain and tenderness in the epigastrium as well as the right hypochondrium. Again, the cause is usually obvious from the history and physical examination.

Bornholm disease (see also Thoracic pain, p. 43)

This acute viral infection is associated with both upper abdominal and thoracic pain. In young children the characteristic stabbing or 'vice-like' pain is felt more often in the epigastrium than in the chest. During paroxysms there will be splinting and rigidity of the abdominal wall. Malaise, fever, headache and a recent upper respiratory infection will point to the correct diagnosis.

PSYCHOGENIC CAUSES

It was said in the chapter on abdominal pain that the alimentary canal is readily played upon by the emotions. Dyspepsia of nervous origin is very common in anxiety states, depression and in neurotic subjects. The complaint is usually of vague epigastric discomfort not clearly related to meals and often accompanied by belching from aerophagy. Suggestive accompanying symptoms and the patient's description and history often point to a psychological origin. The irritable bowel syndrome has already been referred to earlier in this chapter.

In anorexia nervosa dyspeptic symptoms are not infrequent and sometimes lead to fruitless investigations of the gastrointestinal tract before the true nature of the condition is appreciated. Severe weight loss and amenorrhoea in the adolescent female is seldom due to intra-abdominal disease.

CHAPTER 6
Umbilical pain

SYNOPSIS OF CAUSES*

INFLAMMATORY
Enteritis; Appendicitis; Mesenteric adenitis; **Acute peritonitis**; Haemoperitoneum; Tuberculous peritonitis.

OBSTRUCTIVE
Strangulated hernia; Adhesions; Intussusception; Volvulus; **Crohn's disease**; Meckel's diverticulum; Diverticulitis; Neoplasm; Drugs; Impaction of faeces, gallstones or food bolus.

VASCULAR
Aortic aneurysm; Mesenteric ischaemia; Henoch-Schönlein purpura; Polyarteritis nodosa; Sickle cell disease.

METABOLIC
Lactose intolerance; Addison's disease; Porphyria; Lead poisoning; **Irritable bowel**; Periodic syndrome.

* Bold type is used for causes more commonly found in Europe and North America.

PHYSIOLOGY

The umbilical region is bounded laterally by the midclavicular lines, and vertically it occupies the middle third of the linea alba. Umbilical pain is nearly always of intra-abdominal origin and mainly arises from spasm or obstruction of the small bowel. It is carried by afferent sympathetic fibres to the ninth to eleventh thoracic segments of the cord.

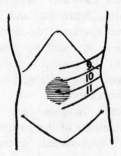

FIGURE 6

Spasm may arise from inflammation of the wall of the gut, ischaemia, metabolic disorders or distension caused by interference with the onward passage of its contents. Intestinal obstruction may result from extramural causes such as strangulation of a hernia or adhesions; mural causes, as in neoplasia, intussusception or volvulus; or rarely from intramural causes such as a large gallstone or an impacted food bolus.

The distinction, which may depend upon the patient's memory, between epigastric and umbilical pain and also between umbilical and hypogastric pain, may not be clear-cut and must not be laboured. In practice umbilical pain is that felt around and centred upon the umbilicus.

DIAGNOSTIC APPROACH

Acute central abdominal pain permits of no delay in diagnosis. In practice the diagnostic approach is modified by the presence of accompanying symptoms and also by consideration of the age of the patient, for certain disorders are commoner in, and may indeed be restricted to, particular age groups.

Thus diarrhoea with or without vomiting points to an inflammatory cause, as a rule gastroenteritis. Here the existence of other cases in the family, at school or in the neighbourhood should be enquired for. The presence of constipation with umbilical pain and perhaps vomiting raises the question of intestinal obstruction, of which strangulated hernia is the commonest cause.

In children, apart from enteritis, one must be alert for the possibilities of appendicitis, intussusception, Henoch–Schönlein purpura, Meckel's diverticulum, lactose intolerance and the periodic syndrome. In young adults appendicitis remains common, irritable bowel is frequent and Crohn's disease a possibility. In middle age hernias and adhesions from previous operations are common causes of acute intestinal obstruction, while in the elderly neoplasia, volvulus and colonic diverticulitis become increasingly frequent. It is in this latter age group that vascular conditions such as mesenteric ischaemia and aortic aneurysm are seen.

Rarities include porphyria, lead poisoning, Addison's disease, sickle-cell anaemia and polyarteritis nodosa. Unless there are suggestive clues in the history or examination to draw attention to their presence they should not be considered until the more common causes of central abdominal pain have been excluded.

INFLAMMATORY CAUSES

Enteritis (see also Diarrhoea, p. 130)

In enteritis pain only arises if there is any hold-up of intestinal contents. Diarrhoea is the more prominent symptom and there may be vomiting if there is an accompanying gastritis. In *Shigella* and *Salmonella* infections colicky pain is marked. Giardiasis may affect children in endemic areas and is seen in returning tourists. There is abdominal discomfort with attacks of explosive diarrhoea and the pale stools of steatorrhoea. In typhoid pain is not prominent whilst in cholera it is overshadowed by the intense diarrhoea and collapse.

Appendicitis

Aetiology
Appendicitis is so common in Europe and America that it should be suspected as being the most likely cause of acute abdominal pain. It must be the first thought in children, however young, in whom it is about ten times as common as mesenteric adenitis and intestinal obstruction. In old people appendicitis is apt to progress rapidly and with little complaint to gangrene or perforation with abscess formation.

Clinical features
At onset the pain is usually felt in the umbilical area but it can begin in the right iliac fossa. It is persistent but may vary in intensity and is accompanied by anorexia and nausea and sometimes vomiting. When the appendix lies behind the caecum or in the pelvis diarrhoea or frequency of micturition may be present. There is then a risk, particularly in young children, of attributing the symptoms to gastroenteritis or urinary tract infection. After some 6–12 hours the peritoneal surface of the appendix becomes involved and contact with the anterior abdominal wall causes the pain to shift to the right iliac fossa.

On examination the temperature and pulse may be normal at first but rise later. Furring of the tongue and an offensive breath occur early in the illness. The abdomen is rarely distended and maximum tenderness is usually elicited about 5 cm from the right anterior superior iliac spine on a line drawn from that point to the umbilicus (McBurney's point). Muscle guarding develops in the right iliac fossa and rebound tenderness, which occurs in about two-thirds of cases, is a reliable sign.

These findings may be minimal when the appendix is retrocaecal or in the pelvis. In the former case the right thigh may be flexed as a result of psoas spasm and passive straightening may be painful; when the organ lies in the pelvis flexion and internal rotation of the right hip may increase the pain, and tenderness will be elicited on rectal examination.

Investigations
The urine must be examined to exclude urinary tract infection. A polymorph leucocytosis is often present by the time the patient is seen. In suspected appendicitis the most important investigation is a prompt laparotomy and a surgical opinion should be sought without delay.

Mesenteric adenitis (see also Lateral abdominal pain, p. 86)

This condition cannot always be distinguished from appendicitis in child-hood. It is usually associated with an upper respiratory infection.

Acute peritonitis

Aetiology

The peritoneum may become infected:

1. From a penetrating wound, during peritoneal dialysis or in the course of an abdominal operation
2. In acute salpingitis, following a septic abortion or puerperal infection, or the rare pneumococcal peritonitis seen in young girls
3. Most commonly from appendicitis, perforated peptic ulcer or acute pancreatitis

Less common conditions causing perforation include cholecystitis, typhoid fever, fulminating ulcerative colitis and the gangrenous gut of unre-lieved obstruction or mesenteric thrombosis. In diverticulitis and Crohn's disease peritonitis may occur but more often the inflammation remains localised and forms an abscess. The use of corticosteroids in Crohn's disease and ulcerative colitis increases the risk of perforation; more importantly they may mask the clinical features.

Clinical features

The initial presentation will depend upon the underlying cause. The pain of a perforated peptic ulcer will be epigastric and sudden in onset whilst that of a pelvic infection will begin low down and progress steadily upwards. With the onset of peritonitis pain becomes widespread, vomiting is frequent and the pulse rate rises. Abdominal distension, rebound tender-ness and guarding are present and no bowel sounds are audible. This is in contrast to intestinal colic or the early stages of obstruction when borbor-ygmi are marked. In a day or two the rigidity subsides but the diagnosis should have been made long before this stage is reached.

Investigations

A blood count will show a polymorph leucocytosis and straight X-rays of the abdomen may reveal dilated loops of bowel and fluid levels. An early laparotomy is indicated provided that pancreatitis has been excluded as far as this is possible.

Haemoperitoneum

Blood in the abdominal cavity is very irritant and can mimic the signs of peritonitis. In young women it can arise from a ruptured ectopic pregnancy. Other causes include a lacerated spleen following injury, and a leaking aortic aneurysm in an elderly atherosclerotic subject. Intra-abdominal bleeding should always be considered if there is a history of fainting at the onset. Shoulder-tip pain is commoner than in inflammatory conditions and blood in the peritoneal cavity should be considered if the patient is more comfortable in the sitting position. The presence of fever does not exclude this diagnosis, and the pulse rate and blood pressure may be normal despite extensive haemorrhage.

Tuberculous peritonitis

Aetiology
Tuberculosis of the bowel is now rare in the UK but is still relatively common in the Middle East, India and Asia. Tuberculous peritonitis should not be forgotten as a possible cause of unexplained fever and abdominal pain in immigrants from these countries. It may arise as a blood-borne infection from a pulmonary focus or directly from a tuberculous lesion in the intestine, mesenteric lymph nodes or fallopian tubes.

Clinical features
The condition appears insidiously over a period of months with lassitude, loss of weight, intermittent fever and night sweats. Vague central abdominal pain may be accompanied by a complaint of abdominal distension and sometimes diarrhoea. On examination the characteristic doughy feeling may be elicited on palpation. Ascites is a late development.

Investigations
A chest X-ray should be done to exclude pulmonary disease. The ESR is likely to be raised and a normocytic normochromic anaemia may be present. The white count may show a relative lymphocytosis. A positive Mantoux test is helpful if BCG has not been given in the past but laparotomy is usually necessary to confirm the diagnosis.

OBSTRUCTIVE CAUSES

Strangulated hernias and adhesions from previous surgery or pelvic sepsis account for the majority of cases of intestinal obstruction. In Britain about 2000 patients die annually from this common and dangerous surgical emergency, the mortality being highest at the extremes of life. In young children intussusception is a frequent cause whilst in the elderly colonic growths and diverticulitis become increasingly common. Volvulus is an unusual cause in Western Europe but is said to be exceedingly common in Eastern Europe and parts of Africa and India; the reason for this geographical variation is unknown.

Small bowel obstruction presents with sudden colicky or continuous umbilical pain, vomiting and abdominal distension. When it is complete constipation is absolute and no flatus is passed, though an initial bowel action may occur; with incomplete obstruction there may be normal stools or diarrhoea. Augmented bowel sounds will be heard on auscultation and

X-rays of the abdomen may show distended loops of bowel with multiple fluid levels.

Colonic obstruction differs from that of the small bowel in the order of the onset of symptoms and signs. Progressive constipation often alternating with spells of diarrhoea are seen in the two most common causes, cancer and diverticulitis. The constipation may be accompanied by attacks of abdominal pain and increasing distension; vomiting is often absent. Abdominal palpation sometimes discloses a mass and impacted faeces may be evident on rectal examination.

Strangulated hernia

Aetiology

Inguinal hernia is much commoner than the femoral type and affects males more frequently than females. It is seen in infancy and childhood as well as in adults and incarcerated inguinal hernia is, with intussusception, the commonest cause of intestinal obstruction in the first 2 years of life. Femoral hernia is said to be commoner in women and rarely appears before puberty. Umbilical hernia can occur at any age but is particularly prone to develop in obese middle-aged women. It should not be forgotten that hernial protrusions may occur elsewhere than at the hernial orifices; through abdominal scars, at the site of a colostomy or in the midline above or below the umbilicus (para-umbilical hernia).

Clinical features

The symptoms and signs of a strangulated hernia are those of acute intestinal obstruction. A palpable lump will usually be felt at one or other of the hernial orifices unless the hernial sac is very small or the patient is very obese. Local pain and tenderness may be absent even when gangrene is present. Intestinal obstruction developing a few days after an abdominal operation is likely to be due to herniation from partial disruption of the abdominal wound; a serosanguineous discharge from the incision may be its only local manifestation.

Investigations

X-rays of the abdomen may show fluid levels but this is not invariable and there are no radiological or laboratory tests to indicate the presence of gangrene. Blood should be taken for cross-matching and routine biochemistry whilst the patient is being prepared for emergency surgery.

Adhesions

These are the late sequels of abdominal surgery and pelvic infection and form an increasing proportion of cases of intestinal obstruction; they usually involve the lower ileum. The colon is rarely obstructed by bands or adhesions except in the vicinity of the ileocaecal angle.

Intussusception

Aetiology
The great majority of cases occur during the first two years of life. They are usually ileocaecal or ileocolic, the latter being more lethal. Adenoviral infection of the bowel is thought to be a factor in initiating the process. In adolescence it is rare and nearly always due to a Meckel's diverticulum; in adults it is occasionally caused by a cancer or large polyp.

Clinical features
A hitherto healthy infant is suddenly seized with severe colicky pain and may scream, with knees drawn up. This occurs in bouts between which the child is listless and pallid. Vomiting follows and straining may produce blood from the rectum or the extrusion of the intussusceptum. The passage of 'redcurrant-jelly stools' is typical. The abdomen is distended and unless the intussusception has reached the hepatic or splenic flexure it is likely to be palpable as a sausage-shaped lump; the apex is sometimes felt in the rectum and blood will be present on the examining finger.

Investigations
A barium enema provides confirmation of the diagnosis and may effect reduction, thus avoiding operation.

Volvulus

This uncommon cause of obstruction in the colon is seen most often in the elderly. It usually involves the sigmoid and is likely to be of sudden onset with umbilical or hypogastric pain, vomiting, constipation and marked distension. A mass may be palpable in the lower abdomen and X-rays will show a loop of bowel grossly distended by gas and fluid levels.

Crohn's disease (see also Lateral abdominal pain, p. 86)
Attacks of partial obstruction with colicky umbilical pain and vomiting lasting a day or two are not uncommon.

Meckel's diverticulum

This congenital anomaly, situated a short distance above the ileocaecal valve, is present in about 2% of people and is commonly silent. When it does give rise to symptoms these are apt to occur in children and young adults. As a diverticulum of the bowel it may become infected or cause obstruction from torsion or intussusception. Since some diverticula contain ectopic gastric mucosa peptic ulceration may lead to perforation or haemorrhage. All these abnormalities can give rise to severe central abdominal pain. The diagnosis is seldom made pre-operatively. Painless, massive rectal bleeding is a not uncommon mode of presentation in young children.

Diverticulitis (see also Lateral abdominal pain, p. 87)

Adhesions or stricture may complicate diverticulitis of the colon with increasing constipation leading to obstruction.

Neoplasm

In the small intestine cancer is rare and accounts for less than 5% of growths in the alimentary canal. The Peutz–Jeghers syndrome occurs anywhere in the gut as multiple polypi which initiate obstruction from intussusception; it is associated with freckles around the mouth. Carcinoid tumours secrete serotonin which stimulates the smooth muscle of the bowel and has long been held responsible for the recurring attacks of diarrhoea, abdominal pain, bloating and severe tenesmus which are characteristic of this disorder. Serotonin also stimulates fibroblastic activity and this is probably the cause of the fibrous strictures which lead to intestinal obstruction. Its conversion to 5-hydroxyindole acetic acid accounts for the large quantities of 5-HIAA which may be found in the urine. The flushing and tachycardia associated with carcinoid tumours is thought to be due to the secretion of other chemicals such as bradykinin and prostaglandins. By the time the patient is seen the liver is usually enlarged from hepatic metastases.

Neoplasms are much commoner in the colon than in the small bowel, but seldom give rise to obstruction. This is seen chiefly in the sigmoid colon from the accumulation of faeces behind a constricting cancer. Constipation or 'spurious' diarrhoea are the main complaints though they may be followed by spasmodic bouts of umbilical pain. Vomiting is distinctly uncommon.

Drugs

The possible role of drugs in causing umbilical pain should not be forgotten. For example, potassium salts given with diuretics, especially when combined in one tablet, may cause ulceration and stricture formation in the small bowel. This should be borne in mind in elderly patients with congestive cardiac failure complaining of mid-abdominal pain.

Impaction of faeces, gallstones or food bolus

In the old and bedridden faeces may become hardened and impacted in the rectum, with symptoms of obstruction. On rare occasions a large gallstone may ulcerate through the walls of the gall-bladder and adjacent duodenum and become impacted in the narrowest part of the ileum, a short distance above the ileocaecal valve. In the edentulous a food bolus, such as a large portion of orange pulp, can similarly become arrested in its passage down the bowel.

VASCULAR CAUSES

Aortic aneurysm (see also Epigastric pain, p. 60)

Dissection or rupture of an aneurysm of the abdominal aorta in an elderly atherosclerotic patient will often give rise to intense epigastric or central abdominal pain, particularly if it is leaking from its anterior surface. When the split occurs in its posterior wall the predominant symptom will be low backache which may be mistaken for 'lumbago'; abdominal pain may then be minimal or absent. In more than 90% of cases a pulsating mass will be felt in the upper abdomen. This is a surgical emergency and delay of only a few hours may be fatal.

Mesenteric ischaemia (see also Epigastric pain, p. 60)

Reference has already been made to superior mesenteric ischaemia as a cause of epigastric pain. Occlusion of the superior mesenteric artery and its branches results in ischaemia of the small bowel and ascending colon so that pain may be referred also to the umbilicus. It results from atheromatous narrowing, thrombosis or small emboli arising from a fibrillating heart; it is therefore seen mainly in the elderly. Before the occlusion is complete, umbilical pain may occur in bouts over many months without any physical signs. It finally becomes persistent and is accompanied by vomiting and loss of weight. When infarction occurs the bowel sounds disappear and there may be gastrointestinal haemorrhage; rigidity is usually absent until peritonitis has set in.

Occlusion of the inferior mesenteric artery also causes colicky midabdominal pain but is less often diagnosed as infarction of the colon is rare. Spontaneous resolution is the rule and rectal bleeding is seldom seen.

Henoch-Schönlein purpura (see also Purpura and bleeding, p. 193)

This uncommon vasculitis is seen most often in children in whom it occurs acutely with fever, a palpable purpuric rash and painful joints. In about half the cases there is central abdominal pain, vomiting and bloody diarrhoea.

Polyarteritis nodosa (see also Fever, p. 328)

When the vessels of the intestinal tract are involved there will be multiple small infarcts in the bowel which may bleed or perforate. It is a very rare cause of umbilical pain but should be thought of if there are signs of arterial occlusion in other organs.

Sickle-cell disease (see also Anaemia, p. 221)

This congenital disorder of the red cells is seen mainly in Black people. Dramatic episodes of sudden severe abdominal pain with fever may occur during haemolytic crises and be mistaken for appendicitis or other intra-abdominal emergencies. Clumping of red cells leads to thrombosis and rupture of capillaries in the gut. The usual features of a haemolytic anaemia will be found in the blood and a raised leukocyte count is common during an attack.

METABOLIC CAUSES

Whilst lactose intolerance, Addison's disease, lead poisoning and porphyria are legitimately described as metabolic conditions the aetiology of the irritable bowel and periodic syndromes remains obscure. Their inclusion in this section is of course open to challenge.

Lactose intolerance (see also Loss of weight, p. 270)

This is an important cause of umbilical pain in children. In Britain it is seen chiefly in immigrants from Cyprus, Africa and Asia, in whom the levels of intestinal lactase are too low to deal with the large amounts of milk consumed in this country. Frequent bouts of colicky pain are accompanied by bloating, diarrhoea and the passage of frothy stools. Whilst a lactose tolerance test may provoke an attack, the only sure way of confirming the diagnosis is by demonstrating the absence of lactase activity in a jejunal biopsy.

Addison's disease (see also Loss of weight, p. 283)

It is not uncommon for an acute adrenal crisis to present with severe abdominal pain and vomiting. A history of previous episodes within the past year or two may be obtained from the patient or a relative. The pain is poorly localised but more often than not it is felt in the umbilical region. The absence of any convincing abdominal signs and the presence of profound weakness, pigmentation and low blood pressure should point to the correct diagnosis. A dramatic improvement will follow the administration of corticosteroids and intravenous saline.

Porphyria

Aetiology

The term 'porphyria' is used to describe a group of rare inherited metabolic disorders in which there are defects in the enzyme systems controlling haem synthesis. These result in the excessive production of intermediate metabolites in the liver, and their excretion in the bile and urine. Why the presence of high levels of these substances should cause the abdominal, neurological and skin manifestations is still unexplained. The administration of enzyme-inducing drugs such as alcohol, barbiturates, griseofulvin, rifampicin, sulphonamides and oestrogen-containing contraceptives are known to precipitate attacks in affected individuals.

Clinical features

These vary according to which particular metabolites are present in excess. Acute intermittent porphyria is inherited as a dominant trait and presents with recurring attacks of abdominal pain and neurological disturbances. It is commoner in women and rare before puberty, usually making its appearance in the third to fourth decade of life. Attacks range in severity from mild abdominal discomfort to agonising colic with vomiting and persistent constipation. Neurological manifestations include a peripheral neuropathy mainly affecting the upper limbs, generalised muscle weakness, cranial nerve palsies, confusion and even madness. Sinus tachycardia is common during an attack and there may be a transient rise in blood pressure. Loss of consciousness is probably due to cerebral oedema for it is accompanied by hyponatraemia and other evidence of inappropriate ADH secretion.

In variegate porphyria the patient may also present in early adult life with attacks of abdominal pain and neurological symptoms, but in this form the skin is also affected and light-sensitive rashes appear on the exposed parts of the body. Similar skin lesions are also seen in porphyria cutanea tarda which, as its name implies, presents later in life. Abdominal pain and neurological symptoms are however absent in this type which is seen mainly in middle-aged men with liver disease.

Investigations

The diagnosis depends upon finding increased amounts of amino-levulinic acid and other porphyrin metabolites in the faeces and urine. The latter, when voided, may be the colour of port wine or colourless until after standing. This darkening is due to the conversion of porphobilinogen to porphyrins and other pigmented derivatives.

Lead poisoning

Aetiology

Such gross manifestations of plumbism as painter's colic, wrist drop or the convulsions of lead encephalopathy are now seldom seen. Small children are, however, still at risk from sucking lead-containing toys or the flaking paint in old houses.

The use of *surma* to decorate the eyes of Asian children is another potential source; although it is illegal to sell lead-containing *surma* in Britain it is brought in from the Indian subcontinent by friends and relatives.

The elimination of lead pipes in domestic water supplies has removed this source.

In industry, despite stringent regulations, about 100 cases of lead poisoning are notified annually in Britain. The hazard exists from the mixing of lead pigments, exposure to tetra-ethyl lead in petrol, the burning of car batteries and the burning off of lead paint. It is still an occupational hazard amongst potters and artists using lead paints. Lead is present in trivial amounts in the blood of most city workers from pollution of the atmosphere by car exhausts.

Clinical features

In acute lead poisoning copious vomiting and obstinate constipation are accompanied by abdominal colic which may be so severe as to suggest intestinal obstruction requiring immediate surgery. Abdominal tenderness and rigidity will however be absent. In one case at operation the gut was seen to be in intense spasm. These unpleasant symptoms may be followed by bone pain, paralysis of the upper limbs and encephalopathy. In chronic poisoning symptoms are milder and intermittent in the form of occasional abdominal pain, tiredness and lethargy. A blue or black line of lead sulphide on the gums is rarely seen but should be sought.

Investigations

The serum and urinary lead levels will usually exceed those currently regarded as acceptable in city dwellers, namely 2.0 μmol/l (40 μg/dl) and 400 nmol/24 h (80 μg/24 h) respectively. The striking similarity between the clinical picture of lead poisoning and porphyria may not be a coincidence, for lead is known to interfere with haem synthesis and increased amounts of aminolevulinic acid and coproporphyrin are also found in the urine in this condition. In chronic poisoning a normochromic microcytic anaemia is common but basophil stippling of the red cells is rarely found.

Irritable bowel (see also Lateral abdominal pain, p. 90)

This, after gastroenteritis, has been described as the commonest cause of abdominal pain. It may be felt in any region but in adults is located as a rule in the left iliac fossa or the hypogastrium.

Periodic syndrome

Babies and young children often experience brief episodes of colicky abdominal pain which may be accompanied by vomiting. In the absence of a defined cause this has been termed the periodic syndrome. The tendency to such attacks may persist into adolescence and adult life and there is often a positive family history. In a group of 34 adults reviewed 30 years after a complaint in childhood of recurring abdominal pain, 18 continued to have 'troublesome abdominal symptoms'; 16 suffered from 'irritable colon' with or without peptic ulcer and 11 were subject to migraine, headaches, back pain or 'bad nerves'.

CHAPTER 7

Hypogastric pain

SYNOPSIS OF CAUSES*

COLON

Flatulence; Irritable bowel; Colitis; Ischaemic colitis; **Diverticulitis**; Obstruction; Schistosomiasis.

BLADDER

Cystitis; Calculus; **Acute retention**; Neoplasm; Rupture.

GENITAL TRACT

Dysmenorrhoea; Endometriosis; Labour; Neoplasm; Fibromyoma; Epididymo-orchitis; Torsion of testis; Prostatitis.

* Bold type is used for causes more commonly found in Europe and North America.

PHYSIOLOGY

This is the lowest of the three central regions of the abdomen. It is bounded laterally by the mid-clavicular lines and below by the inguinal ligaments. In the vertical plane it occupies the lower third of the linea alba. The twelfth thoracic and first lumbar nerves supply the skin, muscle and parietal peritoneum of the belly wall. The first lumbar nerve also innervates the skin of the adjacent inner thigh, testis and labium major. Within the pelvis afferent sympathetic fibres supply the lower colon and rectum, bladder, uterus, overies and fallopian tubes.

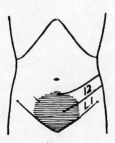

FIGURE 7

Hypogastric pain arises for the most part from the pelvic organs. Pain from the uterus or bladder is felt centrally, whilst pain from disorders of the ovary or fallopian tube begins laterally but may spread to the hypogastrium. In the colon the site of the pain depends upon the part of the large gut which is involved. Disorders of the lower colon causing obstruction, such as a volvulus of the sigmoid, result in pain referred to this region. In irritable bowel, diverticulitis or cancer of the sigmoid colon the pain is more often felt in the left iliac fossa.

DIAGNOSTIC APPROACH

As elsewhere in the abdomen the approach to diagnosis differs according to the mode of onset of the pain. This may be abrupt and severe, as in acute retention of urine, but is more often chronic and intermittent in nature. The duration and incidence should be determined and whether the pain is related to the periods.

Aggravating and relieving factors must be established, such as the effect of a bowel action or the passage of flatus. Associated symptoms include diarrhoea, constipation, frequency of micturition, dysuria, haematuria and the passage of clots during the menstrual flow. The presence of any one of these will direct attention to the most likely source of the pain.

While disorders of the fallopian tube and ovary usually give rise to pain in the iliac fossa this may spread to the hypogastrium, emphasizing the importance of determining where the pain began. When a colonic cause is suspected the appearance of the stools should be ascertained, and whether they contain blood or mucus. A freshly passed urine sample should be examined for evidence of infection and the presence of blood. Finally, a rectal examination should never be omitted and a vaginal examination will be necessary in appropriate cases.

CAUSES IN THE COLON

Colonic pain is poorly localised and may be felt in the hypogastrium or in the lateral abdominal regions.

Flatulence

This term is used to describe the distension of the stomach and intestines by swallowed air or gases produced by bacterial fermentation in the bowel. A small amount of air is normally swallowed with meals and trapped in the stomach; it is unlikely to pass onward into the duodenum unless the individual is recumbent. Air swallowing is increased by pain and anxiety, by heavy smoking and by the gulping of food or fluids. In adults it may cause gastric distension with upper abdominal discomfort which is eased by belching; it rarely produces lower abdominal pain. In infants, on the other hand, the swallowed air passes into the intestines and hasty feeding often results in colicky abdominal pain which is relieved by passing wind from either end.

The main constituents of intestinal gas are hydrogen and methane derived from the breakdown of unabsorbed carbohydrates by bacteria in the large bowel. Distension of the colon by excessive quantities of gas is a common cause of hypogastric pain which is colicky in nature and is often accompanied by borborygmi and bloating of the abdomen. The pain is relieved by expulsion of flatus from the anus.

Excessive flatus may be due to the nature of the diet — a wide variety of fruit and vegetables, particularly beans, contain large amounts of non-absorbable carbohydrates which provide an ample substrate for bacterial gas production. Similarly, lactose intolerance results in a great increase in undigested carbohydrate and excessive gas formation. The reason that stools float in patients with intestinal malabsorption is not due to their fat content but to the presence of trapped methane which reduces their density below that of water.

Irritable bowel (see also Lateral abdominal pain, p. 90)

In this common disorder pain in the hypogastrium, left iliac fossa or elsewhere in the abdomen may be persistent or colicky and accompanied by constipation or diarrhoea. The stools may be fragmented or 'bitty' on examination. Extensive investigations fail to reveal any structural abnormality in the colon.

Colitis (see also Diarrhoea, p. 139)

Recurrent colicky pain in the hypogastrium or left iliac fossa is usually mild except in an exacerbation of colitis. Diarrhoea is invariably present and the stools will contain both mucus and blood. The pain is often relieved by defaecation. Tenesmus is present if there is an accompanying proctitis.

Ischaemic colitis (see also Lateral abdominal pain, p. 89)

This is occasionally seen as a complication of atherosclerosis in the elderly. It usually begins acutely and may be mistaken for ulcerative colitis, diverticulitis or pseudomembranous colitis unless it is borne in mind. Pain in the left iliac fossa or hypogastrium is sometimes accompanied by bloody diarrhoea.

Diverticulitis (see also Lateral abdominal pain, p. 87)

Diverticula of the colon become increasingly common with advancing age and tend to develop in the sigmoid colon. Diverticulitis usually gives rise to pain in the left iliac fossa unless there is a pericolic abscess or perforation occurs when the pain may spread to the hypogastrium. Vomiting may follow the onset of the pain, the temperature is usually elevated and a tender mass may be palpable in the lower abdomen.

Obstruction

Small bowel obstruction has been considered in the previous chapter, under Umbilical pain. Colonic obstruction differs from it in the age incidence, mode of onset and site of the pain. Carcinoma of the colon, sigmoid diverticulitis, volvulus and impaction of faeces account for the great majority of cases and are seen mainly in the elderly. In colonic obstruction the onset is likely to be gradual with increasing constipation accompanied by aching or colicky pain in the hypogastrium or left iliac fossa. Vomiting, if it occurs, is late in onset.

Schistosomiasis (see also Diarrhoea, p. 141)

The symptoms are those of colitis. The frequent stools contain bloodstained mucus in which the cercariae may be found.

CAUSES IN THE BLADDER

Cystitis

Aetiology

It is generally accepted that the colon is the main reservoir for most of the organisms which invade the urinary tract. The bladder is usually infected via the urethra from the perianal region. It is therefore hardly surprising that acute cystitis is a common complication of an indwelling catheter, particularly in diabetics. The female urethra is shorter than that of the male and is more exposed to infection; this probably accounts for the much higher incidence of acute cystitis in women of all ages. *Esch. coli* is the commonest organism involved, but when instrumentation of the urethra and bladder are performed other coliform organisms and even staphylococci may be found.

Clinical features

In most cases there will be frequency of micturition, a burning sensation on passing urine and suprapubic discomfort. The patient may complain of a foul odour to the urine which will be cloudy and occasionally tinged with blood. Fever is rarely evident unless the infection has spread upwards to involve the kidneys. Recurrences are not uncommon despite apparently adequate antibiotic therapy.

Investigations

Microscopic examination of a freshly passed specimen of urine is the quickest way of establishing the diagnosis. Pus cells will be present in large numbers and motile organisms may be seen. A midstream urine sample should be collected and sent to the laboratory for culture; this should be done before any antibiotics are given.

Calculus

Bladder stones may grow to a considerable size without producing symptoms. Hypogastric pain is usually absent until infection occurs from obstruction to the flow of urine from the bladder. Bladder stones are an uncommon cause of acute cystitis in the UK.

Acute retention

Acute retention of urine is extremely painful and is seen mainly in men with prostatic hypertrophy or urethral stricture. It may follow operations or be precipitated by the administration of short-acting diuretics such as frusemide to elderly males with heart failure. It has been seen as a complication of anorectal herpes simplex infection in homosexual males, and is a rare complication of herpes zoster infection of the sacral ganglia. Obstruction to the urinary outflow by blood clot is a major complication of transurethral resection of the prostate or haemorrhage from a vesical neoplasm. In women a pelvic mass such as a large ovarian cyst or retroverted gravid uterus may cause retention.

The clinical picture is quite characteristic. The patient, usually a man, is in great distress at being unable to micturate and in severe pain localised to the hypogastrium. The bladder is tense and tender and readily palpable except in the very obese. Relief will rapidly follow the insertion of a catheter by the urethral or suprapubic route.

Neoplasm (see also Haematuria, p. 186)

Haematuria is the presenting symptom in most cases of bladder cancer. Pain is often absent in the early stages but becomes intense and unremitting with invasion of the bladder wall.

Rupture

Rupture of the bladder can follow any injury to the abdomen, pelvis or perineum. The diagnosis should be suspected in every patient with a fractured pelvis or other lower abdominal injury, particularly if the patient is unable to micturate or complains of strangury. There may be hypogastric tenderness, swelling and rigidity. The passage of small amounts of blood-stained urine will support the diagnosis.

CAUSES IN THE GENITAL TRACT

Pain of uterine origin is felt in the hypogastrium but may be referred to the sacrum and the inner aspects of the thighs. Its chief cause, menstruation, is self-evident. Salpingitis causes lower abdominal pain which is usually felt first in one or other iliac fossa; it is therefore discussed in the chapter on lateral abdominal pain.

Dysmenorrhoea

Aetiology

Many women have pain at the menstrual periods. In a small number it is intense and disabling. Primary dysmenorrhoea is not associated with organic disease and occurs mainly in adolescent girls and young women with regular ovulatory cycles. Its cause is obscure though it has been suggested that it is due to ischaemia of uterine muscle produced by sustained contractions leading to the accumulation of pain-producing substances such as prostaglandins. Secondary or congestive dysmenorrhoea is seen in older women and is thought to be due to generalised venous congestion in the pelvis. It is usually associated with endometriosis, chronic pelvic inflammatory disease or fibroids.

Clinical features

Primary dysmenorrhoea begins as a rule a day or two before the onset of the period and rarely lasts for more than 3 or 4 days. The pain begins in the lower abdomen and may spread to the back. It is colicky in nature and may be accompanied by fainting, headache, nausea, vomiting and sometimes diarrhoea. It rarely persists after childbirth and does not occur if ovulation is suppressed by the combined contraceptive pill. Emotional factors such as unhappiness at work or discord in the home may potentiate the discomfort.

Secondary dysmenorrhoea commences as a dull aching pain in the hypogastrium some 3–4 days pre-menstrually and may last throughout the period. When it is associated with endometriosis the pain becomes worse as the period progresses and the patient may also complain of dyspareunia, menorrhagia or infertility.

Investigations

Pelvic examination will usually exclude an organic cause in the primary form. In secondary dysmenorrhoea a full gynaecological examination will be necessary under an anaesthetic, including a diagnostic curettage and laparoscopy.

Endometriosis

Aetiology

In this condition ectopic endometrium is implanted in adjacent pelvic organs and may involve the ovaries, fallopian tubes, uterosacral ligaments, vagina, sigmoid colon, rectum, ureters or bladder. The endometrial cells are thought to reach the pelvic cavity either by retrograde flow of menstrual blood along the fallopian tubes or by dissemination through the lymphatics or blood vessels. The latter theory would explain the rare occurrence of endometrial tissue in such distant sites as the lungs, pericardium and skin. Lesions vary in size from scattered small dots to large cystic masses filled with altered blood (chocolate cysts); the ovaries are most frequently affected. Although this disorder can occur at any time after menarche until the onset of the menopause its peak incidence is in multiparous women between the ages of 30 and 45.

Clinical features

Endometriosis is the commonest cause of secondary dysmenorrhoea. Backache and lower abdominal pain usually commence a few days before the period and continue throughout the menstrual flow. The pain may be referred to the rectum or perineum if the rectovaginal septum is involved. Menorrhagia is common and there may be dyspareunia. Involvement of the bowel results in diarrhoea, rectal pain, blood in the stools and even intestinal obstruction. Enlarged tender ovaries may be palpable on rectal or vaginal examination and hard fixed nodules may be felt in the uterosacral ligaments or pouch of Douglas.

Investigations

Examination under anaesthesia and laparoscopy are necessary to confirm the diagnosis; these patients should be referred to a gynaecologist without delay.

Labour

Uterine pain is of course felt in the hypogastrium during labour and spontaneous abortion. The diagnosis may not be immediately obvious in the obese female who denies the possibility of pregnancy despite several months of amenorrhoea!

Neoplasm

Pain is not usually a conspicuous feature of cancer of the body or cervix until the growth has spread beyond the uterus and invaded the parametrium. An earlier symptom is a bloodstained discharge or postmenopausal bleeding which may be provoked by coitus. It is hoped that the widespread use of cervical cytology, being aimed at diagnosis in the pre-invasive stage, will diminish the number of inoperable cases of cervical carcinoma.

Leiomyoma (fibroid)

This is ordinarily painless but if red degeneration or torsion takes place the pain is acute and severe. Hypogastric pain is also felt during the extrusion of a polypus through the cervical canal.

Epididymo-orchitis

Acute inflammation of the epididymis and testis is seen in adults as a complication of urinary tract infection. In younger men it is frequently associated with sexually transmissible disease and preceded by a urethral discharge. The commonest organisms involved are the gonococcus and *Chlamydia trachomatis*. In older men epididymo-orchitis is usually due to coliform organisms and is a complication of cystitis, instrumentation of the urethra and prostatic surgery. Pain in the scrotum and inguinal region may be accompanied by malaise and fever. The epididymis is always more involved than the testis and will be swollen and tender, with reddening and oedema of the overlying skin. The swelling may extend up to the external inguinal ring and a secondary hydrocele sometimes develops.

Epididymo-orchitis also appears after puberty as part of a more generalised disease such as mumps, coxsackievirus infection or brucellosis. In mumps it usually presents acutely some 5–10 days after the onset of the illness when the parotid swellings are subsiding. Symptoms vary in severity from a mild discomfort to severe testicular pain, high fever and vomiting. The epididymis and testis will be swollen and tender and there may be a secondary effusion. In a minority of cases both testes are involved. Although some degree of testicular atrophy may be detectable when the condition has subsided it rarely leads to gonadal failure.

Chronic epididymo-orchitis occurs in syphilis, tuberculosis, leprosy and some other tropical diseases and is usually painless. Tumours of the testis sometimes present with pain and swelling and should not be forgotten in the differential diagnosis of an enlarged swollen testis, particularly if there is no evidence of a urinary infection or systemic illness.

Torsion of testis

Torsion of the spermatic cord with consequent ischaemia of the testis is seen mainly in infants and around puberty. In one published series 81% of 243 patients who had undergone emergency scrotal exploration were under 20. When it does occur in older men there is often a history of intermittent attacks of testicular pain. Testicular torsion is commonly mistaken for epididymo-orchitis, which is rare in childhood and adolescence, and treated ineffectively with antibiotics. In Britain some 2000 infarcted testes are removed each year, apparently from failure to make the diagnosis in time.

Typically the onset is abrupt and may waken the patient from sleep. Severe pain in the testis, external inguinal ring or iliac fossa is accompanied by nausea and sometimes vomiting. Fever is absent at first but may appear later when infarction occurs. In atypical cases there may be little more warning of impending disaster than a dull aching pain in the groin or hypogastrium.

On examination the tender enlarged testis will be retracted into the upper part of the swollen scrotum and the epididymis will not be palpable as a separate structure. If an effusion develops, or if it is impossible to get above the testis, the condition may resemble that of a strangulated inguinal hernia. In either case the correct treatment is prompt surgical exploration of the inguinoscrotal region under general anaesthesia. Untreated, the pain settles in a few days and the swelling disappears in about a fortnight. Only later will the presence of an atrophic testis draw attention to the missed diagnosis.

Prostatitis

Inflammation of the prostate gives rise to pain which is felt in the suprapubic region, the groin and one or both testes. The pain may radiate to the perineum or inner thigh or be felt in the urethra or meatus at the beginning and end of micturition. It is often accompanied by dysuria, urgency, frequency of micturition and painful ejaculation. Malaise, fever and sometimes rigors occur in an acute attack but are absent in the more chronic case. On rectal examination the prostate is likely to be firm and tender. Although the condition is commonly associated with sexually transmissible disease it is not always possible to isolate the causative organism. The urine should be examined for *Esch. coli* and urethral smears taken for gonococci, *Chlamydia, trichomonas vaginalis* and herpesvirus.

CHAPTER 8

Lateral abdominal pain

SYNOPSIS OF CAUSES*

INTRA-ABDOMINAL

INTESTINE

Appendicitis; Mesenteric adenitis; **Crohn's disease**; Acute ileitis; **Diverticulitis**; **Neoplasm**; Colitis; Ischaemic colitis; **Irritable bowel**.

LIVER, BILIARY TRACT AND SPLEEN

Hepatitis; Hepatic abscess; **Gallstones**; **Cholecystitis**; Hepatic neoplasm; Biliary tract cancer; Splenic infarct and rupture.

RENAL

Calculus; **Blood clot**; Papillary necrosis; **Pyelonephritis**.

GENITAL TRACT

Salpingitis; **Endometriosis**; Ectopic pregnancy; **Mittelschmerz**; Polycystic ovaries; Torsion of ovarian cyst; Oophoritis.

EXTRA-ABDOMINAL

Muscular strain; **Pleurisy**; Herpes zoster; Spinal lesions.

* Bold type is used for causes more commonly found in Europe and North America.

PHYSIOLOGY

The lateral regions of the abdomen lie outside the midclavicular lines and are bounded above by the rib margins and below by the pelvic brim. While the abdominal regions are defined anatomically in this way, the distinction in practice lies between pain which is central, whether precise or vague in location, and pain which is felt definitely to one side or the other and is thus lateral. Such pain may be due to causes lying within the abdomen or referred from extra-abdominal structures.

The ninth to the twelfth thoracic and first lumbar nerves supply the skin, muscle and parietal peritoneum of the region. The abdominal organs are supplied by afferent sympathetic fibres which terminate in the same segments of the cord. The stomach, pancreas, biliary tract, gut, uterus and

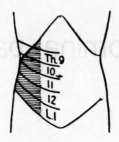

FIGURE 8

bladder have a bilateral nerve supply and pain from these organs will tend to be felt centrally unless the overlying parietal peritoneum is involved.

The diaphragm, gall-bladder, liver, spleen, kidney, ureter, fallopian tube and ovary on the other hand have a predominantly unilateral nerve supply and pain from these organs tends to be felt laterally, though this is not invariable. The diaphragm is supplied by the lower seven intercostal nerves and inflammation in the adjacent lung or pleura may give rise to pain which is felt as low as the iliac fossae. The parenchyma of the liver, spleen and kidneys is apparently insensitive to pain-producing stimuli and pain arising from these organs is probably due to distension of their capsules, particularly if this occurs rapidly. In renal disease obstruction to the flow of urine by inflammation, calculi or blood clot causes distension of the smooth muscle of the pelvis and ureter with pain referred to the loin or iliac fossa. When severe this may radiate to the thigh, testis or labium major for these structures are also innervated by the first lumbar nerve.

DIAGNOSTIC APPROACH

Once it becomes obvious from the preliminary enquiries that the patient is complaining of lateral abdominal pain the level at which this is felt should be determined. Pain arising from the liver, gall-bladder, spleen or kidneys will be felt in the upper abdomen beneath the costal margins. Pain arising from the pelvic organs will present in one or other iliac fossa.

The character of the pain, whether somatic or visceral in type and its severity, may throw more light on its probable aetiology. Well-localised burning, aching or stabbing pain in the abdominal wall is likely to be due to local causes or be referred from the spine or thorax. If the latter is suspected the patient should be asked if the discomfort is made worse by movements of the spine, deep breathing, coughing, sneezing or blowing the nose. A positive answer to one or more of these questions should focus attention outside the abdomen. Failure to ask them or to interpret them correctly may result in needless surgery. For example, cholecystectomy has been performed in error for pain arising from collapse of a thoracic vertebra. Local tenderness and rigidity are not always due to intra-abdominal disease.

It is also important to determine whether this is a solitary attack or if there have been previous episodes. Sudden severe pain, often agonising in its intensity, is typically seen with obstruction of both the biliary and renal tracts. The chronic intermittent aching or griping pain of the sufferer from an irritable bowel is in a different league. Changes in the position of the pain with time should also be noted, for shifting pain is seen when a diseased intra-abdominal organ comes into contact with the overlying parietal peritoneum. Thus the pain of a typical attack of appendicitis shifts from the umbilicus to the right iliac fossa in a matter of hours, and that of acute cholecystitis may start in the epigastrium but soon moves to the right hypochondrium. In addition, as the intensity of the pain increases there may be radiation into adjacent segments of the spinal cord. It is this phenomenon which accounts for the spread of pain from 'loin to groin' in renal disease, and for the shoulder-tip pain associated with gall-bladder disease and peritonitis in the upper abdomen.

Finally, account should be taken of any aggravating or relieving factors and of any accompanying symptoms. Mention has already been made of some of these when discussing referred pain from the spine but movement may also aggravate the pain of intra-abdominal disease, particularly when the peritoneum is inflamed. Such patients are apt to lie still in bed in marked contrast to the restlessness of the sufferer from renal colic or an impacted gallstone. Sweating, nausea and vomiting may accompany any severe pain of visceral origin but diarrhoea would point to an intestinal cause. In females a menstrual history is essential if such disasters as an ectopic pregnancy are not to be overlooked whilst in both sexes altered bowel habit, frequency of micturition, dysuria or haematuria may indicate the probable site if not the nature of the underlying pathology.

INTRA-ABDOMINAL CAUSES

Abdominal pain felt in the lateral regions is most often due to intra-abdominal conditions. It mainly arises in organs with a predominantly unilateral nerve supply unless the overlying parietal peritoneum is involved.

INTESTINAL CAUSES

Appendicitis (see also Umbilical pain, p. 64)

Whilst the initial pain of obstruction or inflammation of the appendix is visceral and felt centrally, with the onset of inflammation of its peritoneal coat the pain settles in the right iliac fossa. The possibility that this may arise, not from the appendix, but from gravitation of fluid from a perforated peptic ulcer down the right paracolic gutter, must be borne in mind. It is an example of the importance in the analysis of the symptom of the question 'Where did the pain begin?'.

Mesenteric adenitis

This is not uncommonly seen in school children and may be mistaken for appendicitis. It is thought to be due to an adenoviral infection and is often associated with upper respiratory symptoms and cervical adenitis. Pain in the umbilical region or right iliac fossa is accompanied by slight fever.

Crohn's disease

Aetiology

The small intestine, particularly the terminal ileum, is the most common site for this disease but any part of the gastrointestinal tract from the stomach to the anus may be involved. Work with mice supports the theory that the condition may be due to a transmissable agent which has yet to be identified. Crohn's disease, or regional enteritis as it is sometimes called, can appear at any age but is most common in young adults; the sexes are equally at risk.

The affected gut becomes chronically inflamed and greatly thickened with narrowing of the lumen and ulceration of the mucosa. These changes are often patchy in distribution with multiple 'skip' lesions separated by segments of apparently normal bowel. Fistulae occasionally develop between loops of bowel and adjacent organs such as the bladder, vaginal or skin of the perianal region.

Clinical features

The disease may begin acutely but an insidious onset is commoner, with bouts of abdominal pain and the passage of several semi-formed stools a day. The pain, which is often colicky and is probably due to partial intestinal obstruction, is felt in the umbilical region, hypogastrium or right iliac fossa. It may be provoked by eating and is sometimes relieved by the passage of flatus or a stool. In a severe attack vomiting and abdominal distension are seen. Between attacks the bowel action may be described as normal, although close questioning may reveal that the stools float and stick to the lavatory pan. Frequency of micturition is an uncommon but important symptom and arises when the inflamed bowel lies in contact with the bladder. Systemic complications of this disease include iritis, arthritis and a slowly progressive hepatitis. Loss of weight is usual and malabsorption is not uncommon.

On examination there may be little to find apart from some tenderness in the right iliac fossa, although a mass may be palpable if the terminal ileum is extensively involved. The perineum should be examined for the characteristic skin tags, fistulae or perianal abscesses; the involved skin is usually of a dusky purple colour.

Investigations

During an acute attack the stools will be semi-formed and contain mucus and occasionally frank blood. Occult blood may be found even when the stools appear to be normal. If the rectum is involved sigmoidoscopy will show some reddening and possibly ulceration of the mucosa; biopsies rarely show the characteristic histological picture of Crohn's disease but merely the changes of non-specific inflammation. When the large bowel and rectum are involved it is very difficult to distinguish this condition from ulcerative colitis.

An iron-deficiency anaemia or less commonly a macrocytic anaemia due to B_{12} or folate deficiency may be found. The ESR is often moderately raised when the disease is active. Abnormal liver function tests may return to normal during remissions. A small bowel meal and barium enema should be administered to try to establish the extent of the disease. The characteristic radiological signs are narrowing and rigidity of the bowel, mucosal irregularities and fistulae; these changes may, however, be minimal even when the disease is widespread.

Acute ileitis

An acute ileitis is occasionally seen in a child or young adult. The symptoms and signs resemble those of acute appendicitis, for which it is often mistaken. It appears to be due to infection of the terminal ileum by *Yersinia enterocolitica* or *Yersinia pseudotuberculosis*, which together account for about 80% of cases. The diagnosis is usually made by culturing the bacteria from the stool or from the inflamed tissues at laparotomy, and may be confirmed by a rising titre of antibodies to these organisms in the blood. It is sometimes associated with erythema nodosum and polyarthritis in patients with the HLA-B27 tissue antigen. Without specific treatment the condition is likely to resolve spontaneously but a small proportion of patients go on to develop Crohn's disease. Other infections which give rise to a similar clinical picture include tuberculosis, tularaemia, amoebiasis, actinomycosis and schistosomiasis, but all of these are rare in Britain.

Diverticulitis

Aetiology
In Western countries hernial protrusions in the colon, particularly in the sigmoid region, become increasingly common with advancing age. This is in striking contrast to the rarity of the condition in rural communities in Africa and Asia where the diet is largely composed of unmilled flour and unrefined carbohydrates. The high prevalence in Europe and the United States is thought to be due to the low fibre content of the diet. This results in small hard stools which require a high intracolonic pressure to propel them through the large bowel. Over many years this high pressure leads to hypertrophy of the muscular wall of the sigmoid colon, segmentation of the bowel and herniation of the mucosa through the gaps between the segments. Diverticular disease can give rise to symptoms from colonic spasm even in the absence of inflammation but stasis in the diverticula encourages infection with coliform organisms. The resulting inflammation

may cause local abscesses, perforation, obstruction or the development of fistulae between bowel, bladder or vagina. Diverticula in the caecum and ascending colon are less common than in the distal part of the colon and are usually symptomless.

Clinical features
Painful diverticular disease without inflammation is sometimes difficult to distinguish from diverticulitis for they both give rise to colicky pain in the left iliac fossa and constipation. The pain may be exacerbated by meals and temporarily relieved by the passage of flatus or a stool. When inflammation is present, however, the pain persists and is accompanied by fever. Vomiting is unusual in the absence of peritonitis or obstruction. On examination there will be tenderness and possibly guarding in the left iliac fossa and a tender mass may be palpable on rectal examination. Diverticulitis in the caecum or ascending colon is indistinguishable from acute appendicitis. A minority of cases present with profuse rectal haemorrhage from erosion of a vessel in a diverticulum. Frequency of micturition or a vaginal discharge is indicative of impending fistula formation, and gas or faeces will be passed in the urine or from the vagina when this has occurred.

Investigations
Acute diverticulitis can be differentiated from uncomplicated diverticular disease by the presence of a polymorph leukocytosis and a raised ESR. Laparotomy will confirm the diagnosis if the condition does not subside with more conservative treatment. When the acute episode is over a co-existent neoplasm should be excluded by sigmoidoscopy and a barium enema. The latter will show diverticula wholly or partly filled with barium which may still be visible some weeks after the examination on plain films of the abdomen.

Neoplasm

Aetiology
In Britain adenocarcinoma of the colon and rectum accounts for about 14% of all cancer deaths. In the United States it is said to be the commonest malignancy after skin cancer. The high prevalence of this disease in these countries, like that of diverticular disease, is in striking contrast to the low reported incidence in Africa, Asia and South America. The reason for this is unknown but has been blamed on the carcinogenic properties of food additives in Western food. Most of these cancers appear to arise in pre-existing adenomatous or villous polyps which may account for the very high incidence in patients with familial polyposis coli. They are a common complication of long-standing ulcerative colitis and may co-exist with diverticulitis. About 70% of growths occur in the sigmoid colon or rectum, the remainder being evenly distributed throughout the rest of the large bowel. While these tumours are seen most often after 50 years of age they occur occasionally in much younger people.

Clinical features

Abdominal pain is the commonest presenting symptom in colonic cancer, its position being determined by the site of the growth. In left-sided lesions it may be felt in the left hypochondrium but more often in the left iliac fossa. The pain is usually accompanied by increasing constipation, or constipation alternating with diarrhoea, and there may be mucus and blood in the stools. A small proportion of cases present with signs of acute intestinal obstruction or pelvic peritonitis. The less common carcinomas of the caecum and ascending colon are silent in the early stages and may present with an unexplained iron-deficiency anaemia due to occult bleeding. Later there may be dyspepsia and loss of weight. This has been said to occur in one third of cases of right-sided cancer, and there is a danger of being satisfied with a normal barium meal and omitting to investigate the colon. On examination an abdominal mass is palpable in about half of patients. There may be anaemia and, in advanced cases, weight loss and hepatomegaly due to liver secondaries.

Rectal bleeding is the commonest sign of a carcinoma of the rectum, occurring in about three-quarters of patients. It may be associated with some alteration in bowel habit; involvement of the lower third of the rectum is accompanied by hypogastric pain and tenesmus. Annular growths of the rectosigmoid junction often cause obstruction. The presence of a rectal neoplasm is usually evident on digital examination and is confirmed by sigmoidoscopy; a high proportion are within reach of the examining finger.

Investigations

If a rectal growth is seen on sigmoidoscopy a biopsy will confirm the diagnosis. Most lesions of the colon can be shown by a double-contrast barium enema with sufficient certainty to satisfy the surgeon. Fibreoptic colonoscopy, if available, may be helpful in equivocal cases and will enable biopsies to be taken.

Colitis (see also Diarrhoea, p. 139)

Colitis may be specific as in bacillary, amoebic or schistosomal dysentery or of undetermined aetiology. In non-specific ulcerative colitis pain is usually felt in the left iliac fossa and precedes the passage of loose stools.

Ischaemic colitis

Aetiology

Ischaemia of the large bowel is usually due to localised occlusive disease of the inferior mesenteric artery or to interruption of the colonic blood supply during aortic surgery or abdominoperineal resection. Rarely it is associated with an obstructing colonic cancer.

Clinical features

Most patients are elderly with pre-existing vascular disease. Atrial fibrillation, when present, will suggest an embolic cause. The onset is usually abrupt with cramp-like pain in the left iliac fossa, diarrhoea and rectal bleeding. In some patients the onset is less acute and there will be a history of similar episodes over the preceding weeks or months. When fever and signs of a left-sided peritonitis are present the condition may be mistaken for acute diverticulitis. If ischaemic colitis follows abdominal surgery it usually presents within a few days of the operation. Many patients will be managed conservatively on antibiotics and the condition will often subside without surgical intervention.

Investigations

Sigmoidoscopy may show a non-specific proctitis if the rectosigmoid area is involved. A barium enema often shows the characteristic picture of intra-mural haemorrhages and oedema with thumb-printing, tubular narrowing, saw-tooth irregularities and sacculations. Angiography is of little value for it will only show occlusive lesions in the larger vessels.

Irritable bowel

Aetiology

Hyperactivity of the bowel in the absence of an organic lesion is probably the commonest cause of recurrent abdominal pain. A recent survey of 300 apparently healthy adults revealed that no less than 20% had experienced bouts of abdominal pain in the previous year, but few had sought medical advice. This condition occurs at all ages but seems to be particularly prev-alent in adolescents and young adults undergoing stressful situations. Although much of the pain can be explained on the basis of colonic spasm, abnormal contractions of the oesophagus and a reduction in the lower oesophageal sphincter pressure have been demonstrated in some cases. These findings suggest that there may be a widespread disorder of smooth muscle or its innervation in this syndrome which is not confined to the colon. This may explain why some patients complain of upper abdominal discomfort, heartburn and occasionally dysphagia. In a small minority the irritable bowel syndrome follows an attack of food poisoning or dysentery.

Clinical features

Abdominal pain is present at times in most patients. It may be felt anywhere in the abdomen but is most common in the hypogastrium and left iliac fossa. The pain is usually griping in nature, being aggravated by the intake of food or cold fluids and relieved by defaecation and the passage of flatus. It varies widely in intensity, duration and time of onset but rarely wakens the patient from sleep. When there is epigastric discomfort, heart-burn, nausea or dysphagia the condition may be mistaken for oesophagitis, peptic ulceration or biliary tract disease. A careful history will reveal that exacerbations coincide with periods of stress or emotional tension, and it may become apparent during the interview that the patient is unduly anxious or depressed.

The prolonged retention of faecal material in a spastic sigmoid colon leads to excessive absorption of fluid and the infrequent passage of small, hard, pellet-like stools. This constipation may alternate with episodes of diarrhoea accompanied by urgency and tenesmus. The semi-formed stools will contain mucus but no blood and are more likely to be passed around breakfast time and in the evening. On examination the sigmoid colon is sometimes tender and easily palpable but a rectal examination will be normal.

Investigations
The irritable bowel syndrome can mimic a wide variety of gastrointestinal disorders. The diagnosis should only be accepted when organic disease has been excluded as far as possible by examination of the stools, sigmoidoscopy and a barium enema. Upper abdominal symptoms may call for a barium meal, gastroscopy, cholecystogram or ultrasonography of the biliary tract.

CAUSES IN LIVER, BILIARY TRACT AND SPLEEN

Hepatitis (see also Jaundice, p. 149)

In acute viral hepatitis, epigastric or right hypochondriac pain, anorexia and nausea are more prominent and earlier symptoms than jaundice. The liver is usually tender and the serum transaminases will be elevated. Discomfort over the liver is a feature of chronic persistent hepatitis which may follow a viral infection or result from alcohol abuse.

Hepatic abscess

Pyogenic abscesses in the liver are rare. They may result from penetrating abdominal wounds, ascending cholangitis secondary to biliary obstruction or from portal pyaemia complicating appendicitis, chronic peritoneal dialysis or diverticulitis. The patient is gravely ill with a dull aching pain in the right hypochondrium, a spiking fever, rigors and sometimes jaundice. There will be a polymorph leukocytosis and blood cultures should be done in the hope of identifying the responsible organism. The serum bilirubin, alkaline phosphatase and transaminases are likely to be raised. Scanning with isotopes, ultrasound or computed tomography may be helpful in establishing the diagnosis. The prognosis is poor even with prolonged antibiotic therapy and laparotomy is usually necessary to effect adequate drainage.

Amoebic abscess of the liver is also rare in Britain but may develop in those who have lived in tropical countries. The most frequent site is the right lobe and the abscess may attain a great size without giving rise to symptoms until it becomes secondarily infected or reaches the liver surface. A dull aching pain in the liver area is accompanied by intermittent fever, rigors and sweating. On examination the liver will be enlarged and tender. Warm, freshly passed stools must be examined for *Entamoeba histolytica* or its cysts, whilst sigmoidoscopy may reveal evidence of amoebic infection in the rectum. X-ray screening of the chest sometimes shows a high deformed right diaphragm moving little on inspiration, or a pleural effusion. Scanning of the liver with isotopes, ultrasound or computed tomography will reveal the site and extent of the abscess whilst a liver puncture will confirm its nature. A positive fluorescent antibody titre of more than 1:256 in the blood is confirmatory evidence of amoebic infection.

Gallstones

Aetiology

Gallstones are a common disease of affluent societies living on low-fibre diets containing an excess of refined carbohydrates. They are found in about 15% of autopsies in Britain. Women are more frequently affected than men and there is an association with obesity, diabetes mellitus, multiple pregnancies and the oestrogen-containing contraceptive pill. Large solitary stones are composed almost entirely of cholesterol and this substance is the main constituent of the much commoner mixed or multifaceted stones.

Cholesterol is secreted in the bile and concentrated in the gall-bladder where it is kept in solution by the combined action of bile salts and phospholipids. If these mechanisms fail to keep it in solution it will be deposited as microcrystals on epithelial debris or particles of calcium bilirubinate. Eventually these crystals will coalesce and grow to form gallstones. This situation may arise as a result of increased cholesterol synthesis in the liver so that the bile is saturated with this steroid, or from a deficiency of bile salts.

Oestrogens and a high carbohydrate diet both promote synthesis of cholesterol in the liver which may explain the higher incidence of gallstones in obese multiparous middle-aged women.

Pigment stones contain very little cholesterol and occur in association with chronic haemolytic anaemias and cirrhosis of the liver. Although their aetiology has still to be elucidated it must have something to do with the increased excretion of bilirubin in the bile. Gallstones rarely give rise to symptoms unless they become impacted in the cystic or common bile duct.

Clinical features

Though its accuracy has been questioned the term 'biliary colic' is still used to describe the pain resulting from obstruction by calculi in the biliary tract. The onset is abrupt and the pain often agonisingly severe, being felt first in the epigastrium. It soon passes to the right hypochondrium and may be referred to the interscapular region or tip of the right shoulder. It is accompanied by nausea and vomiting, sweating, tachycardia and pallor. The pain is steady rather than intermittent and may increase in intensity for the first hour or two. It often persists for several hours, ceasing as abruptly as it began. Relief of pain occurs with the falling back of the stone into the gall-bladder or its passage onward through the common bile duct. On examination there may be little to find beyond tenderness in the right hypochondrium. A history of previous attacks at irregular intervals may be elicited.

Persisting impaction in the cystic duct for 6 hours or more leads to acute cholecystitis. The pain continues and is accompanied by fever and rigors. Prolonged obstruction of the common bile duct will result in jaundice, cholangitis or acute pancreatitis. On rare occasions a large stone may ulcerate into the adjacent bowel, pass down and give rise to intestinal obstruction.

Investigations

During an attack there will be a transient elevation of the serum conjugated bilirubin, alkaline phosphatase or transaminases. X-rays of the abdomen will show radio-opaque gallstones in about 10% of cases. In the absence of jaundice an oral cholecystogram which fails to visualise the gall-bladder is very suggestive of cystic duct obstruction. Ultrasonography is very useful in demonstrating the presence of calculi in the gall-bladder, while endoscopic retrograde cholangiopancreatography will disclose impacted stones in the common bile duct.

Cholecystitis

With the rare exception of cholecystitis occurring as a complication of typhoid or paratyphoid fever, inflammation of the gall-bladder is almost always associated with the presence of gallstones. Acute cholecystitis follows an attack of biliary colic when the cystic duct is obstructed for several hours. The initial inflammation is probably due to the irritant action of the imprisoned bile salts, but this is usually followed by secondary infection with coliform or anaerobic organisms from the bowel. Pain, often felt initially in the epigastrium, shifts to the right as the hours pass. It is accompanied by anorexia, fever and sometimes vomiting. Some tenderness and guarding is usually evident in the right hypochondrium and palpation may produce pain and inspiratory arrest when the patient takes a deep breath (Murphy's sign). The inflamed gall-bladder is felt in about one third of patients, particularly if this is their first attack.

X-rays of the abdomen or ultrasonography may show stones and there will be a polymorph leukocytosis. The attack subsides in a few days, as a rule, with appropriate antibiotic therapy; otherwise necrosis of the gall-bladder wall, empyema or even perforation ensue. Chronic cholecystitis results from repeated attacks of acute inflammation and may give rise to bouts of nausea and indigestion.

Hepatic neoplasm

Primary cancer of the liver is rare in Britain but common in Africa, Asia, Italy and Greece. It is seen chiefly in men, and pre-existing cirrhosis is common. A close if not causal relationship between chronic hepatitis-B virus infection and subsequent hepatocellular carcinoma is evident from epidemiological studies and the presence of hepatitis-B antigens in the liver cells of patients with this neoplasm. It usually presents with right hypochondriac pain, anorexia and loss of weight; the diagnosis is made on liver biopsy.

Another rare primary tumour is angiosarcoma, which presents with abdominal pain and swelling, fatigue, anorexia and gastrointestinal haemorrhage. Hepatosplenomegaly and ascites are usually found. The importance of this cancer lies in its association with the manufacture of polyvinyl chloride (PVC), which is widely used to make roofing, food and liquid containers, footwear and waterproof clothing. Like other industrial hazards there is a long latent period of years between the first exposure to vinyl chloride and the appearance of the tumour.

In temperate climates these rarities are eclipsed by secondary deposits from neoplasms arising in the alimentary tract, pancreas, breast, bronchus or pelvic organs. Although the liver may be palpably enlarged such growths seldom give rise to pain, but when they do so it will be felt in the right hypochondrium.

Cancer of the biliary tract

Cancer of the gall-bladder is uncommon; it is seen as a rule in elderly women with pre-existing gall-bladder disease. Epigastric and right hypochondriac pain are usually gradual in appearance but in about 25% of cases the onset is acute. If the common duct is involved jaundice appears early but if the growth is restricted to the fundus jaundice may appear late or be absent. A palpable mass is felt in the right hypochondrium in about half the cases. A cholecystogram will fail to outline the gall-bladder and gallstones may be visible on ultrasonography. Cancer of the extrahepatic ducts is rare. Pain is common and may be colicky in nature; jaundice is usually present by the time the patient is seen. The gall-bladder may be distended and palpable. The diagnosis of cancer of the biliary tract is rarely made without laparotomy.

Splenic infarct and rupture

Enlargement of the spleen from whatever cause is ordinarily painless. Perisplenitis may give rise to pain in the left shoulder from irritation of the diaphragm, and in the left hypochondrium from involvement of the parietal peritoneum; the commonest cause is a splenic infarct in bacterial endocarditis. The onset of pain is sudden and the spleen will be palpable and tender. In rupture of the spleen agonising pain is felt locally, with shock from intra-abdominal haemorrhage.

RENAL CAUSES

Calculus

Aetiology

Stones in the renal tract result from precipitation of crystals of relatively insoluble salts and acids from saturated urine. Kidney stones, in contrast to those in the bladder, are much commoner in the richer industrialised countries and this may be due to their higher dietary intake of animal protein.

Cystine stones are rare and confined to a few individuals with a congenital defect which prevents the tubular reabsorption of cystine and other amino-acids.

Uric-acid stones occur in patients with gout and myeloproliferative disorders who excrete an excessive amount of this substance in their urine.

Calcium-containing stones are by far the commonest variety and have a peak incidence in middle-aged males. They are associated with upper urinary-tract infection, idiopathic hypercalcuria, primary hyperparathy-roidism, prolonged immobility, Paget's disease and medullary sponge kidneys. They occasionally complicate such disorders as renal tubular acidosis, the milk–alkali syndrome, sarcoidosis or Cushing's syndrome. Like biliary calculi renal stones vary in size from staghorn calculi, filling the renal pelvis and often associated with pyelonephritis and hydrone-phrosis, to the size of a grain of wheat or coarse sand. They may long be symptomless but ultimately are likely to give rise to obstruction or infection.

Clinical features
When a calculus is present in the renal pelvis pain in the loin may be intermittent, dull but increased by jolting movements. If however a stone enters and obstructs a ureter the onset of pain is abrupt and often agonising in its severity. Renal colic is felt as a rule over the renal angle or in the lateral abdominal region anteriorly, and classically radiates from loin to groin. It may reach as far as the inner thigh, labium or scrotum. The attack usually lasts some hours and is often accompanied by frequency of mictur-ition, nausea and vomiting.

On examination the patient will be sweating, restless and unable to lie still, in contrast to the immobility associated with other intra-abdominal crises. There may be little else to find apart from tenderness of the kidney on the affected side.

Investigations
Microscopic haematuria is common and a chemical test for blood is often positive. Pus cells may be seen in freshly passed urine and a specimen should be sent for culture. X-rays of the abdomen will usually show calculi in the kidney — most are radio-opaque — but small stones in the ureter may be obscured by gas shadows or overlie some bony structure and so be missed. Immediate intravenous urograms are rarely helpful, for the kidney involved may fail to excrete dye, and these should never be done if there is any possibility of renal failure. Blood should be taken routinely for serum creatinine, urea, calcium, phosphate and uric-acid estimations. If the calcium is raised a further sample should be sent for ionised calcium and parathormone levels with hyperparathyroidism in mind; the urinary calcium excretion may be elevated in this disorder as it is in idiopathic hypercal-

curia. Any stones which are passed should be sent for chemical analysis, which will provide an important clue as to their likely aetiology. If cystinuria is suspected an early morning urine specimen should be examined for excess amino-acids. Further investigations may be left until the acute attack has subsided but in any case patients should be referred for a urological opinion.

Blood clot

Haemorrhage from a kidney may result in the formation of blood clots in the pelvis and ureter and give rise to pain similar to that seen in calculus obstruction. This is a common complication of anticoagulant therapy when the prothrombin time is unduly prolonged. Very occasionally an otherwise silent hydronephrosis may present in this way.

Papillary necrosis

Necrosis of the renal papilla, accompanied by interstitial nephritis, is a not uncommon complication of analgesic abuse and an important cause of chronic renal failure. It is seen mainly in patients with chronic painful arthritis who have taken large amounts of aspirin and other non-steroidal anti-inflammatory drugs for many years. It is rare under 30 years of age and occurs most often in middle-aged women, particularly if they are also diabetic. Some of these patients present acutely with renal colic, haematuria and deteriorating renal function due to ureteric obstruction by papillary fragments. This condition should be suspected if there is a history of analgesic abuse and the urine is heavily infected but abdominal X-rays show no calculi. Each specimen of urine must be carefully inspected for fleshy material as soon as it is passed; the necrotic tissue rapidly disintegrates and becomes unrecognisable if the urine is kept for any length of time before examination.

Papillary necrosis is also seen in sickle-cell disease, in renal transplants and occasionally in chronic liver disease. It is a rare complication of shock and severe dehydration in young children.

Pyelonephritis (see also Fever, p. 322)

Loin pain is common in acute pyelonephritis but is usually overshadowed by high fever, rigors and vomiting. Both kidneys are affected, but the pain and tenderness may be localised to one flank. Urinary symptoms may be absent unless there is an accompanying cystitis. The condition is much commoner in women, particularly during pregnancy. The urine will be opalescent and contains pus cells and numerous organisms. Outside hospital the majority of these infections are still due to *Esch. coli*. Most attacks subside within a few days on appropriate antibiotic therapy.

CAUSES IN THE GENITAL TRACT

Salpingitis

Aetiology

Most cases of pelvic inflammatory disease are due to an ascending infection from the uterus or vagina. Salpingitis is therefore associated with sexual activity, retained products of conception, the insertion of intra-uterine contraceptive devices and diagnostic curettage. It is still common due to a gonococcal infection but *Chlamydia trachomatis* is being increasingly recognised as an important primary cause. Secondary infection occurs when the initial organism is replaced by bacteria, such as *Esch. coli*, *Bacteroides*, staphylococci and streptococci, which inhabit the normal vagina. In a few cases infection spreads from an inflamed appendix or sigmoid diverticulitis. In tuberculous salpingitis the organism is carried in the blood from other foci in the body, notably the lungs.

Clinical features

The most prominent symptom of acute salpingitis is pain which is usually felt as a broad band across the lower abdomen. It may be more marked on one side than the other and when on the right somewhat resembles acute appendicitis. It is continuous in nature and accompanied by fever and sometimes vomiting. The pain may radiate to the back and is made worse by movement, micturition, defaecation and intercourse. A purulent vaginal discharge is not uncommon and uterine bleeding, described by the patients as 'the period coming early', may accompany the pain.

On examination the patient will be flushed and feverish and there will be guarding and rebound tenderness in the lower abdomen. Vaginal examination may be difficult for there is often marked tenderness of the adnexa, but pyosalpinx or tubo-ovarian abscess may be palpated as a mass which is distinctly separate from the uterus.

Chronic salpingitis is a sequel of acute salpingitis and is characterised by bouts of vague lower abdominal pain, dyspareunia and sterility. Tuberculous salpingitis often takes this form and should be borne in mind in a young woman with no history of any previous acute episodes.

Investigations

Swabs should be taken from the cervix and vagina and sent to the laboratory in Stewart's medium for culture. *Chlamydia* is difficult to grow but many laboratories are now able to isolate this organism, using monoclonal antibodies to make a positive identification. In acute salpingitis the polymorph leukocyte count is usually raised and the ESR may be elevated.

Laparoscopy is being increasingly used in the investigation of pelvic pain in women and often enables a confident diagnosis to be made. It has the great advantage that swabs can be taken directly from the infected fallopian tubes. When chronic inflammatory changes are present a diagnosis of tuberculosis may only be excluded by examination of tissue removed at laparotomy. A persistently negative Mantoux or Heaf test, however, makes this diagnosis unlikely.

Endometriosis (see also Hypogastric pain, p. 79)

This often begins in one ovary and spreads to other pelvic organs. It is a common cause of secondary dysmenorrhoea and the pain may at first be localised to one iliac fossa.

Ectopic pregnancy

As a rule one or more periods will have been missed before the ectopic pregnancy makes its presence felt. In the classical case rupture of the fallopian tube occurs suddenly with the onset of severe unilateral pain in one iliac fossa and signs of shock from haemorrhage into the peritoneal cavity. As the blood spreads the pain becomes generalised and, when it reaches the diaphragm, will be referred to one or other shoulder. An ampullary pregnancy, on the other hand, may be more insidious in onset with episodes of pelvic pain accompanied by a vaginal discharge or bleeding. A unilateral tender pelvic mass in a young woman with amenor-rhoea or vaginal bleeding is very likely to be an ectopic pregnancy; a rapidly falling haemoglobin level should arouse suspicion.

Mittelschmerz

As this pain is due to ovulation it is felt in the middle of the menstrual cycle and is not uncommon. It is probably due to rupture of a follicular cyst. The pain is usually felt in one or other iliac fossa and seldom lasts more than 24 hours. It may be mistaken for appendicitis but there is no vomiting, soiled tongue or fever. There is often a history of previous attacks around the time of ovulation. Very occasionally significant haemorrhage occurs and the signs and symptoms may then resemble those of an ectopic pregnancy. Only laparotomy will enable the distinction to be made.

Polycystic ovaries (see also Obesity, p. 296)

This condition was first described by Stein and Leventhal in 1934. It is not uncommon in young women and occasionally gives rise to severe iliac fossa pain, especially on the right side. It may then be mistaken for appendicitis and, unless the ovaries are inspected at operation, the diagnosis will be missed. The aetiology is unknown but it is usually associated with irregular periods and some degree of hirsutism. Obesity is present in about 40% of cases. The diagnosis is best confirmed by laparoscopy as the enlarged ovaries are rarely palpable on vaginal examination. Ultrasonography of the ovaries will usually demonstrate the multiple cysts, but does not prove that they are the source of the pain.

Torsion of ovarian cyst

Torsion of an ovarian tumour or cyst results in acute lower abdominal pain which may start on one side but soon spreads to the other. Vomiting is not uncommon and there may be difficulty in micturition, culminating in acute retention. On examination there will be guarding and tenderness in the lower abdomen and a swelling arising from the pelvis may be palpable on bimanual examination.

Oöphoritis (see also Fever, p. 308)

Inflammation of the ovaries is an occasional complication of mumps occurring after puberty. It usually presents acutely about a week after the onset of the illness, when the parotid swellings are subsiding, with pain in one or both iliac fossae. Symptoms vary in intensity from a mild discomfort to severe pain, fever and vomiting. The condition usually subsides within a few days and does not appear to impair subsequent fertility.

EXTRA-ABDOMINAL CAUSES

Muscular strain

A dull ache may be felt in the lateral abdominal wall following unaccustomed use of the abdominal muscles in sport or other vigorous activities. Stitch is the name given to a sharp, stabbing pain below one or other of the costal margins which is exacerbated by movement; it is thought to be due to spasm of the diaphragm or an intercostal muscle. There is usually little difficulty in distinguishing these superficial discomforts from pain arising from within the abdomen.

Pleurisy (see also Thoracic pain, p. 30)

Inflammation of the diaphragm or pleura supplied by the eighth to the twelfth thoracic nerves may cause pain which is felt in the hypochondrium or even lower in the lateral abdominal wall. It is characteristically stabbing in nature and made worse by coughing and deep inspiration. The lungs must be examined with embolism and pneumonia in mind. Bornholm disease should not be forgotten as a cause of severe paroxysmal upper abdominal pain in children and young adults.

Herpes zoster (see also Thoracic pain, p. 43)

Involvement of the ganglia of the lower thoracic nerves by this viral infection will give rise to pain in the corresponding dermatomes. It may vary in character from a superficial tingling or burning sensation to a severe deep pain resembling that of appendicitis or cholecystitis. It is usually preceded by a few days of malaise and fever and followed 4–5 days later by the appearance of the typical vesicles on the back and abdominal wall. The diagnosis may be in doubt until the rash appears.

Spinal lesions

These are uncommon but potentially very serious causes of lateral abdominal pain. Collapse of one or more of the lower thoracic vertebrae from trauma, osteoporosis, myelomatosis, metastatic deposits or tuberculosis of the spine can cause agonising pain in the abdominal wall. It is often sudden in onset, stabbing in nature and made worse by coughing, sneezing, blowing the nose and movements of the trunk. There may be local tenderness and guarding. The segmental nature of the pain is usually obvious from the history and a lateral X-ray of the thoracic spine will show the typical wedge-shaped vertebra. Further investigations will be necessary to determine the underlying cause.

Rarely a slowly growing spinal tumour involving the posterior roots of the eleventh or twelfth thoracic nerves will cause iliac fossa pain and nothing else; this may precede any neurological signs in the lower limbs by months or even years. Needless to say, such cases are not easily diagnosed but persistent pain which is worse at night should arouse suspicion.

Osteoarthritis and disc protrusions of the lumbar spine ordinarily result in lumbago or sciatica, but back pain may be minimal or absent and pain may be felt instead in the groin or iliac fossa.

CHAPTER 9
Dysphagia

SYNOPSIS OF CAUSES*

OROPHARYNGEAL
Tonsillitis; Pharyngitis; Ludwig's angina; **Foreign body; Neuromuscular disorders**; Myasthenia gravis; Polymyositis; Neoplasm; Diverticulum.

OESOPHAGEAL
Oesophagitis; Stricture; Paterson-Brown-Kelly syndrome; Foreign body; **Neoplasm**; Achalasia; **Neuromuscular disorders**; Scleroderma; Diverticulum.

EXTRINSIC
Thyroiditis; Neoplasm; Aortic aneurysm.

* Bold type is used for causes more commonly found in Europe and North America.

PHYSIOLOGY

The oral cavity and pharynx are separated from the oesophagus by the cricopharyngeal or upper oesophageal sphincter. These structures are supplied by the ninth to twelfth cranial nerves. The oesophagus itself is a muscular tube containing both voluntary and involuntary muscle, the latter being innervated by sympathetic fibres from the fourth to the sixth thoracic segments of the cord. The upper third is mainly skeletal muscle continuous with the fibres of the inferior pharyngeal constrictors, the middle third is mixed, whilst the lower third is composed entirely of smooth muscle.

The act of swallowing occurs in three stages of which only the first is under voluntary control. In this stage the mouth closes and the bolus of food or fluid is forced backwards through the isthmus of the fauces by the contraction of the cheek muscles and pressure of the tongue against the palate. When the bolus strikes the sensory nerve endings in the posterior pharyngeal wall it triggers off a series of complex reflex activities via the 'deglutition centre' in the brain stem.

During the second stage the oral cavity remains closed off by firm approximation of the tongue against the palate, and the naso-pharyngeal sphincter closes so that the bolus is directed downwards into the lower pharynx towards the oesophageal entrance. At the same time, the larynx is elevated beneath the base of the tongue so that the bolus passes more directly from the pharynx into the oesophagus. The laryngeal sphincter also closes. The bolus is grasped by the constrictor muscles of the pharynx and, having nowhere else to go, is squeezed downwards through the upper oesophageal sphincter which relaxes in order to allow it to pass into the oesophagus. Respiration is momentarily arrested as the bolus passes to prevent food being aspirated into the lower airway.

In the third and final stage the bolus is propelled to the lower oesophageal sphincter by peristaltic waves, taking about 6 seconds to traverse the whole oesophagus. This sphincter is a 'physiological' one in which a section of the circular smooth muscle coat extending above and below the diaphragm is maintained in tonic contraction and helps to prevent gastro-oesophageal reflux. It is innervated by the vagus nerve and relaxes upon arrival of the oesophageal peristaltic wave from above to permit the bolus to enter the stomach.

Dysphagia may result from disordered function of the pharyngeal muscles or the upper oesophageal sphincter, narrowing of the oesophageal lumen from intrinsic or extrinsic causes, or from failure of the lower sphincter to relax.

DIAGNOSTIC APPROACH

Dysphagia is by definition difficulty in the act of swallowing. There is a feeling that what has been swallowed has not gone down properly and is sticking in the throat or gullet. Factors to be considered in the differential diagnosis are the age of the patient, the level at which the difficulty occurs, accompanying symptoms such as the regurgitation of fluids or undigested food and the presence or absence of pain.

Disorders which give rise to a sensation of food sticking in the back of the throat include inflammation or obstruction in the oropharynx and neuromuscular diseases affecting the coordination of the tongue, pharynx and upper oesophageal sphincter. Inflammatory causes may occur at any age but are commoner in childhood and are usually obvious from the history and examination. Swallowing is painful although fluids may pass without too much difficulty. Neuromuscular diseases on the other hand are painless and give rise to difficulty in swallowing both solids and liquids. In the elderly this is commonly due to cerebrovascular disease; in younger patients, particularly women, the possibility of myasthenia gravis or poly-myositis should be considered. In these patients there may be evidence of muscular weakness elsewhere.

Once the food has been swallowed it may stick on its way down the oesophagus and the patient can sometimes indicate the approximate level at which the obstruction occurs. Regurgitation of undigested food is seen in old men with a pharyngeal pouch and in younger patients with achalasia; in the latter dysphagia is often preceded by intermittent chest pain. There may be a history of recurrent chest infections in both disorders as a consequence of aspirating oesophageal contents into the lungs.

Reflux oesophagitis causes spasm at the lower end of the oesophagus and interferes with the normal action of the lower oesophageal sphincter. Food appears to stick at the xiphisternum and produces substernal pain which may radiate into the neck or through to the back. It is by far the commonest cause of dysphagia in adults and is characteristically eased by antacids and histamine H_2-antagonists. Most importantly, when confronted with a short history of painless dysphagia in or after middle-life the clinician's first thought should be of neoplasia. Regrettably many oesophageal cancers are already inoperable by the time they are referred to a thoracic surgeon.

Something may be said here concerning the discomfort in the throat due to contraction or spasm of the cricopharyngeus muscle. This has been experienced by many people in moments of emotional stress, being commonly described as a 'lump in the throat'. A persistence of this discomfort has long been termed 'globus hystericus' and may be mistaken for dysphagia; it is in fact temporarily relieved rather than induced by swallowing food or drink. As it may have an organic cause this term should be abandoned.

OROPHARYNGEAL CAUSES

Lesions confined to the mouth cause discomfort in eating rather than difficulty in swallowing; they should be visible on inspection. Spread of infection to the pharynx, larynx or oesophagus may, however, be inapparent though giving rise to dysphagia.

Tonsillitis

Inflammation of the tonsils causes pain on swallowing, especially if the infection has spread to the pharynx. It is commonly due to streptococcal or viral infections and infectious mononucleosis is a frequent cause in young adults. Acute ulceration of the tonsils occurs in leukaemia and agranulocytosis; the latter may be due to medication so that a drug history is necessary in appropriate cases. Peritonsillar abscess (quinsy) is an occasional complication of tonsillitis.

Pharyngitis

In acute pharyngitis each act of swallowing is painful. The buccal mucosa and pharynx are inflamed and the temperature may be raised. Acute retropharyngeal abscess is now rare in Britain. This suppuration of the retropharyngeal lymph nodes can, however, follow an upper respiratory infection in infants and young children and presents with high fever, painful dysphagia and stridor. The head is extended in an attempt to improve the airways and the bulging mass is easily seen unless there is trismus.

Candidiasis is common in debilitated elderly patients on antibiotic or corticosteroid therapy. It usually starts in the mouth but the characteristic soft white plaques on the palate may be seen only when the dentures have been removed. Spread of the fungus to the pharynx, larynx or oesophagus causes painful dysphagia.

Ludwig's angina

This occasionally arises from a root abscess in a lower molar tooth producing a sublingual cellulitis. The tongue is elevated and there is a severe pain and dysphagia. The swelling may increase rapidly and produce respiratory obstruction. The causative organism is usually a haemolytic streptococcus and prompt antibiotic therapy will often avoid the necessity for surgery.

Foreign body

Small objects, such as fish or chicken bones, may become embedded in a tonsil, pillar of the fauces or in the pyriform fossa causing much pain and discomfort. In young children in particular a toy from a Christmas cracker or a peanut may be held up at the glottis but usually passes into the trachea and bronchi. Such obstruction of the larynx is not uncommon in the elderly when inadequate mastication with poorly-fitting dentures allows a bolus of food to become impacted. Total obstruction of the glottis obviously leads to death from asphyxiation within minutes. More often the obstruction is incomplete and the difficulty in swallowing is relieved either- by coughing the object up or by its passage down the oesophagus.

Neuromuscular disorders

A minor degree of incoordination of the skeletal muscles involved in the initiation of the act of swallowing is a not uncommon cause of intermittent dysphagia in the elderly; it is probably the result of 'little strokes' affecting the ageing brain. Grosser examples are seen in pseudobulbar palsy or from lesions of the medulla oblongata causing true bulbar palsy. The latter is seen as a complication of poliomyelitis, pharyngeal diphtheria and motor neurone disease. A similar impairment of the local mechanisms of swallowing occurs in myasthenia gravis and polymyositis which are considered below.

The patient has difficulty in transferring food from the mouth and pharynx into the oesophagus because the upper oesophageal sphincter fails to relax at the proper time. Fluids, and to a lesser extent solids, may spill over into the airway, causing coughing. In the elderly there will be a history of deteriorating mental function and, in the case of pseudobulbar palsy, evidence of past or present strokes.

Myasthenia gravis

Aetiology

This autoimmune disease is a rare cause of painless dysphagia. It is seen mainly in women and may be associated with other autoimmune disorders such as thyroiditis, pernicious anaemia, rheumatoid arthritis or systemic lupus erythematosus. The underlying defect in neuromuscular transmission is probably due to the production of antibodies to the acetylcholine receptors in striated muscle. These have now been demonstrated in many cases. It seems likely that these antibodies originate from the thymus for hyperplasia of this gland is commonly found at autopsy and some 10–15% of cases harbour a thymoma. Removal of the thymus may lead to a prolonged remission.

Clinical features

The patient, usually a young woman, presents with dysphagia, choking and nasal regurgitation of fluids. There may be difficulty in finishing a meal and the symptoms are often worse at the end of the day. If these are the only manifestations a diagnosis of hysteria may be entertained. Other signs of a generalised muscle weakness should be sought such as difficulty in rising from a chair or climbing stairs; ptosis and diplopia are not uncommon. The symptoms often remit in pregnancy and may be exacerbated by an intercurrent infection.

Investigations

The intravenous injection of 10 mg of edrophonium (Tensilon) will produce a dramatic increase in muscle strength lasting a few minutes; a positive response to this test is virtually diagnostic. Ideally the serum should be tested for the presence of acetylcholine-receptor antibodies but this procedure is only available in a few centres. Tomograms and, where available, computed tomography of the anterior mediastinum may reveal a thymoma.

Polymyositis

Aetiology

Polymyositis is an uncommon but important cause of generalised muscular weakness in adults. Dysphagia is frequently seen and is secondary to weakness of the pharyngeal muscles and hypotonicity of the upper oesophagus. When the muscular weakness is accompanied by a rash the term dermatomyositis is used to describe the condition. It is rare in childhood, and women are more usually affected than men. Its aetiology is obscure but it can follow a viral infection. Recently coxsackie-B virus RNA has been found in the affected muscles of some patients, which suggests that a persistent viral infection may be responsible for the patchy inflammatory changes found on muscle biopsy. In the elderly it is sometimes associated with malignant disease.

Clinical features

Profound weakness is the most striking feature of this disease, affecting mainly the proximal muscles of the hip and shoulder girdles. It may present acutely, as in dermatomyositis, or appear insidiously over a period of weeks or even months. Aching and tenderness of the affected muscles often accompany the loss of power. In a severe case there may be a total inability to swallow either fluid or solids. Depending on the mode of onset and the age of the patient it may be mistaken for the Guillain–Barré syndrome, motor neurone disease or myasthenia gravis. In those cases associated with a neoplasm the tumour may be apparent at the onset or escape detection for a year or two.

Investigations

The diagnosis is usually confirmed by serum enzyme estimations, electro-myography and muscle biopsy. In those patients with dysphagia a barium swallow will show pooling of the contrast media in the vallecular and pyriform sinuses. In the elderly a diligent search should be made for an occult neoplasm in the lung, alimentary tract, breast, kidney and pelvic organs.

Neoplasm

Malignant growths of the larynx comprise about 2% of all cancers in Britain. They are seen as a rule in men over 60 and particularly in cigarette smokers. Like the now rarely seen tuberculosis of the larynx they may cause no more than huskiness or hoarseness. Only when large do laryngeal tumours cause dysphagia. Pain on swallowing appears when the spread of the growth has led to perichondritis and may be accompanied by pain referred to one or other ear. At this stage in the disease enlarged lymph nodes may be palpated in the neck. Hoarseness in an elderly man persisting for several weeks calls for laryngoscopy for the growth can be cured at an early stage.

Diverticulum

A pharyngeal diverticulum or pouch is an unusual cause of painless dysphagia in the elderly. It consists of a protrusion of the mucosa of the posterior pharyngeal wall just above the cricopharyngeus muscle. It is prob-ably the result of some incoordination of muscular activity during the second stage of swallowing so that the cricopharyngeus muscle fails to relax at the right moment, leading to excessively high intrapharyngeal pressures. The pouch enlarges downward into the mediastinum and, when filled with food, compresses the oesophagus and may appear as a swelling on the left side of the neck. Regurgitation at night may cause cough and respiratory infection. Its presence is revealed by a barium swallow and confirmed by endoscopy.

OESOPHAGEAL CAUSES

The sensation of food sticking in the throat or at the xiphisternum is usually due to oesophageal abnormalities, of which the commonest are mucosal inflammation and squamous cell carcinoma. Both give rise to organic strictures requiring surgical intervention.

Oesophagitis (see also Thoracic pain, p. 37)

Reflux oesophagitis is by far the commonest cause of painful dysphagia at all ages. It is particularly common during pregnancy and in the elderly and is often associated with an hiatus hernia. The damage produced in the lower oesophagus by excessive exposure to gastric juices ranges from minor changes in the mucosa, visible only under the microscope, to gross ulceration, scarring, and stricture formation. Reflux and the discomfort which it provokes occurs after meals, during physical exertion or bending and on retiring to bed. The pain, which may spread up into the neck or through to the back, is normally relieved by the taking of antacids or a glass of milk. A certain diagnosis can be made only by oesophagoscopy; this procedure enables the severity of the damage to be assessed and biopsies to be taken. In practice many patients are not investigated to this extent. A typical history and a good response to antacids or histamine H_2-antagonists is often taken to be sufficient evidence of its existence, particularly if a barium meal shows the presence of a hiatus hernia or reflux of the contrast media.

In the elderly oesophagitis may be due to the downward spread of oral candidiasis and the mouth should be inspected carefully with this in mind. In such cases a barium swallow will show a shaggy outline to the oesophageal wall. Herpetic oesophagitis is sometimes confused with oesophagitis due to *Candida* — both occur in debilitated patients on antibiotic or immunosuppressive therapy. An even more insidious cause in old age is the ingestion of certain drugs in tablet form which may be held up at the lower oesophageal sphincter, particularly if they are taken at bedtime with insufficient fluid to wash them into the stomach. These include aspirin and other non-steroidal anti-inflammatory drugs, antibiotics, ascorbic acid, emepronium bromide, ferrous sulphate and Slow-K tablets. Finally, it should not be forgotten that a very painful oesophagitis and consequent stricture formation will follow the swallowing of a corrosive taken accidentally or with suicidal intent.

Stricture

Narrowing of the oesophageal lumen from cancer and achalasia is discussed later in this chapter, but by far the commonest cause of stenosis is ulceration of the lower oesophagus from long-standing reflux oesophagitis. Benign strictures may also result from clumsy instrumentation, an impacted foreign body, candidiasis and inflammation produced by corrosive chemicals.

In the newborn infant congenital atresia of the oesophagus occurs once in some 5000 births. It presents within a few hours or a day or two with an accumulation of frothy mucus, cough and cyanosis. Although it certainly gives rise to difficulty in swallowing a complaint of dysphagia has yet to be recorded!

Paterson–Brown–Kelly syndrome

Sideropenic dysphagia is occasionally seen in middle-aged women with hypochromic anaemia and atrophic glossitis. Koilonychia is sometimes present. Iron deficiency leads to atrophic changes in the pharyngeal and upper oesophageal mucosa, submucosal fibrosis in the postcricoid area and stricture formation. On oesophagoscopy a concentric stricture is visible whilst a barium swallow discloses the characteristic web appearance. Some 15% of such cases develop a postcricoid carcinoma.

Foreign body (see also Dyspnoea, p. 239)

When there is failure to eject a foreign body from the glottis it may pass on into the bronchial tree, as so commonly happens with small children, or into the oesophagus. From the latter it usually passes on into the stomach but an angular-shaped object or a coin may be held up at the level of the thoracic inlet, aortic arch or lower oesophageal sphincter. When this occurs there will be localised substernal discomfort increased by swallowing. If the object is not removed stricture, perforation and mediastinitis may ensue. The accident is often overlooked or forgotten and it is important to obtain a definite history if possible. A chest X-ray will disclose a radio-opaque body; otherwise a barium swallow is necessary prior to endoscopy.

Neoplasm

Aetiology
Cancer of the oesophagus accounts for about 4000 deaths annually in Britain and is nearly always squamous in type. It was noted to be a frequent cause of dysphagia by Avicenna as long ago as the tenth century. In Europe it is mainly a disease of the elderly and is seen most frequently in male smokers, although postcricoid carcinoma is more commonly found in women with iron-deficiency anaemia as indicated above.

Oesophageal cancer is particularly prevalent in parts of Africa and China. This may be due to dietary deficiencies or to the presence of high concentrations of tannin in their diet. There is an increased risk of this disease in patients with hereditary tylosis, achalasia, sideropenic dysphagia, gluten enteropathy and chronic reflux oesophagitis.

Squamous cell carcinoma of the oesophagus is one of the most lethal neoplasms of the alimentary tract and arises at three main sites — the postcricoid region, at the level of the aortic arch, and just above the cardia. It spreads locally by direct invasion of adjacent structures or through submucosal lymphatics.

Clinical features
The only hope of survival in this grave disorder is early diagnosis. A mild and occasional sensation of food sticking behind the sternum in an elderly subject is frequently ignored or leads to the adoption of a semi-fluid diet. This may fatally delay the seeking of advice until dysphagia becomes troublesome and discourages eating, with consequent loss of weight. A short history of only a few weeks' duration is not uncommon. When obstruction develops regurgitation results in inhalation, cough and respiratory infection.

Investigations
Although a barium swallow may show a typical lobulated intraluminal mass some growths produce a smooth narrowing which is easily mistaken for a benign stricture. Multiple biopsies taken at oesophagoscopy are essential for the diagnosis.

Achalasia

Aetiology
This rare disorder is seen equally in men and women and most often between the third and sixth decades of life. In the normal act of swallowing the lower oesophageal sphincter relaxes as each peristaltic wave thrusts against it. In achalasia this relaxation fails to occur, and passage of food into the stomach is only accomplished by vigorous contractions of the oesophagus and the weight of food or fluid trapped at its lower end. Atony and dilatation of the oesophagus are the inevitable consequence of this obstruction but may take years to develop. The cause is unknown but histological examination has shown degeneration of the ganglion cells in the myenteric plexus. In South America an identical disorder is seen in endemic form amongst patients with Chagas' disease.

Clinical features
Dysphagia is the major symptom but may be intermittent at first. The adoption of a semi-fluid diet and slow eating relieves the discomfort and leads the patient to defer seeking advice for his 'indigestion' until the condition is well advanced.

Cramping retrosternal pain after meals may accompany or precede the dysphagia and is often rapidly eased by drinking cold water. Dilatation of the oesophagus leads to the regurgitation of undigested food, and the aspiration of oesophageal contents into the lungs during sleep may cause recurrent chest infections. There is usually nothing to find on physical examination.

Investigations
An enlarged mediastinal shadow may be seen on a plain chest X-ray but a barium swallow is necessary to reveal the characteristic appearance of a dilated and elongated oesophagus with a smooth tapering stenosis at its lower end. Oesophagoscopy must be carried out to exclude a neoplasm in the oesophagus or fundus of the stomach. Oesophageal motility studies, in

the hands of an expert, may enable the condition to be diagnosed at a much earlier stage before there is any radiological or endoscopic evidence of its existence.

Neuromuscular disorders

Diffuse oesophageal spasm is an uncommon cause of intermittent dysphagia and substernal pain in adults. In some cases it is associated with reflux oesophagitis whilst in others it is provoked by emotional stresses and may be yet another manifestation of the irritable bowel syndrome. The sudden onset of dysphagia during the course of a meal is often overshadowed by intense retrosternal pain which may be so severe as to mimic that of myocardial ischaemia. The pain may occur independently of meals and sometimes wakens the patient at night.

A barium swallow may be normal but characteristically shows trapping of beads of contrast in a spastic lower oesophagus. This appearance has been described by radiologists as the 'corkscrew' oesophagus and is due to uncoordinated segmental contractions. If there is any doubt about the diagnosis oesophagoscopy should be carried out to exclude oesophagitis, achalasia and, in the older patient, neoplasia.

Scleroderma

In systemic sclerosis the alimentary tract, as well as other systems, is often involved. Oesophageal motor function is abnormal in the majority of patients but dysphagia is rarely a problem, being overshadowed by the heartburn and acid reflux in the mouth from reflux oesophagitis. These symptoms sometimes precede cutaneous and other manifestations of the disease. In advanced cases an atonic, non-contracting lower oesophagus can be seen on barium swallow.

Diverticulum

Diverticula of the oesophagus are uncommon. They are located either half way down the gullet or just above the lower oesophageal sphincter. Mid-oesophageal diverticula are wide-mouthed pouches which lie in close proximity to the right bronchus and seldom give rise to symptoms. Those at the lower end are more likely to present with dysphagia because they are often associated with achalasia or diffuse oesophageal spasm. The diagnosis is made on barium swallow.

EXTRINSIC CAUSES

Dysphagia is sometimes due to compression or infiltration of the oesophagus by disease in adjacent organs. A large substernal multinodular goitre for example may grow to a sufficient size to cause some difficulty in swallowing from occlusion of the oesophagus. Other thyroid disorders by contrast involve the pharyngeal mechanisms and are discussed below.

Thyroiditis

Acute bacterial inflammation of the thyroid gland is rare. It may be part of a cellulitis of the neck or arise from an infected cyst in a multi-nodular goitre. The gland is swollen and very tender, swallowing is painful and fever is present. There will be a polymorph leukocytosis and the condition subsides on appropriate antibiotic therapy.

Subacute thyroiditis is not so rare as the acute form and usually appears some 2–3 weeks after an upper respiratory infection. It seems likely that it is due to an abnormal immunological response to certain viruses and cases have been reported following mumps. The gland is enlarged and often extremely tender, the patient being afraid to eat because of the pain induced by swallowing. Hyperthyroidism is occasionally seen and may require treatment. The ESR is often markedly raised, a polymorph leukocytosis may be present and thyroid antibodies will be found in the blood. Untreated, the pain and swelling persist for weeks and even months. Anti-inflammatory drugs will usually suppress the symptoms but relapses are not infrequent when these are withdrawn. The condition is likely to progress to chronic thyroiditis and eventual hypothyroidism.

Neoplasm

Thyroid neoplasms are rare, accounting for less than 1% of all cancer deaths in Britain. They usually present as a slowly growing lump in the neck. Dysphagia and hoarseness are late symptoms due to invasion of adjacent structures. Enlarged lymph nodes may be felt in the neck and biopsies of these or of the thyroid itself are necessary to establish the diagnosis. In medullary cell carcinoma X-rays may show calcification in the gland and the serum calcitonin level will be raised. These tumours secrete a variety of humoral agents which may cause flushing attacks, chronic diarrhoea or Cushing's syndrome.

Occasionally the oesophagus is invaded by a bronchial neoplasm or an adenocarcinoma of the fundus of the stomach. The mode of presentation is very similar to that of a squamous cell carcinoma of the oesophagus, with which they may be confused. Multiple biopsies of the affected area at oesophagoscopy will usually suffice to determine the origin of the tumour.

Aortic aneurysm (see also Thoracic pain, p. 37)

In Britain most aortic aneurysms are due to atherosclerosis and present in old age. Compression of the oesophagus by an aneurysm of the thoracic aorta is a rare cause of dysphagia.

CHAPTER 10
Vomiting

Vomiting is not in itself of much diagnostic value for it occurs in many diseases and is usually overshadowed by other complaints. Only those conditions in which it may be the most prominent symptom are mentioned in this chapter.

SYNOPSIS OF CAUSES*

GASTROINTESTINAL
Gastritis; Viral gastroenteritis; Drugs; Poisons; Congenital abnormalities; **Pyloric stenosis;** Operation sequelae; **Intestinal obstruction**.

METABOLIC
Drugs; Reye's syndrome; **Poisons; Ionising radiation**; Renal failure; Hypercalcaemia.

ENDOCRINE
Pregnancy; Diabetes; Addison's disease; Congenital adrenal hyperplasia.

NEUROGENIC
Ménière's disease; Vestibular neuronitis; Motion sickness; Cerebral tumour.

PSYCHOGENIC
Anxiety state; Anorexia nervosa; Bulimia.

* Bold type is used for causes more commonly found in Europe and North America.

PHYSIOLOGY

The term 'vomiting' means 'the expulsion of gastric contents through the mouth'. It does not include the regurgitation of undigested food from the oesophagus. Vomiting is a reflex act initiated in the vomiting centre in the brain stem, either in response to stimulation of the adjacent chemoreceptor trigger zone by toxic substances in the blood or by stimuli reaching it from further afield. The latter may arise in the brain itself, from organs supplied by the cranial nerves, such as the ear and eye, or from the viscera and their enveloping membranes. As far as the alimentary tract is concerned nausea and vomiting appear to be initiated by impulses arising in receptors in the gastric and intestinal mucosa. These occur in response to chemical stimuli or to changes in intramuscular tension and reach the spinal cord in afferent fibres of the autonomic nervous system.

The act of vomiting is usually preceded by nausea and retching and accompanied by pallor, sweating, faintness and excessive salivation. Co-incident with these unpleasant sensations there is relaxation of the lower oesophageal sphincter and upper part of the stomach with closure of the pylorus. This is rapidly followed by vigorous contractions of the diaphragm and abdominal muscles leading to a sharp rise in intra-abdominal pressure and ejection of the gastric contents upwards through the relaxed oesophagus into the mouth. At the same time the glottis is closed, respiration ceases momentarily and the soft palate rises to shut off the nasopharynx.

Reverse peristalsis in the gut is not necessarily a concomitant of the act of vomiting but, when present, bile and intestinal contents will pass up into the stomach and hence into the vomit. When the vomiting is profuse and prolonged, dehydration, hypokalaemia and metabolic alkalosis will ensue unless the losses of water, sodium, potassium, chloride and hydrogen ions are made good by parenteral therapy. Urgent vomiting, particularly after a heavy meal, has been known to cause oesophageal rupture or, more commonly, bleeding from tears in the gastric mucosa, as is seen in the Mallory–Weiss syndrome. Finally, vomiting in the unconscious patient is particularly dangerous for the glottis may fail to close and the inhalation of gastric contents into the air passages will result in a chemical pneumonia.

DIAGNOSTIC APPROACH

Reference was made in the introduction to the importance in diagnosis of selecting the *significant* sign or symptom. Vomiting can occur in so many illnesses of widely differing aetiology that it is of little diagnostic value in itself. Attention must therefore be directed to accompanying symptoms such as pain, diarrhoea, pyrexia or vertigo. Nevertheless, there are some disorders in which vomiting is the prominent symptom and these are considered in the present chapter.

The time of onset and the possible relationship of an attack of vomiting to a preceding meal, to an emotional upset or to the taking of a drug must be determined and also whether this is a single incident or repeated, and if so over what period of time. An acute onset is likely to be due to gastroenteritis and a history of similar symptoms in another member of the family or others attending the same school or social function would suggest food poisoning or a common viral infection. The latter would be more likely if the attending doctor was aware of other cases in his practice, particularly during the winter months. The presence of vertigo would point to a vestibular cause such as travel sickness, Ménière's disease or vestibular neuronitis.

More prolonged vomiting, occurring in bouts over a period of weeks or even months, is seen in pregnancy, pyloric stenosis and following gastric operations. Occasionally it is due to the metabolic consequences of renal or adrenal failure or to the presence of a cerebral tumour.

The age and sex of the patient have a bearing upon the likely diagnosis. In infancy the commonest cause of repeated vomiting is underfeeding. Careful observation will show that it is associated with excessive air-swallowing and, in the bottle-fed baby, may be cured by enlarging the hole in the teat. Some otherwise healthy infants regularly regurgitate part of their feed which is a source of considerable anxiety to their parents. Spontaneous recovery usually follows the establishment of mixed feeding. Congenital abnormalities are rare causes of vomiting in the first few weeks of life, with the exception of pyloric stenosis in male infants.

In the older child vomiting is usually due to a viral infection, dietary indiscretions, travel sickness or accidental poisoning. On rare occasions it may be the first manifestation of diabetic keto-acidosis, Reye's syndrome or renal failure. Psychological problems of one sort or another may be the cause of cyclical vomiting in childhood, though this is still debatable. There is however no doubt that emotional disturbances play an increasingly important role during the turbulent years of adolescence and early adult life. Self-induced vomiting in the female is the hallmark of anorexia nervosa and bulimia and is often precipitated by stress in the home or in the world outside.

In adult life the number of possible causes increases with each decade as a result of the rising incidence of diseases of the gastrointestinal tract and other organs, and the increased risk of exposure to toxic chemicals at work or in the form of medication. Morning sickness may be a symptom of alcohol abuse or renal failure in either sex but pregnancy is-more likely in a female between the ages of 14 and 40, even if she denies this possibility. In old age vomiting is commonly due to the toxic effects of drugs in patients with impaired renal or hepatic function.

The history should include details of marital status and parity, occupation, menstruation, diet, drinking habits, previous illnesses or operations and any current medication, including the contraceptive pill. Questions should be asked about possible accompanying symptoms, such as abdominal pain, diarrhoea, constipation, deafness, tinnitus, giddiness, thirst or polyuria, which might throw more light on the underlying pathology.

The examination should be thorough and may reveal signs of dehydration, loss of flesh, epigastric tenderness and an abdominal scar or palpable mass. The presence of visible peristalsis or a succussion splash is evidence of obstruction to the gastric outflow. Papilloedema, deafness and nystagmus should be looked for if a cerebral or vestibular cause is suspected from the history. Bilateral conjunctivitis is a most unusual finding but is sometimes seen with high serum calcium levels. In an emaciated young female brady-cardia, hypotension, lanugo hair, acrocyanosis and yellow palms will confirm the diagnosis of anorexia nervosa. In an obscure case of vomiting the skin should be examined for abnormal pigmentation with Addison's disease in mind. The urine should be tested routinely for sugar, ketones, bilirubin and proteinuria.

Inspection of the vomit is sometimes helpful. In erosive gastritis and peptic ulceration it may contain fresh blood or 'coffee grounds'. The presence of bile will give it a greenish colour and indicates an open passage between the stomach and duodenum; it is usually absent in pyloric obstruction. Copious amounts of fluid containing fragments of undigested food some hours after a meal will also indicate obstruction to the gastric outflow. In intestinal obstruction and paralytic ileus the vomit will be brown in colour and have a faecal odour. The extent of any further investigations will obviously depend upon the probable nature of the underlying cause as determined from the history and physical findings.

GASTROINTESTINAL CAUSES

Vomiting is common to many gastrointestinal disorders but in the majority pain is the more prominent symptom. There are however exceptions to this general rule and in the conditions described below pain may be absent or of a relatively minor nature.

Gastritis (see also Epigastric pain, p. 51)

Acute inflammation of the lining of the stomach is a common cause of vomiting of sudden onset and limited duration. It can be produced by a wide variety of agents, which may be ingested or may alternatively reach the gastric mucosa in the blood. Outbreaks of food poisoning may follow the ingestion of bacterial toxins at social functions or in institutions where communal feeding takes place. The vomiting is typically explosive in onset and accompanied by colicky abdominal pain. Diarrhoea may follow if the inflammation spreads to involve the bowel.

The morning nausea and vomiting which follow an overnight drinking bout are probably due to the irritant effect of the alcohol on the gastric mucosa, but this local stimulus to the vomiting reflex may be supplemented by a direct effect of alcohol upon the vomiting centre itself. Acute gastritis due to viruses, drugs and other poisons is discussed in more detail in the sections which follow.

Viral gastroenteritis (see also Diarrhoea, p. 133)

Winter vomiting disease is an acute self-limiting illness which is very common during the winter months and may present sporadically or in epidemic form. It is probably caused by a variety of different viruses but two main groups have been identified in the stools of acutely ill patients. These are the Norwalk-like agents, which are similar to the parvoviruses, and the rotaviruses which have a predilection for very young children. In fatal cases the inflammatory changes are found mainly in the duodenum and upper jejunum.

The onset is abrupt with nausea, vomiting, abdominal cramps and a low-grade fever. Diarrhoea is not always present. The incubation period ranges from 1–4 days and the illness is usually over in about a week. The nature of the infecting organism may be determined by a rise in viral antibody levels in the blood but this investigation is rarely carried out in practice for what, after all, is a minor illness in the majority.

Drugs (see also Diarrhoea, p. 136)

Gastrointestinal disturbances are the commonest unwanted side-effects of many drugs. Where the cause of vomiting is not clear a careful history of all medications, including those obtained without a prescription, must be taken. It is wise in any case to stop all therapy for at least 48 hours. Nausea and vomiting may be due to a local effect of the drug on the gastric or intestinal mucosa or it may act centrally upon the chemoreceptor trigger zone in the medulla. Sometimes, as is the case with alcohol and ipecacuanha, both mechanisms are involved. The central action of drugs is considered under the metabolic causes of vomiting.

Aspirin, in its many proprietary combinations and even in small doses in a susceptible individual, is a well-known gastric irritant and may produce erosions which bleed. Most of the other non-steroidal anti-inflammatory drugs also have this disadvantage. Oral corticosteroids commonly give rise to indigestion and vomiting may occur in patients with a co-existing peptic ulcer; the risk is reduced if enteric-coated preparations or the water-soluble prednisolone phosphate are employed.

Other compounds which are particularly liable to produce nausea and vomiting when taken by mouth include cytotoxic agents such as azathioprine and methotrexate, chloral hydrate, colchicine, dapsone, ferrous sulphate, potassium chloride, tetracyclines and some of the anti-arrhythmic drugs used in heart disease. Quinidine in particular is rarely prescribed in Britain because of its frequent adverse effects on the gastrointestinal tract.

Poisons

Vomiting may result from the ingestion of household products, poisonous plants and mushrooms or industrial chemicals. Poisoning due to eating fish is practically unknown in Britain but is common in the tropics. The ingestion may be accidental or the poison may be taken with suicide in mind or administered with homicidal intent. Most household products are relatively innocuous but nausea and vomiting may occur after their ingestion and the Poisons Information Service should be consulted about their likely toxic effects and what treatment may be indicated.

A wide variety of poisonous plants may be eaten by inquisitive children and occasionally by adults. They include the berries of such common plants as cowbane, holly, white bryony and the wild arum lily and the seeds of laburnum and yew. Although vomiting is an early and prominent symptom it is usually accompanied by abdominal pain or diarrhoea and may be followed by muscle spasms, drowsiness, incoordination, delirium or convulsions. Mushroom poisoning is uncommon in Britain and is usually due to eating a poisonous variety in mistake for an edible species. Most patients suffer a violent but self-limiting attack of vomiting, diarrhoea and abdominal colic some hours after eating the fungus.

In industry the swallowing of the inorganic salts of antimony, arsenic, lead or mercury may all give rise to an acute gastritis from the irritant effect of these chemicals on the gastric mucosa. Profuse vomiting is the rule and is usually accompanied by abdominal cramps and, with the exception of lead poisoning, by diarrhoea.

Congenital abnormalities

Gross malformations of the alimentary tract are fortunately rare, for they are often fatal. Vomiting within the first few days of life may be seen with tracheo-oesophageal fistulae, intestinal atresia and stenosis, midgut volvulus with malrotation and, very rarely, as a result of meconium ileus in an infant with cystic fibrosis. It is usually obvious within a matter of hours that the baby is in serious trouble and the aspiration of inhaled vomit further complicates the situation. Without immediate and skilled surgery the outlook is extremely grave.

The commoner and less lethal disorder of congenital pyloric stenosis presents later between the third and sixth week of life and has a happier prognosis. It is one of the most frequent surgical conditions in the first few weeks of life and is seen predominantly in firstborn male infants. Initially these babies appear to be thriving and feeding well although there may be the occasional regurgitation after food. Vomiting, usually projectile and following a feed, is the prominent symptom. It is accompanied by crying, constipation and loss of weight; bile will be absent from the vomit, which may be blood-stained. During a feed the abdomen will become distended with visible gastric peristalsis and a mass about 2 cm long should be palpable to the right of the umbilicus. A barium meal is confirmatory but not usually necessary — laparotomy followed by pyloromyotomy is the treatment of choice.

Another less common cause of vomiting in the first few weeks of life is a hiatus hernia associated with incompetence of the lower oesophageal sphincter. The vomit is likely to contain excess mucus and altered blood and a barium swallow will confirm the diagnosis. Fortunately, conservative treatment usually leads to functional recovery without the need for surgical intervention.

Pyloric stenosis

Aetiology
This may be congenital or acquired — the former has just been described.

Acquired pyloric stenosis in adults is due, in the majority of cases, to scarring by a duodenal ulcer and, less commonly, to a gastric ulcer or neoplasm.

Clinical features
A long-standing history of intermittent dyspepsia will favour peptic ulceration. The absence of such a story, particularly in an elderly patient with recent loss of weight, should arouse suspicion of a gastric carcinoma. The vomiting of pyloric stenosis is usually delayed for an hour or more after a meal and is copious and ill-smelling. The presence of material eaten more than 12 hours earlier is evidence of obstruction to the gastric outflow. On examination loss of flesh may be evident, gastric peristaltic waves may be seen and a mass is sometimes palpable in the abdomen. A succussion splash is an important physical sign and should be sought.

Investigations
A barium meal is confirmatory but will not necessarily reveal the nature of the obstruction. In some centres fibreoptic endoscopy has therefore displaced it as the first line of investigation. A low haemoglobin level is evidence of chronic blood loss while a raised blood urea and low serum sodium and potassium levels will reflect the degree of dehydration and electrolyte depletion. Occult blood is likely to be present in the stools in active peptic ulceration and cancer.

Operation sequelae

Operations on the stomach for peptic ulcer frequently relieve the original symptoms, but a significant number of these patients suffer from postoperative vomiting in one form or another. The reported incidence in some series after partial gastrectomy has been as high as 25% and even after a highly selective vagotomy as many as 10% may be affected. In its mildest form regurgitation of food or gastric contents occurs readily on stooping, bending or lying down. This is seen particularly after vagotomy and is due to incompetence of the lower oesophageal sphincter; it usually remits spontaneously with time. More serious is the vomiting of food after meals, and if this occurs in the postoperative period it is due to stasis and delay in gastric emptying and will probably improve spontaneously. Appearing for the first time some months or even years later it is likely to be due to mechanical obstruction at the stoma or more distally in the small bowel; this may be caused by recurrent ulceration, band adhesions, volvulus, internal herniation or bolus obstruction.

Bilious vomiting is one of the most disabling complications of gastric surgery and is liable to occur at any time and particularly in the early morning. The patient may be woken from sleep by intense nausea and an unpleasant bitter taste in the mouth, and the vomit will consist of copious amounts of clear bile-stained fluid. In a severe case vomiting may occur some 15–20 minutes after every meal. Pain is not usually prominent unless there is afferent loop obstruction but there may be some epigastric discomfort which is made worse by eating. The most likely explanation for bilious vomiting is a chemical gastritis from the reflux of bile and pancreatic juices into the stomach or gastric remnant.

Intestinal obstruction (see also Umbilical pain, p. 66)

In mechanical obstruction of the small bowel severe colicky pain is likely to be the prominent symptom. Vomiting is usual and if prolonged the vomited matter is brown in colour and will have a faecal odour. In the paralytic ileus which may follow an abdominal operation or peritonitis vomiting is profuse and painless.

METABOLIC CAUSES

A great variety of blood-borne substances cause vomiting by a central action on the chemoreceptor trigger zone in the brain stem. They include numerous drugs and their metabolites, poisons encountered at home and at work, bacterial toxins and the products of endogenous metabolism if present in excess. In some instances, notably renal failure and alcohol abuse, the vomiting reflex is reinforced by an accompanying gastritis. For convenience the metabolic consequences of endocrine disturbances are dealt with separately.

Drugs

Drugs which cause nausea and vomiting as a common side-effect include the digitalis glycosides, apomorphine and the opiate analgesics, cytotoxic chemicals such as the nitrogen mustards and vincristine, levodopa, bromo-cryptine and the oestrogen in the contraceptive pill. Digitalis intoxication is particularly dangerous in the elderly in whom it may cause arrhythmias, conduction block and worsening heart failure. Nausea is the earliest symptom of overdosage and may persist until the drug is stopped; nausea due to levodopa, bromocryptine and oestrogens is also dose-related but will usually disappear when the dose is reduced.

Vomiting after surgery may be due to the anaesthetic agent or to the opiates used to relieve postoperative pain. Drugs which do not normally give rise to nausea and vomiting may readily do so if alcohol is taken at the same time. The potentiation of its action by disulfiram (Antabuse) is well known and has some therapeutic value in the chronic alcoholic. Few doctors, however, appear to be aware of its similar interaction with chloramphenicol, griseofulvin, metronidazole, chlorpropamide and tolbutamide.

Reye's syndrome

In this rare but potentially fatal disorder of childhood profuse and persistent vomiting develops within 3–4 days after the onset of what appears to be a mild viral illness. Influenza-B and varicella virus have been implicated in many cases but other viruses may also be involved, particularly those causing diarrhoea in preschool children. The vomiting is accompanied or rapidly followed by changes in the child's mental state. Irrational behaviour and clumsy movements may progress to delirium, convulsions and coma within a matter of days. The mortality in reported cases is at least 20% and brain death results from medullary coning due to cerebral oedema.

Apart from the cerebral oedema the main pathology is found in the liver. The hepatic cells are full of fat but there is usually no evidence of hepatic necrosis or inflammation. Nevertheless, liver function is grossly disturbed, with raised serum transaminase levels, a raised blood ammonia concentration and a prolonged prothrombin time. In the survivors the liver returns to normal within a week or two.

It is believed that this disorder is due to an acute self-limiting derangement of hepatic mitochondrial function and that similar changes are taking place in the mitochondria of muscle and brain. Aspirin is frequently given to febrile children with suspected viral illnesses and there are strong suspicions that this drug may precipitate this condition in susceptible individuals. In Britain the Committee on Safety of Medicines has strongly recommended that aspirin should not be given to children under the age of 12 unless specifically indicated, as in Still's disease.

Poisons

Toxic substances which cause nausea and vomiting by acting on the gastric or intestinal mucosa have already been discussed in the section on gastrointestinal causes. In industry there are however many other noxious chemicals which can produce these symptoms by acting centrally. Although stringent regulations exist to protect workers from these hazards poisoning may nevertheless occur from accidental overexposure or failure to wear adequate protective clothing. Chlorinated hydrocarbons, for example, are widely used in the manufacture of plastics and pesticides, as solvents in glues and in the dry-cleaning industry, and as vehicles for paints and other industrial coatings. Their inhalation initially results in euphoria, dizziness, headache, nausea and vomiting but if the exposure is prolonged it may lead to stupor, convulsions and eventually coma. The sense of euphoria which they induce is responsible for the widespread habit of glue-sniffing amongst the young, most commonly in adolescent males. Drunken behaviour, unexplained listlessness and the smell of solvent in the breath or vomit should arouse suspicion.

Carbon monoxide is another common and particularly dangerous hazard, for it is a colourless, tasteless and odourless gas which originates from the incomplete combustion of carboniferous material. Accidental exposure may occur during the cleaning of blast furnaces and generating plants, in coal mines and where petrol or diesel engines are run in a confined space. In countless other occupations the workforce may be at risk from the escape of this gas from underground flues. Unexplained vomiting may precede the onset of more serious and potentially fatal complications. In the home or holiday chalet carbon monoxide poisoning may result from a faulty gas water heater or inadequate ventilation in the bathroom.

Ionising radiation

So common is nausea and vomiting after exposure to ionising radiations that it is common practice to prescribe anti-emetic drugs such as metoclopramide or prochlorperazine to patients undergoing radiotherapy. Anorexia, nausea and vomiting are also amongst the earliest symptoms of radiation sickness following a nuclear explosion or the escape of radioactive material from a nuclear energy plant. The cause is usually self-evident from the history.

Renal failure

Renal failure has many causes, of which the commonest in the UK are probably glomerulonephritis, interstitial nephritis secondary to analgesic abuse and diabetic nephropathy. Less commonly, it is due to potentially reversible conditions such as drug nephrotoxicity, hypercalcaemia or obstruction to the urinary tract by retroperitoneal fibrosis or prostatic hypertrophy. In an obscure case of nausea and vomiting the possibility of renal failure must be seriously considered even if there are no other signs or symptoms which direct attention to the kidneys.

A decline in urine output is not always noticed or commented upon either by the patient or nursing staff and proteinuria may be missed unless the urine is being tested daily. A rising blood urea and serum creatinine will confirm the diagnosis and anaemia rapidly develops, particularly in the presence of haemolysis or disseminated intravascular coagulation. Elderly patients are especially at risk from the renal tubular necrosis which may result from the administration of many drugs of which the chief offenders are the penicillins, sulphonamides, aminoglycosides, cephalosporins and diuretics. Both thiazide and loop diuretics have been implicated and there is a very real danger that increasing the dosage of these drugs in an attempt to flog the failing kidney may only make the situation worse.

Hypercalcaemia

Severe life-threatening hypercalcaemia is an uncommon complication of malignancy, primary hyperparathyroidism, vitamin D intoxication and the milk–alkali syndrome. The condition is often only recognised when the patient is nearly moribund. Repeated vomiting with consequent dehydration is the most prominent feature of the biochemical chaos which develops when the serum calcium level approaches 4 mmol/l (16 mg/100 ml). It is rarely possible to get a satisfactory history from the patients themselves for they are likely to be elderly, confused and suffering from severe impairment of both intellect and memory.

Relatives or friends may, however, have noticed the gradual onset of thirst and polyuria, constipation, loss of weight and muscular weakness which preceded the present emergency. Skeletal metastases and myelomatosis come high on the list of possible causes and may already be known to the attending doctor. Hypercalcaemia of this degree is rare in primary hyperparathyroidism but may be the first evidence of this disease in old age.

The milk–alkali syndrome occurs in a younger age group but is seldom encountered now that sodium bicarbonate has ceased to be a fashionable treatment for dyspepsia. In such cases there will always be a history suggestive of chronic peptic ulceration to alert one to this possibility. Vitamin D intoxication is rare in the UK, where high-dosage vitamin D preparations can only be obtained on prescription, but it is occasionally seen in patients on vitamin D therapy for hypoparathyroidism or osteomalacia.

Apart from the signs of dehydration there may be little else to be found on examination, though reddening of the conjunctivae is sometimes seen. Hypercalcaemia of this magnitude damages the kidneys and increases the renal excretion of potassium. The blood urea and serum creatinine will be elevated, and hypokalaemia is not uncommon. This is a medical emergency and treatment to lower the serum calcium level must be started immediately without waiting for a precise diagnosis. Although the plasma levels of parathyroid hormone and vitamin D metabolites may be of some help in elucidating the underlying cause the results of these radioimmunoassays are unlikely to be available for several days. Osteoporosis and vertebral collapse may be seen on X-rays of the spine but do not necessarily enable a distinction to be made between parathyroid bone disease, myelomatosis or senile osteoporosis. If myelomatosis is suspected the urine should be examined for the presence of light chains and serum sent for immunoelectrophoresis.

ENDOCRINE CAUSES

Vomiting in the absence of abdominal pain is not uncommon in pregnancy, diabetes mellitus and adrenocortical insufficiency. Vomiting associated with a hyperparathyroid crisis has already been considered under Hypercalcaemia in the preceding section.

Pregnancy

Nausea or vomiting before breakfast occurs in about 50% of all pregnancies and for this reason can hardly be described as pathological. It commences soon after the first missed period and may be the earliest indication that conception has occurred. This morning sickness is usually mild and ceases by the fourth month. The stimulus to the vomiting centre is unknown but is presumably hormonal in origin for it coincides with a large but transient rise in the serum chorionic gonadotrophin levels during the first trimester.

In less than 1% of pregnancies vomiting takes a more severe course and is then described as *hyperemesis gravidarum*. Intractable vomiting and impaired nutrition leads to marked dehydration, ketosis, loss of weight, liver damage and sometimes a peripheral neuropathy due to thiamine deficiency. Hyperemesis gravidarum endangers the life of both mother and fetus and is more likely to develop if there are twin pregnancies or a hydatidiform mole. In common with the milder forms it tends to disappear by the fourth month.

Pyelonephritis must be considered as a possible cause of vomiting at any stage of pregnancy but will be accompanied by fever, loin pain and a heavily infected urine. In pre-eclampsia vomiting appears in the third trimester but is preceded by headache, oedema, proteinuria and a rise in blood pressure.

Acute yellow atrophy of the liver is a rare but very serious cause of vomiting in late pregnancy. It is often preceded by a brief febrile illness and presents acutely with malaise, nausea, vomiting, abdominal pain and jaundice. The aetiology is unknown but the fatty infiltration of the liver cells which is found at autopsy is similar to that seen in Reye's syndrome, a disorder in which viral infections and aspirin have been implicated as possible causes. Disseminated intravascular coagulation is a frequent complication and death may result from cerebral haemorrhage or hepato-renal failure.

Diabetes (see also Loss of weight, p. 280)

Vomiting is a major feature of diabetic keto-acidosis and leads rapidly to dehydration and electrolyte depletion. Much fluid and several hundred millimoles of sodium and potassium will also be lost in the urine. Vomiting is preceded by increasing thirst and polyuria and is frequently precipitated by an infection in the respiratory or renal tract. In a previously undiagnosed patient the presence of abdominal pain and a rigid abdomen may suggest a surgical catastrophe before glycosuria, heavy ketonuria or the smell of acetone on the breath draw attention to the correct diagnosis. Gastric dilatation with the accumulation of large quantities of fluid in the atonic stomach is an additional hazard, increasing the risk of inhalation pneumonia in the semi-conscious patient. Early gastric aspiration through a nasogastric tube is essential in such cases.

Repeated vomiting after meals may be the only evidence of autonomic neuropathy in an insulin-dependent diabetic. It is usually associated with poor diabetic control over a long period and is often accompanied by anorexia and some loss of weight. Typically the patient will have had the disease for more than 10 years and may also complain of impotence, diarrhoea or constipation. On examination retinopathy and the signs of a peripheral neuropathy in the lower limbs may be found. There is gross delay in gastric emptying in these patients and a succussion splash may be elicited some hours after the last meal. A barium examination will confirm the delayed emptying of the stomach and may show lack of peristaltic waves and the presence of retained gastric contents.

Addison's disease (see also Loss of weight, p. 283)

Bouts of nausea and vomiting are not uncommon in Addison's disease and occurred in 76% of a personal series of 70 proven cases. In only 24% were these symptoms associated with abdominal pain. In some patients fruitless investigations of their gastrointestinal tract were carried out before the significance of their pigmentation and lassitude was appreciated.

Adrenocortical insufficiency as a consequence of hypopituitarism may be precipitated by a relatively minor stress such as an upper respiratory infection or a dental extraction. Similarly, it can follow the abrupt cessation of corticosteroid therapy. In both these situations it may present with nausea and vomiting.

Congenital adrenal hyperplasia

In the infant, repeated vomiting and failure to thrive during the first week of life may occasionally be due to the *adrenogenital syndrome*. Adrenal failure in this rare disorder is the result of inherited enzyme deficiencies in the biosynthetic pathways leading to cortisol and aldosterone production. In response to a low plasma cortisol level in utero the fetal pituitary puts out more corticotrophin which, in turn, causes adrenal hypertrophy and a massive increase in adrenal androgen production. This may cause such enlargement of the external genitalia in the female infant as to mimic hypospadias in the male. The only external evidence of this abnormality in the male is scrotal pigmentation. Affected babies will die unless promptly treated with hydrocortisone and salt-retaining steroids. Hyponatraemia, hyperkalaemia and a raised blood urea will be found to a varying degree but only sophisticated steroid assays will enable the diagnosis to be confirmed.

Nine out of ten cases will have a 21-hydroxylase deficiency and the diagnosis can be confirmed by measuring plasma 17-hydroxy-progesterone levels. This cortisol precursor is produced in excessive amounts in these patients because of the metabolic block, and high concentrations will be found in the blood. Once the appropriate samples have been taken the child should be treated with hydrocortisone and a mineralocorticoid whilst awaiting the results.

NEUROGENIC CAUSES

Although vomiting is common in disorders of the brain and its sensory organs it is frequently overshadowed by the presence of pain, pyrexia or altered cerebral function — as in migraine, meningitis, stroke and glaucoma. There are, however, a few conditions where sickness may dominate the clinical picture. This particularly applies to disorders of the inner ear.

Ménière's disease

This distressing condition is a common cause of recurrent attacks of vertigo and vomiting in middle age. Tinnitus and deafness usually accompany these symptoms but in a small proportion of cases vertigo may be the only presenting symptom. The aetiology is unknown but there is a well-recognised association between Ménière's disease and migraine. In one series of 190 cases migraine preceded the onset of the otological symptoms in one-third of patients.

The paroxysms are thought to be due to fluctuations in the pressure in the inner ear from failure of the mechanisms which control the production and disposal of the endolymph. Obliteration of the endolymphatic duct by fibrosis has been repeatedly reported in autopsy specimens. In 70% of cases only one ear is initially affected, but the condition is likely to affect both ears eventually. The nausea and vomiting are due to the central spread of impulses from the vestibular to the vagal nucleus in the brain stem.

In Ménière's disease attacks occur without warning at any time of the day or night. They may last some hours and during them nystagmus will be present, the quick component being in the direction of the affected side. Between paroxysms the nystagmus disappears but the tinnitus and diffi-culty in hearing remain, and the patient may complain of a feeling of full-ness or tightness in the head. There is at present no cure for this condition and sufferers will be incapacitated in varying degree for the rest of their lives. They should be referred to an ENT surgeon for full otological assess-ment which will include audiometry and caloric tests of labyrinthine function.

Vestibular neuronitis

This disorder consists of a sudden and often complete loss of vestibular function on one side without any evidence of cochlear dysfunction. The aetiology is unknown but it may be due to a virus or some other infective agent for it is sometimes associated with a febrile illness or upper respir-atory infection. In some respects it resembles acute epidemic labyrinthitis which is certainly infective in origin and occurs in small epidemics during the winter months when viral infections are common in the community. Both these disorders are characterised by the sudden onset of vertigo or giddiness which may be exacerbated by movements of the head. The vomiting may be effortless and not preceded by nausea or retching, and may last for several days. Unlike Ménière's disease deafness is absent but tinnitus is sometimes complained of by patients with epidemic labyrinthitis. Symptomatic recovery is the rule within 2–3 weeks but caloric tests of labyrinthine function often remain abnormal for much longer.

Motion sickness

Abnormal stimulation of the labyrinth by the irregular pitching, rolling or vertical movements associated with travel by car, ship or aircraft is thought to be the major factor in producing motion sickness. The vertigo is however reinforced by autonomic stimuli from the frequent alteration of position of the abdominal viscera and the sight, sound and odour of others being sick in close proximity. Seasickness is extremely common and in rough seas even experienced sailors may be affected. Car-sickness, on the other hand, is seen mainly in young children on long journeys. Stress and anxiety may precipitate an attack.

Cerebral tumour

Projectile vomiting, unaccompanied by nausea, is sometimes seen in patients with cerebral tumours, particularly if the intracranial pressure is raised. It is due to stimulation of the vomiting centre and is usually preceded by personality changes, headaches, focal neurological symptoms or fits. Gliomas in particular may present in this way. Papilloedema is found in only about 25% of cases. Computed tomography has revolutionised the diagnosis and management of this dread disease for it not only enables the site of the tumour to be determined with some precision but an experienced radiologist may be able to indicate its probable nature.

PSYCHOGENIC CAUSES

The whole alimentary tract is easily affected by the emotions — a normally stable person may react to distressing news or the sickening sight of an accident by vomiting. In the psychoneurotic subject vomiting may become a conditioned reflex evoked when the individual is placed in circumstances resembling, but not necessarily recalling, the causal experience. Such vomiting may occur alone or be accompanied by other alimentary or vasomotor symptoms such as sweating, faintness and palpitations.

Anxiety state

Vomiting is one of the many ways in which anxiety may express itself. It is likely to occur on waking when the stresses of the day lie before the subject. An instance may be given of an otherwise healthy youth who complained of nausea and vomiting on waking with giddiness and faintness of several months' duration. He recovered on rising and remained well throughout the day, slept well and did not admit to any undue anxiety. These symptoms ceased promptly when he sat his A-level examinations and have not recurred. Mass hysteria seems to be the most likely explanation of some outbreaks of collapse, fainting and vomiting that have occurred in schools and other institutions although an epidemic viral infection cannot be ruled out.

Anorexia nervosa (see also Loss of weight, p. 262)

Self-induced vomiting is one of the means employed by the anorexic subject to achieve and maintain her self-inflicted loss of weight. The patient, usually an adolescent girl or young woman, vomits soon after meals, allegedly to relieve the abdominal discomfort produced by food. About one-quarter of a personal series of 150 cases admitted to being sick soon after meals, although a few denied that this was self-induced. The true incidence is likely to be higher than this — some patients feel extremely guilty about their behaviour and observe such secrecy that neither family, friends, doctors or nurses are aware of what they are doing. Frequent visits to the lavatory immediately after meals, both at home and in hospital, should be viewed with the utmost suspicion.

Vomiting and purgative abuse tend to go together and both can lead to dehydration and electrolyte depletion. Prolonged potassium loss in stools and vomit, together with a reduced intake, is the most likely cause of profound muscular weakness in an anorexic patient even if she denies these practices. The ultimate prognosis is poorer in the vomiters and purgers than in those whose weight loss has been achieved by dietary restriction alone. Self-induced vomiting is more likely to be a feature in an adult than in a teenager and particularly in those with a history going back more than a couple of years. It is claimed that this group are often overweight before they begin to lose weight, are more sexually active than the pure dieters, more prone to be involved in drug or alcohol abuse, more likely to indulge in compulsive stealing, and to have histrionic personalities. The 'total allergy' syndrome is probably an extreme example of this condition, though fortunately few sufferers claim to be completely allergic to the twentieth century!

Repeated vomiting two or three times a day for many months may cause a perioral dermatitis and the acid content of the vomit is injurious to the teeth, producing widespread caries. A raised blood urea and hypokalaemia, with or without alkalosis, are the biochemical indicators of repeated vomiting and laxative abuse.

Bulimia

Bulimia is defined as an abnormal increase in the appetite outside the subject's control, resulting in the episodic ingestion of large quantities of fattening food. That patients with anorexia nervosa may develop a voracious appetite lasting a few days at a time was first noticed by Sir William Gull as long ago as 1874. The amount of carbohydrates consumed in these binges is almost beyond belief. It is not unknown for the victim to eat such vast quantities of bread, biscuits, cake, chocolate and other 'forbidden' food as to increase her body weight by several kilograms in the space of a day or two. Not surprisingly, this irresistible over-consumption is followed by extreme abdominal discomfort and an intense feeling of guilt which can only be relieved by self-induced vomiting, with or without the use of laxatives.

While it is true that some young women who binge in this way are not significantly underweight and may still be menstruating, it is not uncommon to obtain a history suggestive of anorexia nervosa in the past. It is probable that bulimia and anorexia nervosa are not separate syndromes but different facets of the same psychosomatic disorder. Bulimia can however occur, without any previous history of weight-loss, in schizophrenia and occasionally in organic brain disease.

CHAPTER 11
Diarrhoea

PHYSIOLOGY

After a meal the stomach normally empties within 3 or 4 hours, and by the time the intestinal contents reach the ileocaecal valve a few hours later nearly all the food elements have been absorbed. The residue is ejected at intervals into the caecum and churned in the ascending colon by segmental contractions. At the same time occasional waves of peristalsis, particularly following a meal, project the contents onward into the descending colon. During its slow passage through the large bowel the bulk of the fluid and electrolytes is absorbed. The semi-solid residue is then held up at the pelvirectal flexure until this sphincter relaxes and allows faeces to enter and distend the rectum, thereby inducing a call to stool. The act of defaecation is, however, very much a matter of habit or conditioning as regards its relationship to meals, time of day and frequency of occurrence. Some individuals regularly pass more than one stool a day while others may go several days between bowel actions.

Diarrhoea is defined as the passage of semi-formed or watery stools which are usually, but not always, passed more frequently than normal. It may result from stimulation of intestinal ion secretion, inhibition of ion absorption, the presence in the gut of poorly absorbed but osmotically active substances or to some derangement of intestinal motility. In a given disorder it is not always possible to specify precisely which of these mechanisms is involved — they are not mutually exclusive. The first two are often considered together under the heading of *secretory diarrhoea* since many of the conditions which act by excessive stimulation of the bowel simultaneously inhibit absorption.

Secretory diarrhoea may be provoked by hormones, toxins, excess bile acids and some laxatives. It also results when mucosal damage occurs in gluten enteropathy, inflammatory bowel disease and ischaemia of the gut. The local release of prostaglandins is thought to be one of the factors involved.

Osmotic diarrhoea, on the other hand, is caused by the presence of poorly absorbed osmotically active substances in the bowel. These attract and retain a larger volume of fluid than normal in the lumen of the gut. The substances involved may be ingested as food or laxatives or may arise from the bacterial degradation of fatty acids, unabsorbed sugars or amino-acids. This type of diarrhoea is seen in lactose intolerance and ceases when the patient fasts, or when milk is excluded from the diet.

Finally, deranged motility of the gut occurs in the irritable bowel syndrome, hyperthyroidism, diabetic autonomic neuropathy and after vagotomy and other gastric operations. The diarrhoea which results may be due to reduced peristalsis, leading to bacterial overgrowth in the small intestine, or to intestinal hurry. The latter reduces the contact time between the mucosa and intestinal contents and leads to exceptionally large fluid loads reaching the colon.

The metabolic consequences of diarrhoea depend upon its severity and duration. In cholera, for example, salt and water depletion occur very rapidly and may be fatal. Potassium depletion is rarely a problem in short-lived episodes but is more likely to develop in chronic diarrhoea, particularly diarrhoea produced by purgative abuse. An increased output of aldosterone from the adrenal cortex in response to salt depletion reduces the loss sodium from the kidneys and colonic mucosa, but enhances the loss of potassium in the urine and stools. Hypokalaemia and muscle weakness due to intracellular potassium depletion are not uncommon in such patients.

In practice acute and chronic diarrhoea differ in causation and presentation. They are therefore considered separately in this chapter.

ACUTE DIARRHOEA

SYNOPSIS OF CAUSES*

INFECTIVE
Shigella; Salmonella; E. coli; Campylobacter; Staphylococcus; Clostridium; Viruses; Cryptosporidium; Giardiasis; Amoebiasis; Cholera.

NON-INFECTIVE
Food; Drugs; Henoch-Schönlein purpura; Ischaemic colitis; **Anxiety.**

* Bold type is used for causes more commonly found in Europe and North America.

DIAGNOSTIC APPROACH

Diarrhoea of sudden onset in a previously healthy individual is so commonly due to acute inflammation of the bowel produced by a bacterial or viral infection that this should be the first thought when presented with such a patient, particularly if the diarrhoea is accompanied by fever, vomiting and colicky abdominal pain. In a young child, however, it is necessary to exclude infection elsewhere before concluding that it has gastroenteritis. An upper respiratory or urinary tract infection, septicaemia and even meningitis may present in this way. Viral diseases are more prevalent in winter and the doctor may be aware of other similar cases in the district. The diarrhoea rarely persists for more than a day or two and the patient usually recovers within a week.

When a food source is suspected the time interval between its ingestion and the onset of symptoms is important in the differential diagnosis. This is discussed in more detail in the section on infective causes. It should also be determined whether others sharing the meal have been affected and whether similar cases have occurred in the family, school or institution. If an outbreak of diarrhoea appears to be caused by food poisoning the medical officer responsible for environmental health in the local health authority must be informed without delay. Speedy action increases the chances of identifying the responsible agent and its source. Suspected food, vomited matter and stools should be kept and sent to the laboratory. Stool culture is not usually indicated in a sporadic case of diarrhoea unless the attack is unduly prolonged or if there is blood or mucus in the motions.

Travellers' diarrhoea is common in those who travel abroad as tourists or on business. Attacks due to the local enterotoxic strains of *Esch. coli* are usually brief in duration and rarely last more than a few days. This is not the case however with giardiasis, amoebiasis, *Salmonella* and *Campylobacter* infections where the diarrhoea may continue on returning home. In an elderly confused patient who has recently returned from the tropics malaria must not be forgotten as an occasional cause; death may follow within days if antimalarials are not given. This emphasises the importance of always asking the question 'Where have you been recently?' when taking the history.

The ingestion of poisonous plants or fungi is an uncommon cause and the diarrhoea is usually preceded by vomiting and colicky abdominal pains. A drug history should be taken routinely, particularly in the elderly and in patients in hospital. Antibiotics are the chief offenders and it is important to remember that the pseudomembranous colitis which occasionally follows the use of antibiotics may present some days after they have been stopped.

INFECTIVE CAUSES

In Europe acute diarrhoea is commonly due to bacterial or viral infections. The organisms responsible may be conveyed directly by faecal material from a case or carrier, or by the ingestion of contaminated food or drink. Rotaviruses account for nearly half the episodes of gastroenteritis seen in young children under the age of 5, but in older children and adults Norwalk-like agents, *Shigella*, *Salmonella* and *Campylobacter* are more likely pathogens. Cholera, *Esch. coli* infections and intestinal parasites are important causes in tropical and subtropical countries and may afflict the unwary traveller to these parts.

In bacterial food poisoning the source of the infection may be fresh or tinned meat, poultry, eggs, dairy produce, shellfish or contaminated water supplies. The organism may be spread by flies or by a food handler suffering from a skin infection or carrying it in the nose, throat or bowel.

Some organisms cause diarrhoea by invading the wall of the intestine. Such is the case with *Shigella, Salmonella, Campylobacter, Yersinia enterocolitica* and viruses. If the colon is involved the motions will be small, frequent and bloody. Other organisms are non-invasive but adhere to the bowel wall and produce enterotoxins which provoke the secretion of water and electrolytes. Cholera, *Clostridia* and some strains of *Esch. coli* fall into this group. Patients infected with these bacteria produce large watery stools. With both these mechanisms there is an incubation period of 12–48 hours, and even longer in some cases, before the onset of symptoms.

A few organisms, of which *Staphylococcus aureus* is the prime example, manufacture their enterotoxin within the food prior to its ingestion. Absorption of this preformed toxin is rapid and consequently the incubation period following the meal is brief, usually less than 6 hours. *Bacillus cereus*, which sometimes contaminates the fried rice in Chinese 'take-away' meals, is another which behaves in this way. The commoner and more important pathogens in man are now discussed in more detail below.

Shigella

Bacillary dysentery is an acute colitis endemic throughout the world and due to infection by *Shigella sonnei, Sh. flexneri, Sh. dysenteriae* or *Sh. boydii*. It is spread chiefly by the unwashed hands of patients after defaecation or by carriers, particularly food handlers. In the UK outbreaks are common in nurseries, schools, residential institutions and long-stay hospitals where hygiene is inadequate. The causal organism is usually *Sh. sonnei* and attacks are often mild.

In the tropics where sanitation is poor spread commonly occurs by flies or water contaminated by infected excreta. The causal organism is more likely to be *Sh. flexneri* or *Sh. dysenteriae*. Attacks by these varieties are more serious and may readily give rise to dehydration and circulatory collapse.

The incubation period is 1–4 days and the illness begins abruptly with fever, cramping abdominal pain and the passage of numerous watery stools. This acute phase commonly lasts for 2–3 days but in more severely ill patients it will be followed by a second dysenteric phase which, in the absence of effective treatment, may persist for weeks. During this period the stools become less frequent but now contain blood and mucus.

Salmonella

This is a very common cause of food poisoning in Britain. The organism, usually *Salmonella typhimurium*, has its natural reservoir in the intestines of animals, particularly cattle and poultry. It is liable to infect meat, duck eggs, egg powder and shellfish and may survive inadequate cooking and deep freezing. Another important source is the handling of food by a symptomless carrier.

Between 1976 and 1985 there were over 100 000 reported cases of *Salmonella* infections in Britain, including a large outbreak in a psychiatric hospital affecting nearly half the 800 patients and over 100 members of staff. During this decade there were 447 deaths in which salmonellosis was certified as the main cause of death.

Nausea, colic and diarrhoea appear abruptly within 12–48 hours of the contaminated meal. Fever is often present and transient bacteraemia is not uncommon. The watery stools may contain some blood and mucus. The symptoms usually subside within a few days but sometimes persist for a week or two. Other serotypes occasionally invade the bloodstream and produce a severe pyrexial illness with localised abscesses in the meninges, bone, spleen, lung and other sites.

Salmonella typhi and *S. paratyphi* are exclusively human parasites and are responsible for enteric or typhoid fever. Whilst ordinarily commencing with constipation, vomiting and diarrhoea are sometimes the presenting symptoms in children. Typhoid fever is considered in the chapter on fever.

Escherichia coli

Pathogenic strains of *Escherichia coli* are often responsible for outbreaks of gastroenteritis in young children. They may occur in the nurseries of maternity units and lead to their temporary closure. In developing countries toxin-producing strains are a common cause of diarrhoea at all ages and travellers may become infected on arrival. The attack is usually mild and self-limiting but more severe illnesses resembling cholera and dysentery have been reported.

Campylobacter

It was only in 1977 that infection by these small spiral bacteria was first recognised as a major cause of world-wide gastroenteritis. Only one species, *Campylobacter jejuni*, is a common pathogen in man. This organism has been isolated from many wild and domestic animals and birds, but the main source of infection appears to be unpasteurised milk. Some outbreaks have however been traced to inadequately cooked chicken and contaminated water supplies. Person-to-person transmission is uncommon but may occur in institutions. *Campylobacter* infection is the most frequently identified cause of acute gastroenteritis in Britain; 11 000 cases were reported in the first half of 1987.

The incubation period varies from 2–11 days and the disease presents initially as a flu-like illness with fever, malaise, headache and aching limbs; vomiting is rare. This is rapidly followed by colicky abdominal pain and the passage of watery, offensive stools which may be bloodstained. The diarrhoea usually settles within a few days but the symptoms vary greatly in severity and the condition has been mistaken for appendicitis, intussusception, peritonitis and fulminating ulcerative colitis. The diarrhoea and abdominal pain may last for 2–3 weeks and a reactive arthritis, similar to that seen in other inflammatory bowel disorders, sometimes complicates the clinical picture.

Staphylococcus

Staphylococcal food poisoning is caused by certain strains of *Staph. aureus*. These organisms are mainly derived from the nose, throat and skin of food handlers but bovine mastitis has been implicated in some outbreaks involving milk or cheese. If dairy products and cooked meats are kept at room temperature for some hours the organisms multiply and produce a heat-resistant enterotoxin prior to ingestion. Vomiting, abdominal pain and diarrhoea present abruptly within a few hours of the meal. The illness rarely lasts more than 24 hours, often subsiding by the time the patient seeks medical advice.

Clostridium perfringens

Clostridia are present in the bowels of many animals and their heat-resistant spores can survive for a long time in dust and soil. Outbreaks of food poisoning occur when cooked meat is allowed to cool slowly at room temperature. Spores which have survived the cooking or drifted on to the food from the dust in the kitchen may then germinate and produce large numbers of bacteria. There is an incubation period of 12–24 hours before the onset of abdominal pain and diarrhoea, during which the ingested organisms produce their enterotoxin. Fever and vomiting are seldom symptoms. Complete recovery within a day or two is usual. Outbreaks are mainly confined to residential institutions such as schools and hospitals.

Viruses (see also Vomiting, p. 115)

In the absence of proof we must avoid the temptation to assume that anything we do not understand is due to a virus. Nevertheless, there is increasing evidence that some organisms, notably the Norwalk-like agents and the rotaviruses, are a common cause of acute, non-bacterial gastroenteritis at all ages and in many countries. Rotavirus infections are seen almost entirely in young children under 6 years of age, while the Norwalk-like viruses are probably responsible for the winter vomiting disease which affects older children and adults. After an incubation period ranging from 1–3 days there is a short-lived attack of nausea, vomiting, abdominal pain and diarrhoea which may be accompanied by a low grade fever, headache and myalgia.

Cryptosporidium

The cryptosporidia are coccidian parasites which are known to cause diarrhoea in a wide variety of domestic animals and birds. What is not so well-known is that they can also produce an acute enterocolitis in man, especially in immunocompromised individuals. Patients with AIDS and those receiving chemotherapy for malignant disease are particularly at risk and may develop life-threatening diarrhoea.

The organism can be acquired from infected animals, but person-to-person contact is probably commoner. Outbreaks have been reported in nurseries, within family groups and in hospital staff looking after an infected patient. In a previously healthy individual the diarrhoea may last 2 weeks or more and may be accompanied by abdominal pain of sufficient severity to be mistaken for that of appendicitis. Blood in the stools is unusual but has been reported. The condition should be suspected if repeated stool cultures are negative, and can be confirmed by finding oocysts in the faeces. However, these are often scanty in number and may be difficult to find.

Giardiasis

Giardiasis is the name given to infection of the upper reaches of the small intestine by the flagellated protozoon *Giardia lamblia*. This organism is found throughout the world and exists in two forms, the trophozoite and the cyst. Cysts are excreted in the faeces of a carrier and infection is conveyed by the ingestion of contaminated food or water. After passing through the stomach the cysts disintegrate and release the trophozoites which attach themselves to the mucosa of the duodenum and jejunum. Here they multiply and form new cysts which are then excreted in the stools to perpetuate the life cycle.

In the tropics infection is very common but often symptomless. In Europe and North America this parasite is sometimes responsible for outbreaks of diarrhoea and vomiting in such institutions as children's nurseries. It is a common cause of traveller's diarrhoea and, since the incubation period may be as long as 2 weeks, symptoms may not appear until the end of a holiday or after returning home. The onset is usually abrupt with the passage of loose, foul-smelling, greasy stools. The diarrhoea often persists for several weeks and may be accompanied by anorexia, nausea, vomiting and abdominal colic. If the diagnosis of giardiasis is suspected at least three stool specimens, obtained on alternate days, should be examined for cysts. Trophozoites are rarely found in the faeces but have been isolated in duodenal aspirates from fasting patients.

Amoebiasis

Infection with the protozoon *Entamoeba histolytica* is common in countries where the standards of hygiene are low. Like *Giardia lamblia*, *Entamoeba* exists in two forms, a free-swimming fragile amoeba and a more robust cyst which will survive desiccation outside the body for several months. Normally the amoebae are found only in the lumen of the large bowel where, for much of the time, the browse peacefully on faecal debris without producing symptoms. As the intestinal contents solidify on their way to the rectum the amoebae change into cysts which are excreted in the stools. Infection is acquired by swallowing food contaminated by human faeces.

In the majority of carriers the infection is asymptomatic but in some individuals, for reasons which are still obscure, the amoebae invade the bowel wall by secreting lytic enzymes. This leads to the passage of frequent, bloody stools which, in an untreated individual, may persist for several weeks before the amoebae revert to being harmless saprophytes. The diarrhoea is often accompanied by lower abdominal pain or tenesmus but amoebic dysentery, in contrast to bacterial dysentery, is rarely associated with any constitutional upset.

The diagnosis can only be made with certainty if amoebae containing ingested red cells are found in freshly passed stools or in scrapings taken from an ulcer at sigmoidoscopy. In the absence of symptoms carriers may be identified by finding cysts in the stools.

Hepatic abscesses and amoeboma of the colon are serious complications of this disease and every attempt should be made to eradicate the organism with chemotherapy, however mild the initial attack.

Cholera

This disease is endemic in the deltas of great rivers in the Far East, but the El Tor vibrio has spread in recent years to parts of Europe. Cholera is a strictly human pathogen and the organism is spread by faecal contamination of food and water. After an incubation period, ranging from a few hours to as long as 5 days, vomiting and profuse watery diarrhoea lead to grave dehydration which may be rapidly fatal without fluid and electrolyte replacement.

Asiatic cholera has not been seen in Britain since the last century. The last epidemic was in 1866, by which time its relationship to water supplies polluted by human excreta had been firmly established — 30 years before the discovery of the causative organism. Small outbreaks have, however, been reported in recent years in Italy, Portugal and Spain — visitors to these countries may be at risk.

NON-INFECTIVE CAUSES

The most important of these causes is probably drugs — diarrhoea is a common but often unrecognised side-effect of treatment. When a patient in hospital develops diarrhoea it is easy to blame a mythical virus going round the ward. The real culprit may in fact be the drug trolley.

Food

Substances which are poisonous in themselves, such as certain mushrooms and the seeds and berries of common plants, may be eaten by children — and occasionally by adults — causing colic, vomiting and diarrhoea within an hour or two of their ingestion.

A food harmless to most people may cause acute gastrointestinal symptoms in an atopic subject. This possibility should be seriously considered if there is a personal or family history of allergy or if diarrhoea has been thought to be due to certain foodstuffs in the past.

Drugs (see also Vomiting, p. 116)

Diarrhoea is a common side-effect of many drugs, especially those given by mouth. It is particularly associated with the administration of antibiotics, antimitotic drugs, digitalis, iron preparations, mefenamic acid and phenindione. With some drugs, such as colchicine and metformin, the effect appears to be dose-dependent and the diarrhoea ceases when the dose is reduced.

Antibiotic diarrhoea, although common, is rarely serious and may amount only to some looseness of the stools during their administration. It is most frequently seen with ampicillin and the tetracyclines and occasionally persists for weeks after the drug has been discontinued.

In one such case a doctor with cellulitis of the knee was given tetracycline orally for only 5 days. 2 days later colic and the passage of some 20 stools daily began and persisted for 2 weeks, to be followed by three loose stools a day for a further 9 months. In retrospect, this patient probably had a pseudomembranous colitis, now recognised as a serious complication of both oral and systemic chemotherapy. It may follow the use of any broad-spectrum antibiotic but those most commonly implicated are ampicillin, clindomycin and the cephalosporins. The colitis is caused by a cytopathic toxin produced by an overgrowth of *Clostridium difficile* in the bowel.

This potentially lethal condition may occur at any age but is seen more often in the elderly. It is important to remember that it may first present some days after treatment has been discontinued and the role of the antibiotics in its causation may not be appreciated at first. Sigmoidoscopy will reveal the characteristic raised yellowish-white plaques surrounded by normal or inflamed mucosa. The definitive diagnosis usually depends upon demonstrating the presence of the toxin in the stools for the organism, as its name implies, is extremely difficult to grow in the laboratory. Orally-administered vancomycin is active against virtually all known strains and should eradicate it from the colon. The patient should be nursed in isolation whenever possible to reduce the risk of transferring this pathogen to other susceptible subjects.

Henoch-Schönlein purpura (see also Purpura and bleeding, p. 193)

This widespread vasculitis is uncommon, occurring mainly in childhood. It is frequently associated with an upper respiratory infection and may be due to allergy to the infecting organism. Colicky abdominal pain and bloody diarrhoea are accompanied by a purpuric rash, arthralgia and sometimes haematuria.

Ischaemic colitis (see also Lateral abdominal pain, p. 89)

The sudden onset of loose bloody stools and left iliac fossa pain in an elderly subject is sometimes due to the occlusion of a branch of the inferior mesenteric artery by atheroma or clot. The presence of atrial fibrillation would favour embolism. Sigmoidoscopy may reveal non-specific inflammatory changes if the rectum or sigmoid colon are involved.

Anxiety

That anxiety or fear may cause diarrhoea is known to everyone. It happens because of overstimulation of the sympathetic nervous system and may be accompanied by other autonomic manifestations such as sweating, pallor, palpitations, tachycardia and frequency of micturition. That this reaction to stressful situations is not confined to the human race was recognised by Aesop. In Caxton's edition of Aesop's fables it is stated that 'the wolf shate thryce for the grete fere that he hadde.'

CHRONIC DIARRHOEA

SYNOPSIS OF CAUSES*

INFLAMMATORY
Gluten enteropathy; Tropical sprue; **Crohn's disease**; Tuberculosis; **Ulcerative colitis**; Pelvic abscess; Intestinal parasites; **AIDS**.

NON-INFLAMMATORY
Irritable bowel; Purgative abuse; **Operation sequelae**; **Pancreatic disease**; Lactose intolerance; **Neoplasm**; **Faecal impaction**; Metabolic causes.

* Bold type is used for causes more commonly found in Europe and North America.

DIAGNOSTIC APPROACH

Chronic diarrhoea is usually insidious in onset and persists for weeks or months, either continuously or in recurrent bouts. Whilst it is useful in practice to think of the causes of acute and chronic diarrhoea as being different this is not always so. For example, that due to organisms such as *Giardia lamblia*, *Entamoeba histolytica*, *Shigella sonnei*, *Salmonella typhimurium* and *Campylobacter jejuni* may last for weeks or relapse after apparent recovery. The history, examination of the faeces and stool culture should enable these causes to be eliminated. Similarly, diarrhoea due to a drug may not be recognised immediately and, in the case of antibiotics, may continue after the treatment has been discontinued. On the other hand, both Crohn's disease and ulcerative colitis can present acutely although they are listed here as causing chronic diarrhoea.

The age and sex may be of some help in narrowing down the possible causes. Lactose intolerance and gluten enteropathy usually present in childhood, though the latter is not uncommonly encountered in adult life, the diarrhoea being accompanied by anaemia and other manifestations of malabsorption. Its association with dermatitis herpetiformis should be remembered. The irritable bowel syndrome and ulcerative colitis may be met at any age but are most commonly seen in young adults, whilst most purgative addicts are women with an obsession about their bowels.

In the middle-aged and elderly patient the recent development of looseness of the stools should always be taken seriously — it may be the first indication of a neoplasm of the pancreas or colon. Energetic efforts should be made to uncover the cause before it is too late to do anything about it. Faecal impaction as a cause of 'spurious' diarrhoea should not be forgotten in the very old. It is a common occurrence on the geriatric wards.

Diarrhoea following gastric surgery, extensive small bowel resection or ileorectal anastomosis is unlikely to cause any difficulty, but a pelvic abscess resulting from abdominal sepsis may be more difficult to recognise. In the diabetic the possibility of autonomic neuropathy should always be considered as a likely cause, particularly if there is evidence of retinopathy or peripheral neuropathy. Occasionally, loose stools occur in hyperthyroidism but there are usually other signs of the disease to draw one's attention to it. On very rare occasions chronic diarrhoea may be due to such bizarre metabolic disorders as the carcinoid syndrome or medullary-cell carcinoma of the thyroid, but these rarities are likely to be encountered only once in a lifetime.

Tropical sprue, intestinal tuberculosis, chronic amoebiasis and bilharziasis are rarely seen in the UK but should be considered in immigrants from tropical countries or in travellers returning to this country after living abroad.

Sufferers from AIDS or AIDS-related complex may initially present with prolonged diarrhoea and loss of weight.

The nature and number of stools passed daily should be ascertained. Frequent fluid stools containing blood and mucus point to a colonic cause. In small-bowel disease the motions are semi-formed and may amount to only two or three a day; if excess fat is present they may be pale, bulky, offensive and stick to the lavatory pan. Diarrhoea which disturbs the patient at night has, as a rule, an organic origin.

Further investigations will depend upon the most probable diagnosis determined from the history and examination. If a colonic cause is suspected these will include stool culture, rectal examination, sigmoidoscopy and a barium enema.

INFLAMMATORY CAUSES

Crohn's disease and ulcerative colitis are the commonest inflammatory causes of chronic diarrhoea in Britain, although the aetiology is obscure in both.

Gluten enteropathy (see also Loss of weight, p. 266)

An inflammatory reaction in the submucosa of the small bowel in response to the presence of gluten in the diet justifies its inclusion among the inflammatory causes. It begins as a rule in early childhood following the introduction of cereals into the diet with abdominal distension, irritability and retarded growth. The stools are loose, offensive, voluminous and pale from increased fat.

Gluten enteropathy can however present during adult life with anaemia and diarrhoea. Dermatitis herpetiformis is now well-recognised to be associated with this disease and the rash may long precede other symptoms.

Tropical sprue (see also Loss of weight, p. 267)

This uncommon disorder resembles the adult form of gluten enteropathy and is seen in those living in or returning from India and the Far East. It differs, however, in not responding to a gluten-free diet but to broad-spectrum antibiotics.

Crohn's disease (see also Lateral abdominal pain, p. 86)

In regional enteritis diarrhoea is the commonest presenting symptom. It may be intermittent at first, occurring in bouts with anorexia, abdominal pain, loss of weight and the passage of some three to five semi-formed stools a day. When Crohn's disease affects the colon it may be mistaken for ulcerative colitis.

Tuberculosis (see also Fever, p. 326)

Involvement of the intestine is usually secondary to pulmonary tuberculosis and is now rare in Britain except in immigrants from tropical countries. A normal chest X-ray does not exclude the diagnosis and the organism may not be found in specimens taken at laparotomy. Most of the reported cases in this country have initially been mistaken for Crohn's disease.

Ulcerative colitis

Aetiology

The cause of this non-specific ulceration of the large bowel is still unknown. It may begin at any age but is seen predominantly in young adults. It varies in severity from a mild proctitis with little disturbance of general health to a grave fulminant attack in which the whole colon is inflamed. The acute iridocyclitis, arthritis and erythema nodosum which sometimes accompany the bowel symptoms may result from immune complex deposition. This may also apply to the chronic hepatitis which sometimes develops when the disease has been present for some years.

Clinical features

In the majority the onset is insidious with lower abdominal pain, tenesmus and diarrhoea in which blood and mucus are mixed in with the stools. This may last for weeks or months with unaccountable remissions and relapses. There may be little to find apart from some tenderness over the affected colon. Untreated, the condition may grumble on for years. In those who have had the disease for more than 10 years there is a greatly increased risk of developing cancer which can occur anywhere in the colon and may be multiple. Its presence may be unsuspected until the patient presents with intestinal obstruction.

In a minority the onset is much more acute with the frequent passage of watery stools containing blood, pus and mucus. In this fulminating variety there will be fever, dehydration, anaemia and loss of weight. The abdomen is often distended with diminished bowel sounds. These patients are at risk from thrombo-embolism, acute dilatation, perforation or massive haemorrhage. Once toxic dilatation of the colon or perforation has occurred only emergency colectomy, which has a high mortality rate, will save the patient.

Investigations

The stools should be examined to exclude known pathogens, including amoebae and *Campylobacter*, and for the presence of *Clostridium difficile* toxin. Sigmoidoscopy will show a friable oedematous mucosa with shallow ulceration, and rectal biopsy should be carried out to assess the degree of mucosal damage. Plain X-rays of the abdomen may show the dilated empty colon with 'mucosal islands' which is characteristic of toxic dilatation. A barium enema is probably safe, even in fulminating attacks, provided that no bowel preparation is used and the radiologist is aware of the patient's condition. Unless the disease is confined to the rectum it will show shortening, diminished distensibility, lack of haustration and the absence of a normal mucosal pattern in postevacuation films. Other investigations should include a full blood count, blood cultures in the severe case, and liver function tests.

Pelvic abscess (see also Fever, p. 333)

This may develop as a complication of pelvic appendicitis, diverticulitis or salpingitis. The chief symptoms are diarrhoea, with the passage of mucus and a sensation of the bowel having been incompletely emptied. Constitutional symptoms such as fever, sweating and loss of weight may long be absent. A leukocytosis is present and rectal examination may reveal a tender mass.

Intestinal parasites

Ill-health due to infestation of the alimentary canal by parasites is widespread in the world and is a common cause of chronic diarrhoea in developing countries. Giardiasis has already been mentioned as an occasional cause of acute diarrhoea in travellers returning from abroad, but in some individuals it may pursue a more protracted course, leading to malabsorption and loss of weight. Amoebiasis may also follow a fluctuating course of exacerbations and remissions over a period of months or years. Intestinal bilharziasis, which is endemic in Africa, the Middle East, South America and some Caribbean islands, may also give rise to episodes of colicky abdominal pain and bloody diarrhoea. It is due to infection with the blood fluke *Schistosoma mansoni*, which invades the inferior mesenteric veins to reach the colon. The parasite may enter the liver by the portal vein and cause cirrhosis and portal hypertension.

AIDS (see also Loss of weight, p. 272)

Diarrhoea is not uncommon in the acquired immunodeficiency syndrome. It is the result of secondary infection of the bowel by a wide variety of pathogenic organisms. In Europe and North America homosexuals, drug addicts and haemophiliacs given contaminated factor VIII preparations are most at risk. Antibody tests will confirm infection by the HIV virus, whilst stool examination and culture may reveal the causative organism in the gut.

NON-INFLAMMATORY CAUSES

The most serious non-inflammatory causes of chronic diarrhoea are neoplasms of the pancreas and large bowel. Their existence should always be suspected in middle-aged or elderly patients with a history of a recent change in bowel habit.

Irritable bowel (see also Lateral abdominal pain, p. 90)

This common disturbance of intestinal motility can mimic a wide variety of gastrointestinal disorders. Recurrent attacks of colicky abdominal pain are usually accompanied by the infrequent passage of small hard pellet-like stools. This constipation may however alternate with episodic diarrhoea. When this occurs the semi-formed stools will contain mucus but no blood. No abnormality will be found on sigmoidoscopy, colonoscopy or barium enema and the diagnosis is usually inferred from the absence of any demonstrable organic disease.

Purgative abuse

Sufferers from the irritable bowel syndrome may resort to laxatives in an attempt to relieve their obstinate constipation. This, in turn, often leads to the passage of large watery stools with the consequent risk of producing significant potassium depletion. At its worst this will result in widespread muscular weakness and an atonic bowel. These patients, usually female, often deny that they are taking purgatives in excess and go to great lengths to conceal this fact. An independent history from a near relative is often very informative and well worth the effort of obtaining it. Hypokalaemia, hyponatraemia and a low serum magnesium level will confirm the massive loss of ions in the fluid stools. In the habitual offender the sigmoidoscope will slide easily into the lax and dilated rectum.

Another group of patients who indulge in purgative abuse are the adolescent girls and young women with anorexia nervosa or bulimia. Constipation is the rule in anorexia nervosa and laxatives are taken in an attempt to overcome it; the diagnosis is usually obvious from the history and physical examination. In the bulimic patient, on the other hand, the weight is usually normal and the use of laxatives, along with self-induced vomiting, is employed to counteract the weight gain caused by the voracious appetite. Most of these patients will admit to the habit when challenged.

Operation sequelae (see also Vomiting, p. 118)

Chronic diarrhoea may follow any of the traditional operations for peptic ulceration but it is much commoner after vagotomy than after partial gastrectomy. It appears to be due to the rapid emptying of hypertonic fluids from the stomach. This overwhelms the absorptive capacity of the small bowel with the consequent passage of large volumes of unabsorbed water into the colon. The diarrhoea is usually provoked by meals but may occasionally occur at night. In mild cases it usually improves with time but in the more severe cases it persists indefinitely. Extensive resection in Crohn's disease or following infarction of the small bowel may lead to malabsorption and consequent diarrhoea. Not surprisingly diarrhoea is invariable after a colectomy and ileorectal anastomosis for ulcerative colitis. The passage of up to six semi-formed stools daily is usual after this operation, but blood in the motions is indicative of inflammation in the rectal stump.

Pancreatic disease (see also Epigastric pain, p. 58)

In chronic pancreatitis and cancer of this organ diarrhoea results from failure of enzyme secretion with consequent steatorrhoea and loss of weight. An apparently causeless diarrhoea in an old person should suggest the possibility of an adenocarcinoma of the pancreas for this is the second most common neoplasm of the digestive tract after colonic cancer. In the rare Zollinger–Ellison syndrome, due to a gastrin-secreting tumour, epigastric pain is the most prominent symptom. The diarrhoea which often accompanies it is caused by the massive hypersecretion of acid which damages the mucosa of the gut and inactivates the pancreatic enzymes necessary for the absorption of fat. Although this tumour can occur alone it is not infrequently associated with other endocrine disorders, particularly hyperparathyroidism.

Lactose intolerance (see also Loss of Weight, p. 270)

Chronic diarrhoea due to intestinal lactase deficiency is seldom seen amongst native Europeans but a high incidence is reported in Oriental and Black immigrants unaccustomed to milky foods. It is seen mainly in children, in whom bouts of colicky abdominal pain are associated with the passage of loose frothy stools.

Neoplasm (see also Lateral abdominal pain, p. 88)

Growths in the small bowel are rare and are usually carcinoid tumours. Malignant carcinoid tissue produces a variety of chemical substances which stimulate the production of fibrous tissue in the bowel wall and increase the motility of the gut. By the time this occurs the liver is usually enlarged from hepatic metastases and diarrhoea may be accompanied by flushing attacks, colicky abdominal pain, skin rashes and wheezing.

Much more frequent are growths in the colon and rectum in which there is a history, usually in an elderly subject, of a recent change in bowel habit. Constipation is commoner than diarrhoea but the latter may be precipitated by the injudicious use of laxatives. A rectal carcinoma may present with 'spurious' diarrhoea; the diagnosis is usually obvious on rectal examination and sigmoidoscopy.

Familial polyposis coli is a premalignant condition which is inherited as a dominant autosomal trait. In this disorder multiple adenomatous polyps are scattered throughout the colon and rectum. When these are very numerous there may be some looseness of the stools. A family history is obtained in about 80% of cases. Diagnosis depends on barium enema studies and colonoscopy.

Faecal impaction

A 'spurious' diarrhoea frequently develops in the aged as a result of faecal impaction. Leakage of fluid stools past the obstruction results in incontinence and this may be accompanied by urinary incontinence as well. Rectal examination will disclose the cause and manual removal will relieve the symptoms.

Metabolic causes

Chronic, painless diarrhoea in a poorly controlled insulin-dependent diabetic is usually a sign of automatic dysfunction of the bowel. These patients often have retinal changes and a peripheral neuropathy as well. The diarrhoea may be very difficult to relieve despite a low fat diet and an improvement in their diabetic control. In hyperthyroidism increased frequency of the stools is sometimes seen and is presumably due to intestinal hurry. The diagnosis is usually obvious from the history and physical signs.

CHAPTER 12
Jaundice

SYNOPSIS OF CAUSES*

HAEMOLYTIC
Hereditary; Rhesus disease; Drugs; Infections; Blood transfusion.

HEPATOCELLULAR
Viral hepatitis; Drugs and poisons; Alcohol; Leptospirosis; Chronic active hepatitis; **Neonatal jaundice**; Gilbert's syndrome; Wilson's disease.

CHOLESTATIC
Drugs; Primary biliary cirrhosis; **Secondary biliary cirrhosis; Gallstones; Biliary tract disease; Pancreatic disease**.

* Bold type is used for causes more commonly found in Europe and North America.

PHYSIOLOGY

The terms 'jaundice' and 'icterus' are both used to describe the yellow discolouration of the skin, mucous membranes and sclerae resulting from an excess of bilirubin in the plasma and extracellular fluid. This pigment is mainly derived from the haemoglobin of effete red cells broken down in the reticulo–endothelial system; it is a normal constituent of the plasma where it is bound reversibly to albumin. Because of this binding and its low solubility in water this prehepatic form is not excreted in the urine.

On arrival at the liver the bilirubin becomes detached from the protein and passes into the hepatocytes. There it is conjugated to glucuronic acid in a reaction which is catalysed by the enzyme glucuronyl transferase. The conjugated bilirubin, along with other constituents of the bile, is excreted into the biliary tract and enters the duodenum. On reaching the terminal ileum it is converted to urobilinogen by intestinal bacteria. Most of this compound is excreted in the faeces, but up to 20% is re-absorbed and, on arrival at the liver, is promptly re-excreted in the bile. A small proportion of the circulating urobilinogen escapes this fate and ends up in the urine; the amount is usually to small to be detected by routine chemical tests.

The capacity of the liver to handle an increased bilirubin load is considerable and its concentration in the plasma is normally maintained below

17 μmol/l (1.0 mg/dl). Jaundice does not become apparent until the serum bilirubin concentration exceeds 45 μmol/l (2.7 mg/dl). In healthy subjects and in haemolytic disorders virtually all the circulating bilirubin is in the unconjugated form. In hepatocellular disease and biliary obstruction, on the other hand, most of it is conjugated and, being more water-soluble, will pass through the glomeruli and darken the urine.

DIAGNOSTIC APPROACH

In detecting jaundice it should be realised that it may not be seen in artificial light. In mild cases a dilute urine may look normal so that an overnight or concentrated specimen should be examined. If still in doubt a chemical stick test will soon tell if bilirubin is present or not. The absence of urobilinogen points to biliary obstruction.

Factors which may assist in determining its cause include age and sex, occupation, ethnic origin, drugs taken and any accompanying symptoms. In the newborn, particularly in the premature infant, a mild and transient 'physiological' jaundice is common. If it persists beyond a week, however, the possibility of hypothyroidism, infection or a congenital haemolytic disorder should be considered. More rarely, rhesus disease or atresia of the bile duct may be responsible.

In children and young adults viral hepatitis is the most frequent cause of jaundice. The hepatitis-B virus is often encountered in male homosexuals and in drug addicts using contaminated syringes.

Jaundice in young women is occasionally due to the steroids in the contraceptive pill, whilst primary biliary cirrhosis is seen mainly in middle-aged women. In middle and later life biliary obstruction from gallstones and cancer of the biliary tract and pancreas become increasingly common.

In certain occupations workers are exposed to hepatotoxic substances, e.g. in the manufacture of industrial solvents and insecticides. Glue sniffing is another potential hazard. Farmers and sewage workers, miners and fish cleaners can be infected by *Leptospira*, which has its natural habitat in the urinary tract of rodents. Hospital staff are at some risk in the ward, renal unit and laboratory from hepatitis-B virus conveyed by infected blood. An occupation giving ready access to alcohol may point to a chemically-induced hepatitis despite the alcoholic patient's modest estimate of his intake. In Blacks in particular the possibility of sickle-cell disease or glucose-6-phosphate dehydrogenase deficiency should be kept in mind.

Jaundice accounts for about 10% of the drug reactions reported to the Committee on Safety of Medicines. Any drug being or having been taken recently should be suspect. This particularly applies to psychotropic drugs, antibiotics and non-steroidal anti-inflammatory preparations. The elderly are more likely to be affected.

Accompanying symptoms may provide a guide to the nature of the jaundice and its most probable cause. Fever, anorexia, upper abdominal discomfort and nausea are common in viral hepatitis but may also occur in that due to drugs or alcohol. Severe abdominal pain and vomiting would suggest biliary obstruction by gallstones or acute pancreatitis. Pruritus is a prominent feature of cholestatic jaundice but is absent in haemolytic jaundice; in hepatocellular disease the presence of pruritus depends upon the degree of intrahepatic cholestasis. In sickle-cell disease multiple small infarcts may cause bone pain and haematuria.

Investigations

Patients should be asked if they have noticed any change in the colour of their stools, and these should be inspected whenever possible. Pale, clay-coloured motions provide unequivocal evidence of obstruction to the flow of bile into the intestine. If viral hepatitis is suspected from the history and examination a preliminary blood sample, taken with suitable precautions to avoid contamination, should be sent to the laboratory to test for Australia antigen (HBsAg).

This antigen is the excess surface protein of the hepatitis-B virus and is not infectious by itself. It is, however, always accompanied by the complete virus and is therefore an indicator of active infection. If the test is positive the blood of the patient is highly infectious and further samples should only be taken after consultation with laboratory staff.

Other investigations will depend on the most likely cause of the jaundice and are dealt with in due course.

HAEMOLYTIC JAUNDICE

This is the least common type of jaundice and, with the exception of the icterus which develops in a mismatched blood transfusion, its causes are those of a haemolytic anaemia. They are therefore dealt with briefly here, being also considered in the chapter on Anaemia. In paroxysmal nocturnal haemoglobinuria, and the more chronic autoimmune haemolytic anaemias, the rate of haemolysis is rarely sufficient to cause jaundice.

In haemolytic jaundice the excess bilirubin produced by the accelerated destruction of the erythrocytes surpasses the capacity of the liver to dispose of it. There is consequently a rise in the serum level of unconjugated bilirubin — though this rarely exceeds 70 μmol/l (4 mg/dl). The resulting icterus is therefore mild and is not accompanied by any rise in the serum enzymes.

The freshly-passed urine is usually normal in colour, since bilirubin is absent, unlike the urine passed in other types of jaundice. Urobilinogen is however present in excess and may, through oxidation to urobilin, cause darkening on standing. When the haemolysis is gross the presence of haemoglobin may colour the urine red and be mistaken for haematuria. The colour of the stools will be normal. The accompanying anaemia will vary in degree depending upon the rate of blood destruction and this will also be reflected in the raised reticulocyte count.

Hereditary causes

In the congenital haemolytic anaemias there is a defect either in the membrane of the red cell or within its cytoplasm which causes it to have a short life-span. These diseases usually present in early childhood with anaemia, splenomegaly and jaundice.. Exacerbations are often precipitated by intercurrent infections. In adult life there may be an additional element of cholestatic jaundice caused by numerous pigment gallstones resulting from the chronic overproduction of bilirubin. A history of a similar disorder in other members of the family is usual.

Hereditary spherocytosis is due to a defect in the network of fibrous proteins beneath the cell membrane which maintains the shape of the erythrocyte. It is particularly prevalent in northern Europe and is sometimes seen in the UK. The diagnosis is made on the appearance of the blood film and a negative Coombs' test.

Sickle-cell anaemia is rare in the UK. It is due to the inheritance of a gene for structurally abnormal betaglobin chains in the haemoglobin molecule. It is found almost exclusively in Black people. The homozygous form is often fatal, few cases surviving over the age of 30. Acute haemolytic crises occur without warning during which the haemoglobin level falls very rapidly; severe pain may be felt in the bones and abdomen from multiple small infarcts due to clumping of the sickle cells. Haematuria is common during these episodes, along with haemoglobinuria. The characteristic elongated 'holly-leaf' red cells will be seen on a blood film, and haemoglobin electrophoresis will show a band of sickle haemoglobin.

Congenital enzyme deficiencies in the red cells account for many cases of haemolytic anaemia worldwide. The commonest of these is *glucose-6-phosphate dehydrogenase deficiency* which is also seen most frequently in Blacks. Sufferers are usually symptomless until an acute haemolytic crisis is induced by drugs which interfere with the hexose monophosphate shunt within the cells. These include phenacetin, nitrofurantoin, sulphonamides, quinidine and antimalarial drugs. Splenomegaly is unusual in this condition. Favism is a form of the disorder seen in people of Mediterranean origin after eating broad beans.

Rhesus disease (see also Anaemia, p. 223)

Haemolysis in this grave condition is due to the passage across the placenta of maternal antibodies to the infant's red cells. Brain damage is caused by the high serum levels of unconjugated bilirubin, and jaundice is usually apparent within the first 24 hours. Rhesus disease has become rare in the UK since it has become routine to administer anti-D gammaglobulin to non-immunised Rh-negative women immediately after delivery of an Rh-positive child.

Drugs

The role of certain drugs in producing haemolysis in patients with glucose

6-phosphate dehydrogenase deficiency has already been mentioned under Hereditary causes. Other drugs act by stimulating the production of anti-bodies which destroy the red cells. Quinine, quinidine and stibophen may cause jaundice in this way but the haemolysis produced by penicillin, carbromal and methyldopa is less marked and icterus is rarely evident.

Infections

Destruction of red cells by the malarial parasite is one of the commonest causes of haemolytic anaemia in the tropics. Mild jaundice is not uncommon during attacks, particularly in those due to *Plasmodium falci-parum* infection. Occasionally the haemolysis is so severe that there is gross haemoglobinuria and renal failure. Blackwater fever is never seen in the UK but malaria should always be borne in mind in jaundiced patients just back from the tropics.

Other organisms may cause haemolysis by damaging the red cell membrane. The only one of major importance in the UK is *Clostridium perfringens* and infections may follow bowel operations or a septic abortion. Jaundice appears within a matter of hours and is accompanied by haemo-globinuria. Unless the infected tissues are ruthlessly excised the patient will die of gas gangrene. In infants, however, almost any severe infection may cause haemolysis.

Blood transfusion

Serious errors in blood transfusion are rare causes of haemolytic jaundice. Mild haemolysis may occur in patients who have had previous transfusions and where there has been difficulty in cross-matching. Danger still remains of a serious reaction if the wrong blood is given; great care must therefore be taken in identifying both the patient and the donated blood before the transfusion is commenced. Any reaction is likely to appear within the first hour. It is characterised by anxiety accompanied by fever, flushing, low backache and tachycardia. No great harm will ensue provided that the transfusion is promptly discontinued. Jaundice appears within 24 hours and may persist for several days.

HEPATOCELLULAR JAUNDICE

When liver cells are damaged their capacity for conjugating and excreting bilirubin is impaired. In hepatocellular jaundice the serum concentrations of both unconjugated and conjugated bilirubin are elevated but there is more conjugated bilirubin present. The levels of alkaline phosphatase, gammaglutamyl aminotransferase and transaminases in the serum will reflect the degree of liver damage and may be raised before any icterus is apparent. The urine will be darkened by the presence of bilirubin and excess urobilinogen will be found on chemical testing unless the swollen liver cells compress the sinusoids and produce intrahepatic cholestasis. If this happens the stools will be paler than normal.

The commonest cause of hepatocellular jaundice is undoubtedly viral hepatitis, but a toxic hepatitis may complicate many other infections, particularly in infancy and old age. Alcohol, drugs and congestive cardiac failure must also be considered in the differential diagnosis.

Viral hepatitis

Aetiology

In the majority of cases this is caused by the hepatitis-A or -B viruses, but in a minority neither of these organisms appear to be responsible. In most cases of non-A non-B hepatitis no agent can be identified, but a few are due to cytomegalovirus or the Epstein–Barr virus which causes infectious mononucleosis.

The hepatitis-A virus is transmitted mainly by the faecal–oral route and has an incubation period of 2–6 weeks. Infection with this organism is commoner in temperate climates and is seen most frequently in children and young adults. It is usually spread by person-to-person contact but outbreaks have occurred when water supplies have been contaminated by human sewage or when shellfish have been harvested from polluted river estuaries.

Hepatitis-B infection, on the other hand, is much commoner in tropical and subtropical countries and is spread by the inoculation of minute quantities of infected blood, by kissing or sexual intercourse, and possibly by mosquitoes and other blood-sucking insects. Its incubation period is very variable, ranging from 1–6 months, and many people fail to eliminate the virus and become symptomless carriers. It has been calculated that there may be as many as 200 million chronic carriers throughout the world.

Hepatitis-B infection is a common cause of jaundice in male homosexuals and intravenous drug addicts and is a precursor of chronic active hepatitis, cirrhosis and hepatocellular carcinoma.

The hepatitis-D (delta) virus is a small incomplete virus which has only been found in patients with pre-existing hepatitis-B infection; patients harbouring both organisms are more likely to suffer severe liver damage and to develop cirrhosis.

Non-A non-B hepatitis is also associated with a carrier state and may be conveyed by contaminated blood or faeces. Its true incidence and prevalence are unknown, because it can only be diagnosed by exclusion.

Clinical features

Mild cases of viral hepatitis without obvious jaundice may escape detection unless liver function tests are done. The illness usually begins with a few days of malaise, fever, upper abdominal discomfort, anorexia, nausea and sometimes vomiting. In hepatitis-B infections there may also be arthralgia or a rash; the latter may be maculopapular, urticarial or petechial in nature.

These non-specific manifestations are followed by the passage of dark urine and deepening jaundice. On examination the liver is usually tender and palpably enlarged while the spleen is also palpable in about 15% of cases.

The gastrointestinal symptoms usually subside in 3–4 weeks and the liver and spleen return to their normal size as the jaundice disappears. A prolonged period of lassitude is not uncommon following an attack and full recovery may take several months. Acute relapses sometimes occur, particularly with hepatitis-A infections, and may be precipitated by alcohol or violent exercise. Chronic liver disease is a recognised sequel of both hepatitis-B and non-A non-B infections.

Investigations
The diagnosis is usually inferred from the history, physical findings and disturbed biochemistry. In view of the great infectivity of the blood from patients with hepatitis B it is essential to test for Australia antigen at the onset. If this is found it is unjustifiable to ask for any further blood tests because of the risk of infecting laboratory staff. If it is absent serial estimations of the serum bilirubin, gammaglutamyl aminotransferase and transaminases are very valuable in following the progress of the disease. Elevated levels, however, are not diagnostic of a viral aetiology — similar rises will be found in hepatitis due to other causes.

Hepatitis-A infection can be confirmed by demonstrating a rise in antibody titre to this organism in paired sera taken about 10 days apart. However, the presence of hepatitis-A-specific IgM in a specimen taken early in the illness is probably the best single marker of recent infection. Hepatitis-B infection is usually confirmed by detecting the presence of the surface antigen HBsAg in sera collected during the acute phase of the illness or, in the absence of the Australia antigen, by demonstrating a rising antibody titre to the core antigen HBcAg.

Non-A non-B hepatitis is usually diagnosed by exclusion but the presence of a monocytosis and a positive monospot test will detect the occasional case of infectious mononucleosis. Liver biopsy is rarely indicated and may be dangerous, particularly if the prothrombin time is prolonged. It will show degeneration of the cells in the centre of the liver lobules with ballooning of their cytoplasm and obliteration of the sinusoids. These changes are not specific to viral hepatitis and are also seen in hepatitis due to alcohol and drugs. The main value of a liver biopsy is that it can exclude biliary obstruction or chronic active hepatitis when the jaundice is unduly prolonged and the diagnosis is in doubt.

Drugs and poisons

While liver damage from drugs is not uncommon the effects are seldom serious or lasting, provided that the drug is stopped immediately. Continued administration can result in massive hepatocellular necrosis and death.

Hepatocellular jaundice due to a drug may closely resemble viral hepatitis and is usually unrelated to the dose or duration of treatment. One notable exception is jaundice due to paracetamol overdosage in a suicidal patient. Severe centrilobular necrosis almost invariably follows the ingestion of more than 15 g of this analgesic. Acute liver failure develops within 2–3 days unless a protective agent such as N-acetylcysteine is given intravenously within 15 hours of the overdose. A rise in the prothrombin time is probably the earliest indicator of liver damage.

A large number of drugs are now known to produce a toxic hepatitis in some individuals. The list includes such widely used substances as amiodorone, azothiaprine, isoniazid, ketoconazole, methotrexate, methyldopa, monoamine oxidase inhibitors, nitrofurantoin, penicillamine, perhexilene maleate, propylthiouracil, quinidine, tetracycline and several non-steroidal anti-inflammatory drugs. In addition to jaundice there may be other signs of hypersensitivity such as fever, a rash, lymphadenopathy, arthralgia or eosinophilia. When abdominal pain is particularly severe it is said to indicate a poor prognosis.

Workers in industries which manufacture organic solvents and insecticides are at risk from the hepatotoxic effects of these chemicals, but even laboratory technicians may be affected by inhaling them in the course of their work.

Halothane, widely used in anaesthesia, is now recognised to be a rare cause of hepatitis in some patients following repeated exposure, and may be preceded by an unexplained postoperative fever. Obese women over the age of 40 seem to be most at risk, and jaundice from this cause is associated with a high mortality rate.

Alcohol

Alcohol is a potent liver poison and acute alcoholic hepatitis may follow a drinking bout. Anorexia, nausea, vomiting, mild jaundice and upper abdominal pain may be accompanied by fever and mental confusion. The liver is enlarged and tender, the spleen may be palpable and ascites is sometimes present. Liver function tests will be grossly disturbed and there may be a polymorph leukocytosis. Unless the patient abstains from drinking the condition is likely to progress to chronic active hepatitis and eventually to cirrhosis of the liver.

Leptospirosis (see also Fever, p. 309)

This disorder is rare in the UK but is sometimes seen in farmers, sewage workers, miners and fish cleaners. The leptospira are excreted in the urine of infected rodents, cattle or dogs and gain entry to the patient through abrasions or the mucous membranes.

The disease has an incubation period of 1–2 weeks. Jaundice due to hepatitis usually appears at some stage of the illness but fever, along with headache, conjunctivitis and muscle pains, are earlier symptoms. A leukocytosis is often present and a rising antibody titre to the leptospira will confirm the diagnosis.

Chronic active hepatitis

A prolonged low-grade inflammation of the portal tracts in the liver can follow an attack of hepatitis irrespective of the cause. This chronic persistent hepatitis is a benign condition which may grumble on for years after the initial insult with little to show for its presence apart from raised serum transaminase levels.

In striking contrast is chronic active hepatitis in which the inflammation extends into the liver lobule, causing erosion of the limiting plate and piecemeal necrosis of the liver cells. Their destruction is followed by increasing fibrosis, leading eventually to cirrhosis and portal hypertension.

Two main causes of this disorder are recognised. The first is thought to be an autoimmune disease because it occurs mainly in women at puberty or around the menopause and is sometimes associated with diabetes, thyroiditis, inflammatory bowel disease, vasculitis, glomerulonephritis or Sjögren's syndrome. Its onset may resemble an attack of acute viral hepatitis or it may present more insidiously with amenorrhoea and fluctuating jaundice. The liver and spleen are often palpable and spider naevi may be seen. The serum IgG will be raised and smooth muscle antimitochondrial and antinuclear antibodies are frequently found in the blood. In about 15% of cases LE cells are also present, which accounts for its alternative title of 'lupoid' hepatitis.

The second main cause of chronic active hepatitis is a persisting hepatitis-B infection. This is seen mainly in people of African, Mediterranean or Far Eastern origin and more frequently in men. It may present as an unresolved acute attack with persistence of the surface antigen in the blood, or as a chronic illness, with lassitude, anorexia, intermittent jaundice and low-grade fever.

Chronic active hepatitis may also occur as a complication of non-A non-B hepatitis, Wilson's disease, drug-induced liver damage or alcoholism. The diagnosis is made on liver biopsy and, when it is due to hepatitis-B, the viral antigens may be demonstrated in the liver cells by immunofluorescence.

Neonatal jaundice

This is not uncommon, particularly in premature and breast-fed infants. During intra-uterine life bilirubin is largely removed from the fetal bloodstream by the placenta. If delay occurs in the maturation of the enzyme glucuronyl aminotransferase transient jaundice appears about the third day of life, disappearing within a week or two.

Persistence or deepening of the jaundice raises several possibilities. One of the earliest manifestations of cretinism is an unduly prolonged episode of neonatal jaundice; this diagnosis can now be rapidly excluded by estimating the serum thyroxine and TSH in a drop of blood obtained by heel prick. Alternatively the jaundice may be due to alpha$_1$-antitrypsin deficiency, biliary atresia or neonatal viral hepatitis, but all of these are rare in the UK. Finally, it should not be forgotten that any infection in infants may present as jaundice from a toxic hepatitis or gross haemolysis.

Gilbert's syndrome

A mild recurrent jaundice, without impairment of health, is sometimes seen in this uncommon congenital disorder. It is thought to be due to a defect in the conjugation of bilirubin in the liver cells and is usually detected in adolescence. It should be suspected when an elevated unconjugated bilirubin level is found in an otherwise healthy subject. A liver biopsy will be normal. Other inherited diseases which give rise to unconjugated hyperbilirubinaemia, such as the Crigler–Najjar syndrome, are extremely rare but may be fatal in the first year of life.

Wilson's disease

Copper is an essential trace element which is largely excreted in the bile. In Wilson's disease there is an inherited metabolic defect in the liver which prevents this happening. As a consequence toxic levels of copper gradually accumulate in the liver, brain, kidney and eye to produce mainly hepatic and neurological manifestations. In childhood signs of liver disease often precede those in the central nervous system.

Wilson's disease may present acutely and be mistaken for a viral hepatitis or it may appear insidiously with lassitude, jaundice, abdominal discomfort, ascites and hepatosplenomegaly.

Neurological changes are seldom seen before adolescence but may first manifest themselves by behavioural disturbances, deteriorating performance at school, an unusual gait or clumsiness in carrying out manual tasks. The characteristic Kayser–Fleischer rings in the cornea, which are seen only on slit lamp examination, may not be visible in childhood. Occasionally this disease may present as a haemolytic anaemia or with evidence of renal tubular damage.

The diagnosis should be suspected if there is a family history of this disorder. Typically the serum ceruloplasmin concentration will be less than 200 mg/l and the urinary copper excretion greater than 1.6 μmol/24 hours (100 μg/24 hours). Histochemical examination of a biopsy specimen for copper is unreliable but the liver copper content is usually greater than 250 μg/g of dry liver. Lifelong treatment with D-penicillamine will produce a worthwhile remission in what was once an inevitably fatal disease.

CHOLESTATIC JAUNDICE

This type of jaundice is due to obstruction to the flow of bile within the liver substance or in the extrahepatic portion of the biliary tract. In a typical case the serum conjugated bilirubin level will be markedly elevated and may exceed 500 μmol/l (30 mg/dl). The alkaline phosphatase level will usually be higher and the serum transaminases lower than those seen in hepatocellular jaundice, but there are always exceptions to this general rule and too much reliance should not be placed on the biochemical findings. The urine will be darkened by the presence of conjugated bilirubin but urobilinogen will be absent. The stools will be pale from lack of bile pigments and may contain excess fat. The accumulation of bile salts in the blood is thought to be responsible for the pruritus and bradycardia which occur so commonly in this type of jaundice.

Intrahepatic cholestasis may be due to obstruction of the sinusoids by swollen liver cells, as in viral or alcoholic hepatitis, or to inflammation of the portal tracts and occlusion of the bile canaliculi in biliary cirrhosis and drug-induced hypersensitivity reactions. When doubt exists about the underlying pathology a liver biopsy will often settle the question. This should only be considered if the prothrombin time and platelet count are normal.

Posthepatic cholestasis is due to mechanical obstruction of the common bile duct by stricture, gallstones or pancreatic disease. This has been termed 'surgical' jaundice as the possibility of relief exists by operation.

The distinction between 'medical' and 'surgical' jaundice can be very difficult, for gallstones are seldom visible on a plain X-ray and the conventional radiological techniques for outlining the biliary tract are useless when jaundice is present. Ultrasonography, on the other hand, will often demonstrate the presence of gallstones and even distended intrahepatic ducts provided that it is not carried out too early in the illness before they have had time to dilate. Computed tomography, combined with the use of intravenous contrast media, is equally good at demonstrating the dilated bile ducts and better at indicating the site and probable nature of the obstruction. Endoscopic retrograde cholangiopancreatography provides the only means of visualising the pancreatic duct and its branches.

Some of the causes of cholestatic jaundice are now considered in more detail below.

Drugs

Drug-induced hepatitis has already been described under Hepatocellular jaundice. Another type of chemical reaction in the liver causes intrahepatic cholestasis, which may be difficult to distinguish clinically from cholestasis due to extrahepatic obstruction. Many substances have been implicated but those most commonly involved are the benzodiazepines, carbimazole, erythromycin, gold salts, oral hypoglycaemic drugs, phenothiazines, propoxyphene and tricyclic antidepressants. Occasionally cholestasis occurs in patients taking androgens or the steroids in the contraceptive pill. The jaundice is usually mild and appears within a month or two of starting treatment. Provided that this is stopped immediately the icterus is unlikely to persist for more than a few weeks, but much more prolonged episodes lasting many months have been seen with chlorpromazine. It is not surprising that an extrahepatic cause has been suspected in these patients, for the jaundice is sometimes accompanied by severe right hypochondriac pain.

A liver biopsy will show plugs of bile in distended canaliculi and possibly some lymphocytic infiltration of the portal tracts — the presence of eosinophils is very suggestive of a drug reaction. The architecture of the lobules will be normal unless the drug is capable of producing hepatitis as well.

Primary biliary cirrhosis

This is a chronic inflammatory disorder of the intrahepatic bile ducts first described by Hanot in 1882. The cause is unknown but the presence of antimitochondrial antibodies in a high proportion of patients, and its association with thyroiditis, rheumatoid arthritis and Sjögren's syndrome, is very suggestive of an autoimmune disease.

Occurring mainly in middle-aged women, primary biliary cirrhosis is compatible with reasonably good health for some years before the onset of portal hypertension or hepatic failure. Itching is often the first symptom of the disease and may long precede the appearance of jaundice. The pruritus may start in pregnancy or while taking the contraceptive pill, remit for a time and then return spontaneously some years later. As the jaundice deepens the patient's skin develops a greenish hue which in the latter stages changes to a bronzed appearance from an increase of melanin.

As with other liver diseases, primary biliary cirrhosis may be complicated by diabetes. The liver and spleen enlarge and hypercholesterolaemia may lead to the appearance of xanthomas, particularly around the eyes. Clubbing of the fingers and toes is sometimes seen. Steatorrhoea and malabsorption of the fat-soluble vitamins D and K result in osteomalacia and a prolonged prothrombin time.

The diagnosis is based upon the clinical picture, the presence of antimitochondrial antibodies in the blood and the characteristic liver biopsy.

In the early stages of this condition there is inflammation of the intralobular bile ducts, which are surrounded by a dense infiltrate of lymphocytes and plasma cells. At a later stage there is less inflammation but proliferation of bile ductules and a marked reduction in the number of bile ducts in the specimen.

Secondary biliary cirrhosis (see also Fever, p. 321)

This is much more common than the primary form. It results from long-standing partial or complete obstruction of the common bile duct by gallstones, stricture or cancer of the biliary tract and pancreas. Without surgical relief the resulting jaundice deepens, with the development of pruritus, steatorrhoea and ultimately liver failure. The condition may be complicated by an ascending cholangitis which presents with upper abdominal pain, high fever, sweating and rigors. These grave symptoms will be accompanied by a polymorph leukocytosis and a high ESR.

Since this condition is a septicaemia blood cultures are essential to isolate the offending organism and to determine appropriate antibiotic therapy.

Gallstones (see also Lateral abdominal pain, p. 92)

Impaction of one or more stones in the common bile duct is the commonest cause of extrahepatic obstruction. Although this can occur silently it is usually associated with attacks of upper abdominal pain and vomiting. Unless the obstruction is removed by surgery or by the passage of the stone into the bowel it will be followed by secondary biliary cirrhosis and ascending cholangitis. Dilatation of the extrahepatic biliary ducts may be demonstrated by ultrasonography or computed tomography, but most surgeons prefer to rely on pre-operative percutaneous transhepatic cholangiography or endoscopic retrograde cholangiopancreatography to identify the cause of the obstruction.

Biliary tract disease

Atresia of the bile ducts is the chief surgical cause of sustained jaundice in the newborn infant. It is fortunate that this congenital disorder is rare, because the common bile duct is seldom patent and attempts at surgical relief are often unsuccessful. Icterus appears in the first week of life and deepens, with distressing pruritus. Death ensues as a rule from liver failure or intercurrent infection.

In adult life biliary stricture is nearly always due to injury to the common bile duct during cholecystectomy. This condition should be suspected if the operation is followed by signs of cholangitis and a fluctuating jaundice due to intermittent obstruction of the biliary tract.

Unusual causes of extrahepatic cholestasis include choledochal cysts, compression of the common bile duct by neoplastic or inflammatory lymph nodes, invasion of the biliary tract by *Ascaris lumbricoides* and duodenal diverticuli.

Growths in the extrahepatic bile ducts or ampulla of Vater are rare and cannot be distinguished clinically from other forms of obstruction. It is in such cases that the technique of endoscopic retrograde cholangiopancreatography may enable a pre-operative diagnosis to be made. Carcinoma of the gall-bladder may also present with unremitting jaundice from involvement of the biliary tract.

Pancreatic disease (see also Epigastric pain, p. 58)

In acute pancreatitis severe upper abdominal pain and vomiting are the most prominent features but in one series of 250 cases jaundice developed in 25%. It may be due to compression of the common bile duct by the swollen gland or a pancreatic pseudocyst. In chronic pancreatitis jaundice is rare but occasionally arises from entrapment of the common bile duct in scar tissue.

The incidence of pancreatic carcinoma increases with age and is commonest in elderly men. Jaundice is observed in over half the patients by the time they present but is usually preceded by dull epigastric pain, anorexia and weight loss. On examination there may be a palpable distended gallbladder (Courvoisier's sign). The condition is usually suspected from the results of ultrasonography, computed tomography or endoscopic retrograde cholangiopancreatography and confirmed at laparotomy. It has been claimed that ultrasound-guided aspiration of the organ enables a cytological diagnosis to be made in a high proportion of cases before operation.

CHAPTER 13
Blood loss

What follows serves as an introduction to the next five chapters.

Blood loss, however trivial, can be significant for several reasons. Firstly, it will call attention to the presence of organic disease in the respiratory, alimentary, renal and genital tracts. The first three systems are discussed separately in the chapters which follows, but uterine bleeding is considered in the chapter on anaemia.

Secondly, bleeding from the gastrointestinal tract and uterus are responsible for most of the cases of anaemia which are seen in practice. The former may be silent and intermittent whilst the latter may be dismissed as 'heavy' periods. Menorrhagia is, however, the cause of much of the iron-deficiency anaemia which is seen in women of reproductive age. Finally, bleeding at more than one site will draw attention to the haemorrhagic diseases, which are the subject of a chapter on their own.

Epistaxis

Epistaxis is a minor symptom and does not merit a separate chapter to itself. The bleeding is usually unilateral and, in the majority of cases, arises from a ruptured vessel on the anterior part of the nasal septum. A history of previous episodes is not uncommon. It may occur spontaneously or be provoked by a blow to the nose. Whilst epistaxis following a fall or blow is likely to be associated with a clear-cut history of injury, exceptions include the infant who may fall unobserved and the unconscious 'drunk'.

Nose-bleeding occurs occasionally in upper respiratory infections and is a common feature of typhoid fever. In hypertensive subjects it is also common, and profuse bleeding may be followed by a feeling of relief.

In a middle-aged adult repeated nasal haemorrhage may be the first sign of a naso-pharyngeal neoplasm.

Epistaxis and bleeding from the mouth and nasopharynx may appear in haemorrhagic disease. It is most often due to a lack of platelets as in idiopathic thrombocytopenia, leukaemia and hypoplastic anaemia. The last-named is usually due to the toxic effects of certain drugs upon the bone marrow.

Recurrent nosebleeds are the commonest and often the first manifestation of hereditary telangiectasia. A careful examination of the nose, mouth and lips, preferably with a magnifying glass, should be made for the characteristic small, discrete red spots under the mucosa. This is one of the few conditions where the bleeding may be so profuse as to cause anaemia.

CHAPTER 14

Haemoptysis

SYNOPSIS OF CAUSES*

RESPIRATORY TRACT
Bronchitis; Bronchiectasis; Aspergillosis; Neoplasm.

LUNGS
Pulmonary embolism; Tuberculosis; Pneumonia; Abscess.

EXTRARESPIRATORY
Cardiac disease; Trauma; Goodpasture's syndrome; Haemorrhagic Disease.

* Bold type is used for causes more commonly found in Europe and North America.

PHYSIOLOGY

Haemoptysis literally means 'spitting of blood' but in practice the term is reserved for bleeding from the respiratory tract or lungs. It should always be taken seriously, for it is often a manifestation of such grave conditions as a bronchial neoplasm, tuberculosis, pulmonary embolism, lung abscess or pneumonia. The blood is usually bright red in colour and unclotted and the staining of the sputum may persist for several days after the first appearance.

Depending on the size of the vessels involved the haemoptysis may vary in amount from the coughing up of small amounts of blood-streaked sputum to a torrential haemorrhage from a ruptured bronchial arteriole, which can kill the patient in a matter of minutes. In the latter situation the blood may well up into the throat without any accompanying cough to indicate its pulmonary origin.

Blood from the nose or nasopharynx, inhaled during sleep and later coughed up, could mimic haemoptysis but can usually be excluded by a careful examination of the nose and throat. Haematemesis is unlikely to be mistaken for haemoptysis for it is usually copious in quantity, dark red in colour and mixed with stomach contents. There is usually a history of dyspepsia and it is followed in a day or two by blood in the stools.

DIAGNOSTIC APPROACH

The diagnostic approach will depend to some extent upon the severity of the blood loss. Profuse haemorrhage is uncommon, which is just as well because the patient may die rapidly of asphyxiation before a diagnosis can be made. In such cases immediate bronchoscopy is vital — it will enable the airways to be cleared of blood and the source of the bleeding to be identified. In the majority the haemorrhage can then be halted by inflating the balloon on the end of a Fogarty catheter in the affected segment of the bronchial tree. Blood transfusion will be necessary to support the failing circulation.

In young adults the most likely cause of a massive haemoptysis is *pulmonary tuberculosis*; less commonly it is due to a lung abscess or bronchiectasis. In older patients it may arise from a bronchial neoplasm, chronic cavitated pulmonary tuberculosis or a mycetoma. Rarely it may be due to necrotising vasculitis, as in Goodpasture's syndrome, or to haemorrhagic pneumonia, where the infection is accompanied by some gross disturbance of the clotting mechanisms such as occurs with disseminated intravascular coagulation. When the bleeding has been controlled X-rays of the chest, which may include tomography, will help to confirm the nature and extent of the underlying disease. It is however worth remembering that blood inhaled after a major bleed may literally overshadow and obscure the lesion on the initial films. It may be several days before the lung fields clear sufficiently for the lesion to be seen.

Fortunately the haemoptysis is less severe in most patients and may only amount to the expectoration of some blood-tinged sputum. There is time to take a careful history of past illnesses, smoking habits, current state of health and any accompanying symptoms. In the young tuberculosis remains the most likely cause but it and bronchiectasis may both present with malaise, fever, loss of weight and a productive cough. There is often a history of previous respiratory illnesses or contact with a known case of tuberculosis at work or in the family.

During pregnancy and in females on the contraceptive pill the possibility of *pulmonary embolism* should always be borne in mind. The same applies to all postoperative patients and those who have been confined to bed with major illnesses. The haemoptysis is likely to have been preceded or accompanied by pleuritic pain and some shortness of breath. Similar symptoms will be seen in *pneumonia* but frank haemoptysis will favour embolism.

A small haemoptysis in a middle-aged or elderly subject with a smoker's cough may be the first indication of the presence of a *squamous cell carcinoma* or pulmonary tuberculosis; chronic bronchitis should never be accepted as an adequate explanation without further investigation.

Examination of the patient is essential. Dyspnoea at rest may be due to cardiac failure, obstructive airways disease or damaged lungs. Fever, signs of consolidation and a pleuritic rub may be found in pneumonia and pulmonary infarction. Bleeding elsewhere will point to haemorrhagic disease, while clubbing of the fingers is sometimes seen in association with bronchial cancer and chronic suppurative lung disease.

Further investigations will depend upon the most probable diagnosis in the individual case and are discussed in the text. Chest X-rays are often normal, particularly in patients who present with haemoptysis as the only symptom. Even bronchoscopy will fail to reveal the source of the bleeding in a significant proportion. It is a sobering thought that in one such series of 137 cases no cause for the bleeding was found in 56%.

CAUSES IN THE RESPIRATORY TRACT

Bronchial carcinoma is the commonest and most serious cause of bleeding from the respiratory tract in middle-aged or elderly adults. Apart from bronchitis, the other conditions discussed below usually present much earlier in life.

Bronchitis (see also Cough, p. 230)

Blood-streaked purulent sputum is occasionally seen in acute bronchitis and in chronic obstructive airways disease. Bronchitis should not, however, be accepted as the cause until more ominous conditions such as tuberculosis or a bronchial neoplasm have first been excluded. A chest X-ray is mandatory in such cases, particularly in heavy smokers.

Bronchiectasis (see also Cough, p. 231)

In the UK the incidence of bronchiectasis has fallen markedly with the widespread use of antibiotics for chest infections in childhood. It may follow measles, whooping cough and pneumonia and is an inevitable complication of cystic fibrosis. There will be a history of a long-standing productive cough with copious purulent sputum. Haemoptysis is common and may be profuse. In severe cases there may be clubbing of the fingers and toes. Apart from some crowding together of the lung markings at the bases little will be seen on a plain chest X-ray.

Bronchiectasis is one of the few conditions in which bronchography is of value in confirming the diagnosis and in establishing the extent of the disease.

Aspergillosis

In asthmatic subjects *Aspergillus* may colonise the bronchi, especially in the upper lobes, and cause recurrent attacks of wheezing, fever and sometimes haemoptysis. Plugs of mycelium may temporarily block smaller bronchi and lead to saccular bronchiectasis. *Aspergillus fumigatus* is the commonest pathogenic species which is encountered in the UK. It may be cultured from the sputum. Serum levels of IgE are usually elevated and precipitating antibodies may be found in the serum. A eosinophilia is sometimes present in the blood. Serial chest X-rays may show transient pulmonary infiltrates, particularly in the upper lobes.

Neoplasm (see also Cough, p. 232)

A persistent cough in a cigarette smoker is the presenting symptom in the majority of patients with cancer of the bronchus. Blood-streaking of the sputum does, however, occur in more than 70% of cases and even a single episode in an individual who has smoked 15–20 cigarettes daily for more than 20 years should be investigated as a matter of urgency. The rapid development of clubbing of the fingers is highly suspicious of the presence of a neoplasm. A normal chest X-ray does not exclude the diagnosis and bronchoscopy with biopsy of any suspicious area should be done routinely in such patients. Early morning sputum should be examined for malignant cells.

Bronchial adenomas are much less common than squamous cell carcinomas and differ from them in being seen most often before the age of 40. They occur in non-smokers as well as in smokers. Bronchial adenomas are very vascular and are liable to bleed, so that haemoptysis may be profuse and an early symptom. A round shadow is often visible on plain X-rays in the vicinity of one or other hilum and the tumour may be seen at bronchoscopy. Pulmonary angiography is invaluable in confirming the diagnosis and in demonstrating its position in relation to the major blood vessels for the benefit of the thoracic surgeon.

CAUSES IN LUNGS

In Britain the most frequent cause of haemorrhage from the lungs is *pulmonary embolism. Tuberculosis* is however still rife in many parts of the world and there is a much higher incidence of this disease amongst Asian immigrants to this country than in the native population.

Pulmonary embolism (see also Thoracic pain, p. 30)

This is by far the commonest cause of haemoptysis in a medical or surgical ward. It is seen particularly in bedbound elderly patients in cardiac failure or within days of a surgical operation. Outside hospital it may be seen in patients recently discharged from hospital after surgery, during pregnancy or in women on the contraceptive pill.

The onset of pulmonary embolism is usually signalled by the sudden onset of pleuritic pain which may or may not be accompanied by some shortness of breath. A pleural rub may be present at the onset or develop later. Blood-streaking of sputum or frank blood commonly follows within a day or two. The condition is sometimes mistaken for pneumonia through failure of the doctor to inspect the contents of the sputum pot or to ask specifically about the coughing up of blood. It may be preceded or accompanied by thrombophlebitis and the legs should be inspected with this in mind.

Pulmonary embolism is a medical emergency — only prompt treatment with intravenous heparin, preferably by continuous infusion, may prevent the occurrence of a second and possibly fatal embolus.

Tuberculosis (see also Fever, p. 325)

The incidence of pulmonary tuberculosis has fallen dramatically in recent decades in the West. Its course is marked by gradual loss of weight and energy, night sweats and persistent cough. Recurrent small haemoptyses may be the first sign of the infection — patients who experience these are fortunate as the alarm this causes ensures prompt medical attention.

The condition is readily diagnosed on a chest X-ray which will show soft infiltrates in the apices of the lungs and possibly cavitation in the upper lobes. At least three specimens of sputum should be examined for tubercle bacilli and sent for culture on Löwenstein–Jensen media.

Occasionally a chronic cavity may be colonised by *Aspergillus* which aggregates to form a mycetoma. Chest X-rays will show a dense rounded opacity within its lumen and the fungus will be found in the sputum.

Erosion of a dilated bronchial arteriole in the wall of a tuberculous cavity is a well-recognised but fortunately uncommon cause of massive blood loss.

Pneumonia (see also Fever, p. 317)

Viscid pink or rusty sputum is common at the onset of pneumonia, particularly in the lobar variety. A chest X-ray will show abnormal shadowing in the affected lung. Sputum culture will identify the responsible organism and enable its antibiotic sensitivity to be determined.

Leptospirosis, though rare, can sometimes cause a spectacular haemorrhagic pneumonia; the haemorrhage is then so profuse that the patient is in danger of asphyxiation or of bleeding to death.

Abscess (see also Cough, p. 234)

Since the introduction of antibiotics lung abscess has become an uncommon complication of lung infections. Multiple thin-walled abscesses may however occur with staphylococcal and *Klebsiella* pneumonias, with the production of tenacious purulent blood-stained sputum.

EXTRARESPIRATORY CAUSES

Cardiac disease (see also Dyspnoea, p. 248)

In left ventricular failure an increase in pulmonary artery pressure often occurs at night. The patient is wakened by paroxysmal nocturnal dyspnoea of such severity that he may feel that he is going to die and struggles to the open window to get air. The laboured breathing is often accompanied by wheezing; hence the term 'cardiac asthma' which is sometimes used to describe the condition.

During an attack the patient will be pale, sweating, cyanosed and gasping for breath. When the pulmonary oedema reaches the alveoli it will be coughed up as frothy, blood-tinged sputum. The diagnosis is seldom in doubt, because there is usually a history of valvular or ischaemic heart disease and numerous fine crepitations will be audible throughout the lung fields.

In mitral stenosis the raised pressure in the left atrium is transmitted to the lungs and can result in rupture of a venule and a brisk haemoptysis. Such attacks tend to be recurrent and self-limiting. The history, the characteristic murmur and the X-ray appearance of the cardiac shadow will confirm the diagnosis.

Trauma

Coughing of blood may follow blast injuries of the lungs or penetration of the pleura by a fractured rib. It may also result from exploratory needling of the lung when attempting to obtain a biopsy specimen, and is commonly seen after bronchoscopy. The cause is usually self-evident.

Goodpasture's syndrome (see also Haematuria, p. 180)

This rare condition is included for the sake of completeness. It presents acutely with repeated frank haemoptyses and haematuria. Young men are mainly affected and death from rapidly progressive renal failure is the usual outcome. It is thought to be an autoimmune disorder affecting the capillaries in the lungs and glomeruli of the kidney — IgG antibodies to basement membrane have been found in some of the victims.

Haemorrhagic disease

Haemoptysis is rarely due to haemorrhagic disease but this should be suspected if there is evidence of bleeding elsewhere. It can occur in hereditary telangiectasia, Wegener's granulomata and disseminated intravascular coagulation. In thrombocytopenia the bleeding is more likely to be coming from the nose and mouth.

CHAPTER 15
Gastrointestinal haemorrhage

SYNOPSIS OF CAUSES*

UPPER

Oesophagitis; **Oesophageal varices**; Mallory-Weiss syndrome; **Gastric erosions; Peptic ulcer**;
Neoplasm; Aneurysm.

LOWER

Meckel's diverticulum; **Inflammatory bowel disease; Diverticulitis; Neoplasm;
Angiodysplasia**; Ischaemic colitis; Haemorrhagic disease; Schistosomiasis; Haemorrhoids.

* Bold type is used for causes more commonly found in Europe and North America.

PHYSIOLOGY

This chapter is concerned with blood loss from the alimentary tract
presenting as an acute episode. Bleeding may however be occult — this is
dealt with in the chapter on Anaemia.

Upper gastrointestinal haemorrhage occurs from lesions in the oesophagus, stomach or first part of the duodenum in territory supplied by
vessels arising from the coeliac axis. The commonest causes are oesophageal
varices, gastric tears or erosions and peptic ulcers. The blood may be
vomited upwards as a haematemesis or pass down the alimentary tract to
appear in the stools.

A haematemesis may consist of bright red blood mixed with stomach
contents or have the appearance of 'coffee grounds', the blood having been
altered by contact with the gastric juices. It is usually followed by melaena
but occasionally a massive haemorrhage from a peptic ulcer presents as
frank rectal bleeding instead of the more characteristic black, tarry stools.

Bleeding from the small bowel and caecum may appear as melaena, but
bleeding from the colon and rectum usually presents as fresh blood mixed
with faeces. Intestinal haemorrhage may be caused by inflammatory bowel
disease, neoplasms or vascular abnormalities in the bowel wall. Haemorrhagic disease may cause bleeding from any part of the alimentary canal and
is much more likely if there is other pathology in the gut.

Hypovolaemia inevitably follows an acute gastrointestinal haemorrhage of any magnitude. A loss of a litre or more of blood will result in an immediate fall in blood pressure, tachycardia and peripheral vasoconstriction. The haemoglobin level and haematocrit only fall when the circulating blood is diluted by the fluid which diffuses out of the extravascular compartments into the depleted vascular space. This process takes some hours and during this period the blood pressure may return to normal. The degree of shock in the individual patient will largely depend upon the rapidity of bleeding and the amount of blood lost.

DIAGNOSTIC APPROACH

It has been estimated that about 30 000 cases of upper gastrointestinal haemorrhage are admitted annually to hospitals in the UK, amounting to about one in ten of all emergency medical admissions. Despite all the advances in diagnosis and management in recent years the mortality rate is still around 10%. At least half these patients will have bled from chronic peptic ulcers — acute gastric erosions account for many of the remainder.

If the patient has vomited blood the cause must lie in the oesophagus, stomach or duodenum. A history of indigestion or a previous haemorrhage makes peptic ulceration more likely, particularly if a gastric or duodenal ulcer has been demonstrated by a barium meal in the past. The patient must be asked about the recent taking of drugs such as aspirin, indomethacin and phenylbutazone, as most of the commonly prescribed anti-inflammatory drugs can cause acute gastric erosions. Corticosteroids and anticoagulants increase the risk of haemorrhage in the presence of a pre-existing peptic ulcer or when given along with the analgesics just mentioned. Enquiry should also be made about alcohol consumption with the Mallory–Weiss syndrome and oesophageal varices in mind. A bright red haematemesis shortly after a bout of vomiting may well be due to a tear in the gastric mucosa.

While melaena commonly results from bleeding into the upper alimentary tract a massive haemorrhage from a peptic ulcer occasionally appears as frank blood in the stools. As a rule however, this is more likely to have come from a lesion in the colon or rectum.

Serious blood loss from the lower intestine is far less common than bleeding arising from causes in the oesophagus, stomach or duodenum. Nevertheless, it may on occasions be life-threatening and require urgent hospital admission. It is rare in children, in whom it is most likely to originate from a polyp or Meckel's diverticulum. In adolescents and young adults polyps and inflammatory bowel disease are the most frequent causes whilst neoplasms, diverticular disease, ischaemia and angiodysplasia become increasingly common with advancing age.

Patients often overestimate the amount of blood they have lost, but pallor, sweating, tachycardia and hypotension point to a massive haemorrhage and no time should be lost in setting up a blood transfusion. Fortunately the majority stop bleeding spontaneously, and few require immediate surgery to prevent exsanguination. In the UK most patients with gastrointestinal bleeding are initially admitted to a medical ward. Nevertheless, it is a wise precaution to invoke a surgical opinion within a few hours of admission, because about 20% will bleed again.

The history and physical examination rarely provide sufficient evidence to identify the source of the haemorrhage, but splenomegaly will direct attention to the possibility of oesophageal varices and other stigmata of liver disease should then be sought. The rare presence of circumoral pigmentation should remind one of the Peutz–Jeghers syndrome with its multiple polypi in both small and large intestine. The vomit and stools should always be inspected to confirm the presence of blood and to determine whether the bleeding is continuing. Not all black or brown material contains altered haemoglobin and sometimes patients who claim to have vomited blood or passed melaena stools are mistaken or malingering.

Investigations
Blood will have been taken on admission for grouping, and a full blood count is important as a baseline for comparison with later estimations. If the patient is markedly anaemic when first seen it is probable that he has been bleeding for some days or even weeks beforehand. When haemorrhagic disease is suspected the platelets, partial thromboplastin time and prothrombin time must be estimated. These should also be carried out if liver disease is possible.

Where fibreoptic endoscopy is available it has largely replaced radiology in the investigation of upper gastrointestinal haemorrhage. It is particularly valuable in detecting shallow mucosal lesions in the oesophagus and stomach which are likely to be missed by the conventional barium meal. The procedure is well tolerated, even by the elderly. The source of the bleeding can be identified precisely in about 90% of cases, provided that the examination is carried out within 24 hours of admission. The success rate falls to around 60% if it is delayed for more than 72 hours. Coeliac axis angiography should be considered in those cases where active bleeding continues and endoscopy has failed to determine the bleeding site.

When the source of the haemorrhage appears to be in the colon or rectum proctosigmoidoscopy should be followed by a barium enema. Difficulty arises when these investigations are negative. Colonoscopy enables the more proximal parts of the colon to be examined but it is time-consuming and may not be readily available. Selective visceral angiography is another specialised technique which is reserved for obscure cases of intestinal bleeding in which other investigations have failed to produce a diagnosis. It is particularly effective in locating the source if the patient is actively bleeding at the time of the examination, and is the only way to demonstrate lesions in the small bowel apart from laparotomy.

UPPER ALIMENTARY CAUSES

The great majority of patients presenting with haematemesis or melaena have a lesion proximal to the ampulla of Vater. In Britain the commonest causes are gastric erosions and peptic ulceration. In one series of 720 endoscopies for haematemesis 70% were found to arise from a *duodenal ulcer, erosive gastritis* or *gastric ulcer* in that order of frequency.

Oesophagitis (see also Thoracic pain, p. 37)

Haematemesis from severe oesophagitis is sometimes seen in elderly patients confined to bed because of intercurrent illness or recent surgery. The ulceration may be due to the corrosive effect of swallowed tablets which have been held up at the gastro–oesophageal junction. Slow-K tablets, analgesics, emepronium bromide, ferrous sulphate and antibiotics are the prime suspects (and should always be taken with liberal amounts of fluid). A history of heartburn and dysphagia should be sought. The diagnosis can be confirmed by fibreoptic endoscopy but the bleeding usually stops when the patient is propped up and given antacids.

Oesophageal varices (see also Jaundice, p. 152)

Aetiology
Hepatic cirrhosis leads to portal hypertension with distension and some-times rupture of varices in the oesophagus and cardia of the stomach. Cirrhosis was described by the World Health Organization in 1979 as ranking among the five leading causes of death. It has shown a marked increase in incidence during recent years in Europe and America but is still relatively uncommon in the UK. Bleeding varices only account for about 3% of instances of upper gastrointestinal bleeding in this country.

The aetiology of cirrhosis is unknown in many patients but alcohol is probably responsible for at least half the cases. Other recognised but less common causes include chronic hepatitis-B infection, haemochromatosis and Wilson's disease. In tropical countries schistosomiasis is a major cause and death from haematemesis is not uncommon.

Although cirrhosis is the main cause of portal hypertension it is some-times due to thrombosis of the hepatic, portal or splenic veins as a result of sepsis, trauma, malignancy or thrombotic states.

Clinical features
The vomiting of bright red blood may be the first indication of the presence of varices and the underlying liver disease. It is likely to be sudden and profuse. A history of alcohol abuse or of failing health with mild fever, unexplained nosebleeds or ankle oedema may be elicited. On examination hepatosplenomegaly, spider naevi, palmar erythema and gynaecomastia should be looked for. In an advanced case there may be ascites, jaundice and mental confusion from hepatic encephalopathy.

Investigations

Blood should be taken for a full blood count, serum enzyme estimations and prothrombin time. Thrombocytopenia and impaired synthesis of clotting factors in the liver may hinder attempts to stop the bleeding. Fibreoptic endoscopy to determine the bleeding source should be carried out as soon as the patient has been resuscitated and is in a stable condition. This is essential — the haemorrhage may well be occurring from a non-variceal site such as gastric erosions or a duodenal ulcer, particularly in patients with alcoholic liver disease. A barium swallow may demonstrate the presence of varices but will not establish that they are the site of bleeding.

More sophisticated radiological techniques such as splenoportography must be used if an attempt is to be made to relieve the pressure in the portal system by some form of shunt procedure.

Mallory–Weiss syndrome

Linear tears of the mucosa just below the gastro–oesophageal junction were first recognised as a cause of haematemesis by Mallory and Weiss as long ago as 1929. The tears always begin in the gastric mucosa but may extend up into the oesophagus. They are thought to be due to sudden herniation of the stomach through the diaphragm following a sharp rise in intra-abdominal pressure. By far the commonest cause is prolonged vomiting after drinking excessive amounts of alcohol, which probably accounts for the much higher incidence of the syndrome in middle-aged males. Cases have however been reported after strenuous coughing, defaecation, epileptic fits and blunt abdominal trauma. Blood loss is seldom massive and may amount to no more than some blood-streaked vomit a few hours after the initial insult.

The Mallory–Weiss syndrome was found on endoscopy in 13% of a recent Australian series of 121 cases of upper gastrointestinal haemorrhage. Retching and vomiting often preceded the haematemesis and a number of patients had a history of high alcohol consumption. The condition appears to be less common in the UK. However, early endoscopy is essential to make the diagnosis because the lesions usually heal completely within 2–3 days.

Gastric erosions (see also Epigastric pain, p. 52)

Haemorrhage is due, as a rule, to the taking of ulcerogenic drugs such as aspirin, indomethacin, phenylbutazone and naproxen. Profuse bleeding may follow the casual use of any of these non-steroidal anti-inflammatory agents, whilst anaemia from chronic blood loss is common in arthritic patients taking this kind of medication.

Corticosteroids often cause dyspepsia, but the evidence that they produce upper gastrointestinal bleeding on their own is inconclusive; they are frequently taken with other drugs which damage the gastric mucosa.

Acute alcoholism is an occasional cause. Stress-induced ulceration of the stomach and duodenum is sometimes seen in seriously ill patients suffering from postoperative sepsis, severe burns, renal failure or multiple injuries.

The bleeding usually ceases spontaneously after admission to hospital but this is not always the case, particularly in the elderly. Endoscopy provides the only means of confirming the diagnosis. Ideally it should be carried out within 24 hours of admission since these erosions usually heal rapidly.

Peptic ulcer (see also Epigastric pain, p. 52)

Chronic peptic ulceration is the commonest cause of gastrointestinal bleeding. In most published series duodenal ulcers predominate and these are more likely to present with melaena alone. There is usually a history of chronic dyspepsia and sometimes of previous episodes of bleeding but this is not invariable. There is an increased risk of haemorrhage from a peptic ulcer in elderly patients taking non-steroidal anti-inflammatory drugs.

Neoplasm

Dysphagia and anaemia from chronic blood loss are the presenting features of an oesophageal carcinoma; haematemesis is rare. Benign tumours of the stomach such as leiomyomas and polyps may, however, present with bleeding due to ulceration of their mucosal surfaces. Vomiting is a late manifestation of a gastric carcinoma unless the growth is situated near the pylorus; the vomit may be brown in colour from the presence of altered blood.

Aneurysm

These are rare causes of acute blood loss. Submucosal aneurysms on the distal branches of the left gastric artery sometimes rupture into the stomach and present with haematemesis or melaena. Cases have been reported in children and young adults. The diagnosis is difficult for they do not show up on a barium meal and endoscopy may have to be abandoned because of continuous bleeding. Coeliac axis angiography will reveal the site of the aneurysms provided that the dye is injected into the left gastric artery by selective catheterisation.

Haemobilia is sometimes due to rupture of a hepatic artery aneurysm into the biliary tree. More frequently it is due to hepatic injury following trauma. It presents as haematemesis, upper abdominal pain and jaundice. The bleeding site can usually be demonstrated by selective angiography.

Rupture of an aortic aneurysm into the duodenum is inevitably fatal. It should be thought of in any patient presenting with a massive haematemesis who has undergone an aortic graft operation in the past, but it can occur spontaneously in old age.

LOWER ALIMENTARY CAUSES

Profuse bleeding from the bowel distal to the ampulla of Vater is far less common than bleeding arising from lesions in the oesophagus, stomach and duodenum.

In recent years the use of colonoscopy and selective mesenteric angiography has greatly improved the accuracy of diagnosis.

Meckel's diverticulum (see also Umbilical pain, p. 68)

This congenital anomaly is present in about 2% of the population, but it is commonly silent. It is situated a short distance above the ileocaecal junction and contains ectopic gastric mucosa which may occasionally ulcerate and bleed. It is one of the few causes of massive rectal bleeding in children. Mesenteric angiography may define the bleeding site but laparatomy is usually necessary to identify the lesion and to stop the leak.

Inflammatory bowel disease

Massive haemorrhage from ulceration in the small intestine is one of the most dreaded complications of typhoid fever. It usually occurs during the third week of the illness. Typhoid is rare in Britain, though it may be seen in those returning from a holiday or business trip abroad.

A more common cause of rectal bleeding is the colitis produced by *Shigella* and *Campylobacter* infections. This is always associated with frequent, loose stools and the responsible organisms can be found in the faeces. In tropical countries amoebiasis will produce a similar picture.

Ulcerative colitis is the only chronic inflammatory disorder which regularly causes bloody diarrhoea. Blood mixed with mucus in the stools is invariably present in those with extensive disease, along with other symptoms such as left-sided abdominal pain, tenesmus and loss of weight. When the inflammation is localised to the rectum there may be constipation instead of diarrhoea. The diagnosis is usually readily established by proctosigmoidoscopy and rectal biopsy. Crohn's disease rarely gives rise to rectal bleeding unless the colon is involved but occult blood loss frequently leads to an iron-deficiency anaemia.

Diverticulitis (see also Lateral abdominal pain, p. 87)

This common disorder is seen increasingly often in later life. It is perhaps hardly surprising that erosion of a vessel in a diverticulum should occasionally give rise to an acute haemorrhage, but the presence of diverticula on a barium enema film does not prove that they are the source. Polyps, carcinomas and angiodysplasia may all co-exist with diverticular disease in these elderly patients. Acute bleeding may however be localised by angiography or colonoscopy to a particular diverticulum.

Neoplasm

Polyps occur chiefly in the sigmoid region of the colon and may be solitary or multiple. A family history may be obtained in cases of polyposis coli, and circumoral pigmentation should remind one of the Peutz–Jeghers syndrome. Even quite small polyps can bleed profusely and give rise to rectal bleeding. They may be identified and removed by the skilled use of the colonoscope.

Growths in the colon and rectum account for some 17 000 deaths annually in the UK. The blood loss is small as a rule and is easily overlooked. Frank rectal bleeding seldom calls attention to the existence of tumours, but fresh blood on the lavatory paper should not be ascribed to haemorrhoids unless a rectal carcinoma has been excluded by digital examination and sigmoidoscopy.

Angiodysplasia

This term is used to encompass small haemangiomas and arteriovenous malformations in the mucosa of the alimentary tract. The latter may be solitary but are more commonly present as multiple punctate angiomatous lesions similar to those seen in hereditary telangiectasia. There is, however, no evidence to suggest that these abnormalities are congenital in origin, although there is a recognised association with aortic stenosis and chronic pulmonary disease. The commonest site is the ascending colon but similar lesions have occasionally been reported in the small bowel and stomach.

This condition is being increasingly recognised as an important cause of recurrent intestinal haemorrhage in the elderly. It should be suspected if proctosigmoidoscopy, double-contrast barium enemas and clotting factors in the blood are all normal. Selective mesenteric angiography may reveal an area of dilated small vessels or a vascular tuft but surgical resection is often difficult for the lesions are so small that they are unlikely to be seen or felt by the surgeon, even when he knows of their existence. Colonoscopy provides a more logical approach to the problem, because the mucosal lesions should be visible to the operator and treatment with electrocoagulation may enable major surgery to be avoided.

Ischaemic colitis (see also Lateral abdominal pain, p. 89)

Ischaemic colitis is an occasional cause of rectal bleeding in old age. Atrial fibrillation will suggest an embolic cause. It chiefly affects the descending and sigmoid colon, presenting classically with severe lower abdominal pain and bloody diarrhoea. It may be indistinguishable clinically from an attack of acute diverticulitis. The segment of bowel involved is often clearly demarcated at colonoscopy and shows up as a limited area of 'colitis' on a barium enema. In view of the frailty of most sufferers it is fortunate that the condition usually subsides with conservative treatment.

Haemorrhagic disease

This is an uncommon cause of acute blood loss from the intestines. It is usually accompanied by evidence of bleeding elsewhere but this is not always so with vascular defects. In polyarteritis nodosa multiple infarcts in the intestines sometimes cause melaena whilst bloody stools are typically seen in Henoch–Schönlein purpura, along with the characteristic rash and painful joints.

Gastrointestinal haemorrhage is one of the most serious manifestations of hereditary telangiectasia but fortunately this condition is rare. It usually presents in middle age with recurrent epistaxes and characteristic discrete red spots in the mucosa of the nose and mouth.

Schistosomiasis

Infestation by this liver fluke is endemic in Africa, Asia, the Middle East, South America and some Caribbean islands. It invades the colon, producing diarrhoea with blood and mucus and abdominal pain. The parasite passes to the liver and has been referred to earlier as a cause of portal hypertension and oesophageal varices. It is a possible cause of unexplained rectal bleeding in immigrants from countries in which the disease is endemic.

Haemorrhoids

Fresh blood may accompany or follow the passage of a stool and is then visible on the lavatory paper. The diagnosis is made by inspection and direct vision through a proctoscope. The presence of haemorrhoids does not, of course, exclude other sources of bleeding, such as cancer. Profuse bleeding, particularly in an elderly subject, demands a more thorough investigation.

CHAPTER 16

Haematuria

SYNOPSIS OF CAUSES*

KIDNEY

INFLAMMATORY

Acute glomerulonephritis; IgA nephropathy; Henoch-Schönlein purpura; Polyarteritis nodosa; Systemic lupus erythematosus; Goodpasture's syndrome; Leptospirosis; Acute pyelonephritis; Tuberculosis.

NON-INFLAMMATORY

Trauma; Calculi; **Neoplasm; Alport's syndrome**; Polycystic disease; Hydronephrosis; **Anticoagulant therapy**; Haemorrhagic disease; Sickle-cell trait.

BLADDER, PROSTATE AND URETHRA

INFLAMMATORY

Cystitis; Schistosomiasis; Urethritis.

NON-INFLAMMATORY

Trauma; Calculi; **Neoplasm**; Prostatic hypertrophy.

---

* Bold type is used for causes more commonly found in Europe and North America.

PHYSIOLOGY

Blood in the urine may come from any part of the urinary tract and can vary in amount from a slight excess of red cells, visible only on microscopy, to a massive haemorrhage. Although the term 'haematuria' is commonly used to describe both microscopic and macroscopic bleeding it is only the latter which alarms patients and brings them to the doctor. This chapter is therefore concerned mainly with those conditions which cause sufficient haemorrhage for the blood to be visible to the naked eye.

When the kidney, ureter or bladder is the source the blood will be evenly mixed with the urine. Bleeding at the beginning or end of micturition is likely to be due to a lesion of the bladder neck, urethra or prostate. Haemorrhage from uterus or bowel may contaminate the urine so that it is important to exclude this possibility before concluding that the blood has come from the urinary tract.

In macroscopic haematuria the freshly passed urine will have a smoky,

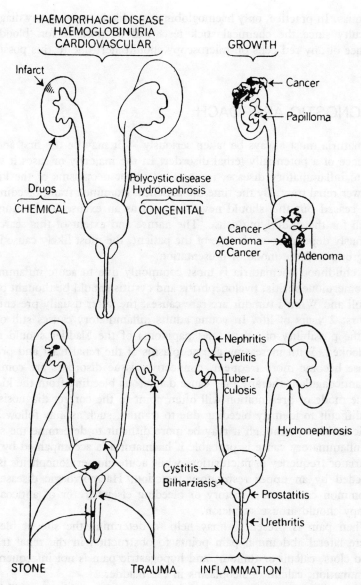

HAEMORRHAGIC DISEASE
HAEMOGLOBINURIA
CARDIOVASCULAR

GROWTH

Infarct

Cancer

Papilloma

Drugs
CHEMICAL

Polycystic disease
Hydronephrosis
CONGENITAL

Cancer
Adenoma
or Cancer

Adenoma

Nephritis

Pyelitis

Tuber-
culosis

Hydronephrosis

Cystitis
Bilharziasis

Prostatitis

Urethritis

STONE

TRAUMA

INFLAMMATION

FIGURE 9

opalescent appearance or be frankly bloody, depending on the severity of the bleeding. On standing, haemolysis takes place and the liberated haemoglobin will impart a brownish colour to acid urine and a reddish tinge to alkaline urine. As little as one millilitre of blood is sufficient to produce this discolouration.

There are a few conditions in which discolouration of the urine may mistakenly be ascribed to the presence of blood. These include the ingestion of certain foods and drugs, the rare disorders of alkaptonuria and porphyria and the haemoglobinuria associated with a variety of acute haemolytic anaemias. In practice, only haemoglobinuria is likely to cause any diagnostic difficulty since the chemical stick tests will be positive for 'blood'; the absence of any red cells on microscopy should alert one to this possibility.

DIAGNOSTIC APPROACH

Haematuria must always be taken seriously — it may be the first and only evidence of a potentially lethal disorder. In the majority of cases it will be due to inflammatory disease, trauma, calculi or neoplasms of the kidneys or lower renal tract. By the time the patient is examined frank bleeding may have ceased but this should never be used as an excuse for putting off a search for the underlying cause. The nature and extent of this search will obviously depend upon the age of the patient, the most likely cause in that age group and the mode of presentation.

In childhood haematuria is most commonly due to acute inflammation, so glomerulonephritis, pyelonephritis and cystitis should be thought of first. Calculi and Wilm's tumour are rare causes, the latter usually presenting in the first 2 years of life. In young adults inflammatory causes still operate but the possibility of calculi and papilloma of the bladder should not be overlooked. With increasing age neoplasms of the renal tract and prostatic disease become more frequent, connective tissue disorders are commoner and anticoagulant therapy may cause dangerous bleeding from the kidneys.

The mode of presentation will often point to the correct diagnosis. It is not difficult to identify bleeding due to trauma, such as may follow a road traffic accident, although it may be more difficult to determine the source. An inflammatory cause is probable if haematuria is accompanied by fever, dysuria or frequency of micturition, while acute glomerulonephritis is often preceded by an upper respiratory infection. Haemorrhagic disease is an uncommon cause but a history of bleeding elsewhere or of anticoagulant therapy should arouse suspicion.

When pain is present it may help to determine the site of bleeding. Severe lateral abdominal pain points to obstruction in the renal tract by blood clots, calculi or tumour, and hypogastric pain is not infrequent with inflammation, calculi or neoplasms in the bladder.

Painless, recurrent haematuria, without any other evidence of ill-health, poses the greatest diagnostic challenge — the cause may remain obscure despite full urological investigations. Between 5 and 10% of cases seen in a urological clinic fall into this category. Proliferative IgA glomerulonephritis is being increasingly recognised as a cause of recurrent haematuria in children and young adults but the diagnosis can only be made by renal biopsy. In older patients neoplasms of the renal tract may escape detection for some time and investigations may have to be repeated at regular intervals if there is to be any hope of a cure. Such patients should be under the care of a specialist.

Investigations

The extent and nature of these will clearly depend upon the most likely cause of the haematuria. Microscopic examination of a freshly passed urine specimen should never be omitted, as the presence of red cell and granular casts will indicate a renal origin, of which the most likely cause is some form of glomerulonephritis. If pus cells are present the urine should be sent for culture.

When phase-contrast microscopy is available the site of the bleeding can be determined with a high degree of accuracy by studying the morphology of the red cells in the urine. Erythrocytes which arise from the glomeruli show a great variation in size, shape and haemoglobin content whereas those coming from a non-glomerular source such as a tumour are uniform in size and shape and, unless the urine is very acid, retain a high haemoglobin content. Casts are also seen more easily by this technique than by ordinary light microscopy.

Plain X-rays of the abdomen are rarely helpful but may show differences in renal size and calculi or calcification in a tuberculous kidney. An intravenous pyelogram will be indicated unless the patient is obviously suffering from glomerulonephritis or there is a previous history of an allergic reaction to the contrast medium. In many centres the non-invasive techniques of ultrasonography and computed tomography are being increasingly used to assess the gross structure of the kidneys and ureters and have the additional advantage that they are not dependant on renal function. Angiography is seldom indicated but may sometimes demonstrate a small renal tumour which has escaped detection by these other imaging procedures. Cystoscopy and retrograde pyelography are reserved for cases where the bleeding is thought to come from the lower renal tract. Biopsies should be taken of any suspicious areas in the bladder, but early cancers may be missed.

Percutaneous renal biopsy is only necessary when some form of glomerulonephritis or Alport's syndrome is suspected, and where other investigations are inconclusive. Biopsy specimens should be examined by immunofluorescence and electron microscopy.

CAUSES IN THE KIDNEY

These have been divided into inflammatory causes, of which the great majority are some form of glomerulonephritis, and non-inflammatory causes, of which the most important is renal cancer.

INFLAMMATORY CAUSES

Acute glomerulonephritis

Aetiology

In the majority of cases glomerulonephritis appears to be due to the deposition of antigen–antibody complexes in the glomeruli. Only rarely is it due to the production of specific antibodies to renal tissue. The damage which results is caused mainly by activation of the complement system, although other factors such as histamine release and intravascular clotting may play a part. The evidence is based on animal studies and on the examination of renal biopsy material by electron microscopy and immunofluorescence. The nature of most of the antigens involved is still unknown but bacteria, viruses, tumours and drugs have all been implicated.

At least seven morphological appearances have been described; the size of the immune complexes and their rate of deposition is thought to determine the type of glomerulonephritis that develops. The disease may present as an acute illness, as recurrent haematuria, as the nephrotic syndrome or with chronic renal failure. Microscopic haematuria may be present in all these forms. However, frank bleeding is usually seen only in the classical type of acute nephritis described below, in IgA proliferative glomerulonephritis presenting as recurrent haematuria, and in glomerulonephritis associated with connective tissue disorders.

Clinical features
Classical acute nephritis is seen most frequently in children of school age but can occur at any time of life. There is often a history of an acute throat, ear or skin infection some 7–14 days beforehand. The pathogen is usually a beta-haemolytic streptococcus but nephritis may follow other bacterial or viral infections.

The onset is abrupt, the child waking with a puffy face, pallor, headache, malaise and frank haematuria. Oliguria is invariable and secondary urinary tract infections are common if the attack is prolonged. The excessive retention of salt and water accounts for the oedema, the elevation of jugular venous pressure and hypertension, which is usually mild in degree. In a severe case there may be dyspnoea from pulmonary oedema and vomiting, drowsiness and fits resulting from hypertensive encephalopathy. Arthralgia is rare and suggests an underlying connective tissue disorder such as Henoch–Schönlein purpura, polyarteritis nodosa or systemic lupus erythematosus.

Acute nephritis follows a benign course in most children and in more than half the adult cases. A diuresis typically occurs within a few days of the onset, although slight proteinuria and microscopic haematuria often persist for months after the attack. A further episode of frank bleeding is sometimes precipitated by exertion. In a small proportion of cases, particularly in adults, there is progressive renal damage leading eventually to death from hypertensive cardiac failure or uraemia.

Investigations
The urine is scanty and will contain protein, blood and casts. Specimens should be sent for culture if the period of oliguria is prolonged. Streptococci may be grown from the throat and the serum antistreptolysin-O titre will be elevated if the initial infection was due to this organism and the case has

not been treated with antibiotics. Low serum complement levels will be found early in the illness but usually return to normal within 2 months. A high ESR is often found but has no prognostic significance. Renal biopsy is only indicated if the course is unduly protracted or if a connective tissue disorder is suspected. In such cases the blood urea and serum creatinine will be persistently raised.

IgA nephropathy

This form of chronic glomerulonephritis is being increasingly recognised as a common cause of macroscopic haematuria in children and young adults. It probably accounts for about one-fifth of all cases of primary glomerular disease. It usually begins in childhood. Episodes of macroscopic haematuria may be precipitated by exertion or infections of the upper respiratory tract or gut. The haematuria may be accompanied by loin pain and dysuria, but oedema and hypertension will be absent. The urine will contain a little protein and microscopic haematuria may be found between attacks. At one time it was thought that this was a relatively benign condition which could persist for years without any obvious deterioration in renal function, but more recent studies have shown that about half the cases eventually progress to end-stage renal failure. The diagnosis of mesangial IgA nephropathy is made on renal biopsy, which shows diffuse deposits of IgA in the glomerular mesangium associated with focal and segmental proliferative glomerulonephritis. The presence of interstitial fibrosis and extension of the IgA deposits to the peripheral capillary loops, together with proteinuria of more than 1 g a day, are associated with an increased risk of developing renal failure. When this condition is associated with non-thrombocytopenic purpura it is part of the Henoch–Schönlein syndrome.

Henoch-Schönlein purpura (see also Purpura and bleeding, p. 193)

This allergic vasculitis is the commonest connective-tissue disorder of childhood. Mesangial IgA glomerulonephritis develops in about half the cases and frank haematuria is frequently seen. The characteristic rash, arthralgia, abdominal colic and bloody stools will point to the correct diagnosis. In children the disease is generally benign and resolves within a few weeks of onset. Renal biopsy is rarely necessary unless the course is unduly prolonged.

Polyarteritis nodosa (see also Fever, p. 328)

The renal tract is frequently involved in polyarteritis nodosa and haematuria may result from extensive vasculitis of the bladder, renal infarcts or focal proliferative glomerulonephritis. An acute onset sometimes follows a respiratory infection with fever, proteinuria and a rising serum level of urea and creatinine. In the variant known as Wegener's granuloma the nephritis is usually preceded by necrotising lesions in the nasal passages or lungs, which may be present months before the onset of renal failure.

Systemic lupus erythematosus (see also Fever, p. 326)

Arthritis, skin lesions, pleurisy and cardiovascular manifestations usually overshadow the renal lesions which may not appear for months or even years after the initial episode. Symptomless proteinuria and microscopic haematuria will be the only evidence of the proliferative glomerulonephritis which may eventually kill the patient; macroscopic haematuria is rare. There is good evidence that the nephritis in this disorder is caused by the repeated deposition of soluble DNA in the glomeruli.

Goodpasture's syndrome

Repeated haemoptyses and frank haematuria are the hallmarks of this rare disease of unknown aetiology. It mainly affects young adult males and may follow a 'flu-like' illness. The lung lesions are similar to idiopathic pulmonary haemosiderosis but an arteritis and necrotizing alveolitis are sometimes found at autopsy. In the kidneys a severe extracapillary glomerulonephritis causes extensive glomerular destruction. IgG antibodies to basement membrane have been identified in the plasma and kidneys of some patients. The outlook is grave and most cases die of rapidly progressive renal failure.

Leptospirosis (see also Fever, p. 309)

An acute glomerulonephritis is not uncommon in leptospiral infections but macroscopic haematuria is rare, occurring in only one per cent of cases. It is an occupational hazard of farm labourers and sewage workers who come into contact with material contaminated by urine from infected rats. The diagnosis can be confirmed by rising antibody titres to leptospira icterohaemorrhagiae.

Acute pyelonephritis (see also Fever, p. 322)

Haematuria is exceptional and suggests that an obstructive cause may be present such as calculus, tumour or enlarged prostate.

Tuberculosis

Renal tuberculosis is an uncommon cause of haematuria, the most prominent symptom being frequency of micturition. It is always secondary to infection elsewhere in the body, usually in the lungs. Tubercle bacilli spread downwards from the kidneys to involve the ureters, bladder and genital tract. The urine will contain pus cells but may appear to be sterile unless secondary infection with other organisms is present. At least three early morning specimens should be sent for Löwenstein–Jensen culture. X-rays may show active or healed lesions in the lungs and calcified areas in one or both kidneys. In the early stages an intravenous pyelogram may be normal; later on the calyces lose their clear-cut outline and become shaggy and clubbed.

NON-INFLAMMATORY CAUSES

The epidemic of jogging which has swept across the western hemisphere has brought with it a number of new syndromes. Prominent amongst them is the haematuria of the long distance runner which appears briefly at the conclusion of the exercise. Once thought to be due to minor repetitive trauma to the bladder wall it now seems more likely that in the majority the bleeding is of glomerular origin. The reason for this glomerular leak remains obscure but the presence of red cells in the urine enables this condition to be distinguished from that of march haemoglobinuria with which it may be confused. The latter is thought to be due to rupture of red cells in the capillaries of the soles of the feet leading to intravascular haemolysis. Other more serious non-inflammatory causes of haematuria are discussed below.

Trauma

A cortical tear produces a haematoma without haematuria; tearing of the calyx has the opposite result but blood may not be passed for 2 or 3 days after the injury because of occluding clot. When renal injury is suspected every specimen of urine passed must be examined. An early intravenous pyelogram may show loss of renal outline or dye leaking into perirenal tissue. Transient haematuria often follows a percutaneous renal biopsy.

Calculi (see also Lateral abdominal pain, p. 94)

Renal calculi form in the calyces and pelvis of the kidney and may long remain silent until pain, infection or haematuria draw attention to their presence. Impaction of a stone in the pelvi–ureteric junction is accompanied by agonising loin pain, nausea, sweating and restlessness. Obstruction in the ureter gives rise to similar symptoms but the pain may then radiate to the groin, external genitalia or inner thigh.

All calcium-containing stones are radio-opaque and will show up on a plain X-ray unless they are very small or overlie a rib, transverse process or sacrum. Uric acid and cystine stones will show up as filling defects on intravenous or retrograde pyelography. Excessive calcium excretion in the urine encourages stone formation so that a 24 hour urine specimen should be collected for calcium estimation; an adult on a normal diet rarely excretes more than 7.5 mmol/24 h (300 mg/24 h). Amounts in excess of this are usually due to idiopathic hypercalcuria but the fasting serum calcium and phosphate should be checked to exclude primary hyperparathyroidism.

Neoplasm

In young children Wilm's tumour usually appears within the first 2 years of life. It presents with abdominal distension, pain and vomiting and a mass is usually palpable in the loin. Haematuria is a common but relatively late manifestation.

Painless haematuria in a middle-aged or elderly adult must always be taken seriously — it may be the first and only symptom of a renal carcinoma (hypernephroma). The bleeding is typically intermittent, each episode only lasting a day or two. Occasionally these tumours present with metastases in bone, but examination of the urine will usually reveal microscopic haematuria. Fever without apparent cause, along with a polymorph leucocytosis, is another mode of presentation. In a more advanced case there may be lateral abdominal pain, a palpable mass, loss of weight and metastases in lung, liver, bone or brain.

The diagnosis can usually be established by ultrasonography, computed tomography or intravenous pyelogram. Occasionally renal angiography may be necessary to demonstrate an early lesion when the other investigations have proved inconclusive.

Alport's syndrome

Aetiology

This hereditary nephritis is one of a number of congenital disorders of the kidneys which cause haematuria in childhood. The underlying abnormality appears to be a defect in the synthesis of the glomerular basement membrane which shows thinning, splitting and fragmentation in an early biopsy. As the disease progresses these changes will be accompanied by glomerular sclerosis, tubular atrophy and interstitial fibrosis. Alport's syndrome is an important cause of persistent haematuria and proteinuria and, in some patients, may be associated with sensorineural deafness and ocular defects. The pattern of inheritance varies from one family to another, but it is commonly autosomal dominant and partially sex-linked. Males are more severely affected than females, become progressively more deaf and usually die of renal failure in early adult life. Most of the females with this disease have a normal expectation of life and severe deafness is unusual.

Clinical features

Recurrent macroscopic haematuria may follow an upper respiratory or urinary tract infection. There may be a family history of renal disease, and protein and red cells may be found in the urine of symptomless relatives. The renal disease often results in hypertension and end-stage renal failure in adult life. Deafness does not usually appear until the child is about 10. Ocular abnormalities such as bilateral anterior lenticonus, cataract, retinitis pigmentosa and nystagmus are present in about 15% of cases.

Investigations

The urine will contain red cells and protein but a definitive diagnosis can only be made by renal biopsy. In one series of 123 children with recurrent haematuria the characteristic changes described above were found in 37%, compared to only 25% with IgA nephropathy. Audiograms may show a partial high tone loss. Thrombocytopenia, giant platelets and hyperlipidaemia have been found in some patients.

Polycystic disease

Aetiology

This congenital disorder makes its appearance either in early childhood or, more commonly, in middle age. The rare childhood form is inherited as an autosomal recessive trait and presents in the first year or two of life with portal hypertension and renal failure. The adult form, on the other hand, is usually silent until the fourth or fifth decades of life and is inherited as an autosomal dominant trait; in large families more than half the members may be affected.

Multiple renal cysts develop slowly over the years and gradually distort and destroy the normal architecture of the kidney.

The aetiology of both forms is unknown but some abnormality of the genetic locus which determines the structure of the collagen in glomerular and tubular basement membrane may be responsible. That this defect is not confined to renal tissue is demonstrated by the frequent presence of cysts in other organs such as the lung, liver, pancreas and spleen and the known association with berry aneurysms in the cerebral circulation.

Clinical features

Loin pain is often the earliest symptom in adults but they may present with hypertension, recurrent renal infections or renal colic due to calculus or blood clot; haematuria is seen in about a quarter of the cases and may be painless. The condition should be suspected in any middle-aged patient with haematuria if the kidneys are easily palpable and there is a positive family history.

Investigations

An intravenous pyelogram will usually show the characteristic elongated pelvis and crescentic calyces, but ultrasonography or computed tomography are more effective in demonstrating the cystic nature of the kidneys and may also reveal cysts in liver, pancreas or spleen.

Hydronephrosis

The congenital form is due most often to narrowing of the pelvi–ureteric junction and sometimes to an abnormal valve at the lower end of the ureter. The enlarged kidney may be palpable in infants and young children. The acquired form is due to obstruction by calculi, tuberculosis, retroperitoneal fibrosis or growth. This predisposes to infection or calculus formation and haematuria is sometimes seen.

An intravenous pyelogram will show a dilated pelvis and delayed emptying of the dye if renal filtration is still maintained, while ultrasonography and computed tomography are invaluable in demonstrating an enlarged, non-functioning kidney in these patients.

Anticoagulant therapy

Haematuria is a serious and not uncommon complication of long-term anticoagulant therapy with phenindione or warfarin. It is due to overdosage and the prothrombin time is likely to exceed 40 seconds by the time the patient is seen. The risk of haemorrhage is increased by the simultaneous administration of drugs, such as phenylbutazone, allopurinol or antibiotics, which prolong the half-life of the anticoagulants by hepatic enzyme inhibition. The bleeding can usually be controlled fairly rapidly by stopping the anticoagulants and by the intravenous administration of vitamin K. In one series of 301 patients seen over a period of 5 years at an anticoagulant clinic, there were 103 episodes of bleeding of which 35 were due to haematuria.

In the majority of cases the bleeding will stop when the prothrombin time has been brought back to normal. If macrocytic or microcytic haematuria persists the possibility that the anticoagulant therapy has unmasked a co-existing lesion in the renal tract should be considered.

Haemorrhagic disease

The importance of anticoagulant therapy, and the vasculitis of connective tissue disorders as causes of bleeding from the kidneys, have already been discussed. Frank haematuria is rare in thrombocytopenia, even when the platelet count is as low as $20 \times 10^9/l$ (20 000/cm^3). It is seen more frequently with coagulation defects, particularly in adult haemophiliacs and in association with disseminated intravascular coagulation.

Sickle cell trait (see also Anaemia, p. 221)

The heterozygous state for the sickle cell gene is characterised by the presence in the red cells of between 20% and 50% of sickle haemoglobin. It has a high prevalence amongst black populations and is a recognised cause of painless haematuria in an otherwise healthy individual. The increased osmolarity, reduced oxygen tension and low pH in the renal medulla are thought to favour clumping of the abnormal red cells, with consequent occlusion and rupture of small vessels.

The presence of the trait can be confirmed by sickling and solubility tests and by the demonstration of major bands of haemoglobin A and S on electrophoresis. These tests should be done in all Black patients, but the sickle cell trait should not be accepted as the cause until full urological investigations have excluded a co-existing renal tract lesion. In the homozygous state of sickle cell anaemia episodes of intravascular clotting lead to infarction of many organs, including the kidneys. There should be no difficulty in recognising the cause of the haematuria in such cases.

BLADDER, PROSTATE AND URETHRA

Haemorrhage from the lower renal tract is mainly due to inflammation or neoplasia in the bladder. The latter can only be excluded by cystoscopy and biopsies of any suspicious areas in the bladder wall.

INFLAMMATORY CAUSES

Cystitis (see also Hypogastric pain, p. 77)
Acute cystitis may accompany acute pyelonephritis but often occurs alone, the coliform organisms reaching the bladder via the urethra. There is usually some predisposing cause such as bladder neck obstruction, calculi, an indwelling urinary catheter, recent cystoscopy or sexual intercourse in the female. The most prominent symptoms are hypogastric pain, dysuria and frequency of micturition. Haematuria is not uncommon and may be profuse. Systemic symptoms such as malaise and fever may be mild or even absent.

Schistosomiasis

Vesical or bladder schistosomiasis, otherwise known as bilharziasis, is the commonest cause of haematuria in Asia, Africa, the Middle East and South America. Millions of people there are infected with the platyhelminth worm *Schistosoma haematobium*, which completes part of its life-cycle in an amphibian snail before being released as a free-swimming larva into paddy fields and irrigation canals. The infection is usually contracted in childhood from working in contaminated water.

Having penetrated the skin the worms mature in the liver before migrating to the bladder wall where the females deposit thousands of eggs. The reaction which they provoke leads to chronic inflammatory changes, secondary bacterial infection and, not infrequently, bladder cancer.

Schistosomiasis should be remembered as a possible cause of haematuria in an immigrant or visitor from these countries.

Urethritis

Urethritis may of course be gonococcal and be accompanied by haematuria, but the majority of cases are seen in young women from *Esch. coli* infection. Haematuria is sometimes seen in Reiter's syndrome.

NON-INFLAMMATORY CAUSES

Trauma

Rupture of the bladder and membranous urethra is a complication of severe injury to the lower abdomen and is usually associated with pelvic fracture and rupture of veins in the prostatic venous plexus. There is retention of urine with extravasation of urine and blood into the peritoneal cavity or extraperitoneal tissues. In the male, rupture of the spongy or extrapelvic urethra is more commonly due to a direct blow or a fall astride a hard object such as a fence or plank. Bleeding into the perineum will cause bruising and swelling. Blood without urine at the external meatus is characteristic of urethral injury.

Calculi

In the UK calculi in the bladder are always secondary to obstruction, infection or foreign bodies which act as a nidus for stone formation. In some Eastern countries calculi are common in otherwise normal bladders and are thought to be due to dietary factors.

Bladder stones may be symptomless until cystitis or haematuria occurs. The urine may be uniformly bloodstained or, if the patient complains of strangury, a few drops of frank blood may appear at the end of an attempt at micturition. Most calculi will show up on a straight X-ray and their presence will be confirmed by cystoscopy.

Neoplasm

Papilloma of the bladder is probably the commonest cause of recurrent painless haematuria in both sexes over the age of 50. They are frequently multiple and are readily seen on cystoscopy. Squamous carcinoma is less common and may present with dysuria and increased frequency of micturition.

The present and previous employment must be noted — the risk of bladder cancer is high in certain occupations. In the dye, cable and rubber industries the main carcinogen has been identified as beta-naphthylamine, a contaminant of some of the ingredients used to make the finished products. Despite stringent precautions small amounts of this chemical may be inhaled or absorbed through the skin and excreted in the urine. The same compound is also a contaminant of alpha-naphthylthiourea, which was widely used as a rat poison in Britain 30 years ago before the introduction of warfarin. A high incidence of bladder tumours has been found in rodent operatives, whose job it was to dispense this substance.

Attempts have been made to provide periodic screening for those at risk but examination of the urine for red cells is not dependable and annual cystoscopy is not always accepted. Exfoliative cytology has, however, proved to be reliable and practical in factories. The continued necessity for this derives from the fact that, as with other industrial forms of cancer, there is a latent interval ranging from 4–48 years after exposure.

Cigarette smoking has also been implicated in the genesis of bladder cancer and vesical schistosomiasis is an outstanding cause of papilloma of the bladder in endemic areas.

Haematuria is uncommon in cancer of the prostate unless disseminated intravascular coagulation is present as a complication of the disease. On rectal examination the gland will feel hard, irregular and fixed. X-rays and bone scans, particularly of the pelvis, lumbosacral spine and lungs may reveal metastases; if these are present the serum acid phosphatase will be raised. The diagnosis will be confirmed by biopsy at cystoscopy.

Prostatic hypertrophy

Benign prostatic hypertrophy is common in elderly men and usually presents with frequency, particularly at night, and difficulty in starting micturition. There will be a poor stream and often terminal dribbling. Acute retention of urine may be precipitated by a urinary infection or the use of a short-acting 'loop' diuretic in cardiac failure. Congestion may lead to the appearance of a few drops of blood at the beginning or end of micturition and is not unusual.

On rectal examination the gland is usually enlarged, firm and smooth to the touch; if only the middle lobe is involved the prostate may feel normal and the diagnosis can only be made on cystoscopy. Occasionally profuse haematuria may be the presenting symptom of prostatic hypertrophy, but this should never be accepted as the cause unless full urological investigations have been carried out to exclude a more serious lesion higher up the urinary tract.

CHAPTER 17
Purpura and bleeding

SYNOPSIS OF CAUSES*

VASCULAR DEFECT
Hereditary telangiectasia; Infections; Drugs; Scurvy; **Henoch-Schönlein purpura**;
Polyarteritis nodosa.

PLATELET DEFECT
Renal failure; Thrombocythaemia; **Thrombocytopenic purpura**; Haemolytic-uraemic
syndrome; Thrombotic thrombocytopenic purpura; Hypersplenism.

COAGULATION DEFECT
Hereditary; Neonatal haemorrhage; Malabsorption; **Drugs; Anticoagulants; Disseminated
intravascular coagulation**.

---

* Bold type is used for causes more commonly found in Europe and North America.

PHYSIOLOGY

The arrest of haemorrhage is brought about by the interaction of three
components; the blood vessels, the platelets and the coagulation factors
present in the blood and tissues.

When a vessel is ruptured the first response is a reduction in the flow
of blood due to contraction of its wall. The platelets then become adherent
to the damaged area and partially or completely occlude the opening. Mean-
while the coagulation factors interact with each other along two distinct
pathways. The intrinsic system is dependent upon the constituents of the
blood alone and is activated by its contact with any surface which differs
from normal vascular endothelium; it is responsible for clotting within
vessels. The extrinsic system, on the other hand, requires the presence of
tissue factors and is responsible for clot formation outside the damaged
wall.

Eventually the two pathways meet to activate factor X, which catalyses
the conversion of prothrombin to thrombin in the presence of factor V and
calcium ions. Thrombin is an enzyme which promotes the release of certain
platelet constituents which cause platelet aggregation, enhances the activity
of other coagulation factors and cleaves the fibrinogen molecule to form

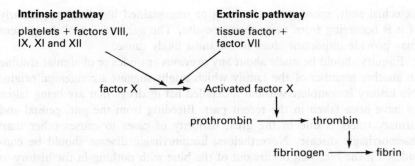

Intrinsic pathway
platelets + factors VIII,
IX, XI and XII

Extrinsic pathway
tissue factor +
factor VII

factor X   Activated factor X

prothrombin ⟶ thrombin

fibrinogen ⟶ fibrin

FIGURE 10

insoluble threads of fibrin. These, with the platelets which adhere to them, become the clot which seals the leak.

The whole process is an incredibly complex cascade of chemical reactions in which the initial interaction of a few molecules becomes enormously magnified in a very short space of time. Many of these reactions probably take place on the surfaces of the aggregated platelets.

A simplified version of events is shown in the diagram above.

The platelets obviously play a major role in regulating normal haemostasis. It is now known that they produce a prostaglandin-like compound called thromboxane A_2 which is a potent vasoconstrictor and causes them to stick together. These properties are inhibited by another arachidonic acid derivative called eprostenol (prostacyclin) which is secreted by the vascular endothelium. It seems very likely that it is the balance between these two substances which prevents the gross clumping of platelets on the healthy vessel wall. Damage to the vascular endothelium, by reducing the local concentration of eprostenol, may upset this balance and trigger off the clotting process.

The production of the coagulation factors VII, IX, X and prothrombin in the liver is dependent on the presence of vitamin K. This fat-soluble substance is present in most green vegetables and is absorbed in the jejunum with the help of the fat-emulsifying bile salts. Some vitamin K may be manufactured by intestinal bacteria but there is no proof that this is an important source in man.

Anything which obstructs the flow of bile will impair the absorption of all the fat-soluble vitamins. Since little vitamin K is stored in the liver it is only a matter of time before a deficiency of these coagulation factors develops.

Disorders of haemostasis may result from interference with the integrity of the vascular wall, the function of the platelets or the mechanisms of coagulation. These will be dealt with in that order in the text.

DIAGNOSTIC APPROACH

A haemorrhagic disorder should be suspected if a patient presents with a petechial rash, spontaneous bruising or unexplained bleeding, particularly if it is occurring from more than one site. The age and sex of the patient may provide important clues to the most likely cause.

Enquiry should be made about any previous episodes or of similar trouble in another member of the family which might suggest a congenital origin. No history is complete without a detailed list of drugs that are being taken or have been taken in the recent past. Bleeding from the gut, genital and urinary tracts is due in the great majority of cases to causes other than haemorrhagic disease. Nevertheless, haemorrhagic disease should be considered if the bleeding occurs out of the blue with nothing in the history to suggest a local cause in one of these systems.

Vascular defects are either immediately obvious, such as the characteristic discrete red spots of hereditary telangiectasia or the inflamed haemorrhagic rash of Henoch–Schönlein purpura, or are concealed from view within the viscera of the chest and abdomen. Constitutional disturbances such as fever, loss of weight, lassitude or abdominal pain may indicate that the bloody diarrhoea or haematuria with which the patient presents is due to a widespread vascular disorder such as polyarteritis nodosa; this diagnosis is frequently missed in the early stages of what often turns out to be a fatal illness.

In a sick, feverish child a widespread petechial rash may be the first sign of meningococcal septicaemia and often precedes the onset of the meningitic symptoms by some hours. Scurvy is a very uncommon cause of spontaneous bruising in Britain but is occasionally seen in geriatric wards and old peoples' homes in frail, elderly patients on inadequate diets; the perifollicular haemorrhages in vitamin C deficiency are usually accompanied by hyperkeratosis of the surrounding skin.

Thrombocytopenia is the commonest cause of a petechial rash and the punctate haemorrhages in the skin may be accompanied by bleeding from the nose and mouth; haemorrhagic bullae in the oral cavity are rarely due to any other condition. In an otherwise well child or young woman the most probable aetiology is the so-called idiopathic variety but thrombocytopenia may be one of the first manifestations of leukaemia, systemic lupus erythematosus or the rare haemolytic–uraemic syndrome.

Drug-induced thrombocytopenia can occur at any age but becomes increasingly common in middle age with the greater use of drugs in treating a wide variety of ailments. It is almost inevitable during intensive cytotoxic therapy and usually appears about 10 days after the last course of treatment.

Coagulation disorders usually present with easy bruising or excessive bleeding from a number of sites. Bleeding due to too much anticoagulant is self-evident and easily remedied. In breast-fed infants haemorrhages during the first few days of life are almost always due to lack of vitamin K. The rare hereditary disorders of coagulation usually present later in childhood and are seen mainly in boys. Disseminated intravascular coagulation is a complication of many serious and potentially fatal diseases and should always be thought of if a patient's condition suddenly worsens with unexplained bleeding from one or more orifices, or the appearance of spontaneous bruises on the trunk or limbs. A similar tendency to bleed excessively in a jaundiced patient or one with steatorrhoea is likely to be due to vitamin K deficiency.

Having decided from the interrogation and examination that haemorrhagic disease is possible the following investigations may help to determine its nature and most probable cause.

Investigations

A full blood count is an essential preliminary investigation. Anaemia, if present, may be due to prolonged bleeding or to marrow suppression. If the latter is the case the neutrophil count is likely to be low as well. The platelets normally vary in number from 150 to 400 $\times$ 10^9/l (150 000–400 000/mm^3), but the range of error in counting is considerable. Thrombocytopenia is defined as a platelet count of less than 150 $\times$ 10^9/l but spontaneous bleeding is seldom seen until it has fallen below 50 $\times$ 10^9/l. There is however no clear-cut relationship between the number of platelets and the appearance or severity of the resulting haemorrhage.

Relatively simple tests are available which will detect a coagulation defect.

The prothrombin time is the interval required for the clotting of blood after the addition of tissue thromboplastin and calcium ions. The normal range is 10–14 seconds and varies with the particular reagent which is being employed; blood from a normal subject is always used as a control. A prolonged prothrombin time points to a deficiency of one or more of the coagulation factors and is found in vitamin K deficiency, liver disease and disseminated intravascular coagulation. The main use of this test is in the control of anticoagulant therapy with phenindione and warfarin.

The partial thromboplastin time is a sensitive test for defective thromboplastin production resulting from a deficiency of factor VIII or IX. The normal range is 34–42 seconds. It is prolonged in the hereditary coagulation disorders. When abnormal it will be necessary to identify the missing factor or factors. These more sophisticated assays are outside the scope of most hospital laboratories and reference must be made to a designated haemophilia centre. In practice the partial thromboplastin time is mainly used to control anticoagulant therapy with heparin; times greater than 120 seconds are associated with a definite risk of haemorrhage.

Plasma fibrinogen deficiency is seen occasionally in liver disease but its commonest cause is undoubtedly disseminated intravascular coagulation. In the latter it will be accompanied by a rise in the fibrin degradation products in the blood. The normal range for plasma fibrinogen is 1.5–4.0 g/l (150–400 mg/dl).

A marrow biopsy is contraindicated in severe coagulation defects though usually permissible and certainly valuable in platelet deficiency. In idiopathic thrombocytopenia, although the platelets are scanty in the blood, the megakaryocytes in the marrow may be normal or even increased in number. Such findings are not diagnostic, however, and the principal value of a trephine biopsy lies in the exclusion of such causes of secondary thrombocytopenia as metastases, leukaemia, myelomatosis and myelofibrosis.

No mention has been made of the traditional clinical tests to measure the bleeding and clotting times since these are rarely employed by the clinician. For the same reason Hess's test of capillary fragility has been omitted.

VASCULAR DEFECT

This type of haemorrhagic disease commonly appears as petechiae or bruises in the skin. Some forms of purpura of vascular origin scarcely merit the title of disease — e.g. the tendency to easy bruising following quite minor trauma which is sometimes seen in young women. The term *orthostatic purpura* is used to describe the petechiae and small ecchymoses on the shins of subjects with varicose eczema. The skin of the elderly becomes unduly mobile from the atrophy of collagen in the subcutaneous tissues so that the capillaries are poorly supported and easily torn; in *senile purpura* multiple bruises appear on the backs of the hands and forearms.

Hereditary telangiectasia

This is a rare, genetically determined, vascular abnormality transmitted to both sexes. The lesions, which consist of dilated capillaries, veins and arterioles lined by a single layer of endothelium, are a millimetre or so in diameter and are distinguished from petechiae in disappearing on pressure. They may occur in the mucosa of the nose, mouth and lips and in the alimentary, respiratory and renal tracts.

The lesions are not present at birth and bleeding seldom occurs until adult life. As age advances the characteristic, discrete red spots under the mucosa increase in size and fragility so that haemorrhage is likely to become more frequent and more severe with consequent anaemia. Epistaxes and haemoptyses are the commonest presenting symptoms whilst gastro-intestinal bleeding and haematuria are much less frequent.

Infections

Purpura fulminans is a rare and often fatal complication of acute infections in childhood, death usually occurring within 2–3 days of onset. It has been reported in chickenpox, measles, streptococcal pharyngitis and meningococcal septicaemia. Bruised areas appear on the lower limbs and rapidly progress to local gangrene; the trunk and upper limbs are usually spared. The child is desperately ill and haematuria and melaena may occur. Histological examination of the affected tissues shows thrombosis of small blood vessels, perivascular infiltration, damage to the vascular endothelium and tissue necrosis. These vascular lesions are sometimes accompanied by thrombocytopenia and coagulation defects so that purpura fulminans is one of the many disorders associated with disseminated intravascular coagulation.

A milder form of this disorder may be responsible for the widespread petechiae which often precede the meningitic signs in meningococcal septicaemia, and may also account for the purpura which is sometimes seen with other infections such as bacterial endocarditis.

Drugs

Petechiae and ecchymoses are exceptional manifestations of allergy to drugs; erythematous, morbilliform or urticarial rashes are more common. The rash usually fades within a few days of stopping the drug. Spontaneous bruising from atrophy of the skin and resulting capillary fragility is not uncommon in Cushing's syndrome and is often seen in elderly patients receiving corticosteroids.

Scurvy

Bleeding is the commonest manifestation of vitamin C deficiency and occasional cases are seen in Britain in ill-nourished children and old people living on a diet lacking in fresh fruit and vegetables. In scurvy the collagen and intercellular cement are defective, leading to the easy rupture of capillaries. Bleeding takes place from the swollen, spongy gums and into the skin. Petechiae develop around hair follicles, along with hyperkeratosis, and bruises appear on the body after relatively minor trauma. In infants haemorrhages occur at the epiphyses and under the periosteum and these babies cry when their limbs are handled. A vitamin C saturation test is sometimes used to confirm the diagnosis in adults.

Henoch–Schönlein purpura

Aetiology

This widespread vasculitis, affecting capillaries and the smaller arterioles, is thought to be caused by circulating immune complexes containing IgA. It is commonly preceded by an upper respiratory infection and in such cases bacterial or viral hypersensitivity may be responsible. A few drug-induced cases have been reported. The peak incidence is in childhood but it is seen in adolescence and very occasionally in adults; it is commoner in males at all ages.

Clinical features

The four cardinal features of this disease are a purpuric rash, abdominal pain with bloody stools, an arthralgia and a focal proliferative glomerulo-nephritis. These manifestations are not always seen together in the same patient nor need they occur simultaneously. The onset is usually abrupt with fever, headache and a rash beginning on the buttocks and outer thighs.

At first this consists of raised urticarial areas, changing within hours to haemorrhagic macules which may later coalesce and even ulcerate.

The rash is usually followed within a few days by colicky abdominal pain, vomiting and the passage of bright red blood or melaena stools. Arthralgia is common and may flit from joint to joint. Proteinuria and haematuria occur in those cases with renal involvement. The disease usually settles spontaneously in 4–6 weeks but may recur. The renal lesions take longer to resolve and occasionally progress to the nephrotic syndrome. In adults the course may be much more insidious with recurring episodes of obscure abdominal pain, fleeting rashes and eventual death from renal failure.

Investigations

The urine should be examined on more than one occasion for protein, red cells and casts. The ESR is raised when the disease is active and a polymorph leukocytosis, sometimes accompanied by a mild eosinophilia, may be found. The platelet count, prothrombin and partial thromboplastin times are normal.

Polyarteritis nodosa (see also Fever, p. 328)

Unlike Henoch–Schönlein purpura this vasculitis involves the larger arterioles, resulting in multiple infarcts in various organs. These may cause melaena, haematuria or haemorrhagic macules and papules in the skin.

PLATELET DEFECT

In platelet disorders haemorrhage may be due to a qualitative defect but is more commonly due to a reduction in the platelet count. Hereditary platelet disorders are so rare that they are hardly worth mentioning here. Thrombocytopenia may result from decreased marrow production, sequestration in the spleen or accelerated destruction in the blood or reticulo–endothelial system.

Renal failure

Excessive bleeding is a common and serious complication of advanced renal disease. The main abnormality lies in a qualitative platelet defect, though a moderate thrombocytopenia is often present as well. Since these abnormalities can be improved by dialysis and corrected by successful renal transplantation it is likely that they are due to the retention of toxic substances in the body.

Thrombocythaemia

This rare disease may occur on its own or in association with the myeloproliferative disorders. Episodes of spontaneous or prolonged bleeding take place despite a raised platelet count. It is seen in middle-aged or elderly patients in whom splenomegaly and thromboses may be found. Morphological abnormalities of the platelets are apparent in some cases.

Thrombocytopenic purpura

Aetiology
There are many possible causes for a fall in the number of the circulating platelets, ranging from an autoimmune disease with the production of platelet antibodies to infiltration or destruction of the marrow by a variety of pathological processes. The so-called 'idiopathic' form is seen predominantly in females; in young children in whom it is usually acute and self-limiting and in pre-menopausal women in whom it tends to run a more protracted course. It is in some of these patients that circulating platelet antibodies have been found. Autoimmunity is also likely to be the mechanism in systemic lupus erythematosus where thrombocytopenia may precede all other manifestations of the disease by several years.

Many drugs cause thrombocytopenia but those chiefly responsible in practice are phenylbutazone, oxyphenbutazone, chloramphenicol, indomethacin and trimethoprim. Together they account for nearly half the reported cases. Others which have been incriminated include the cytotoxic drugs, quinine, quinidine, barbiturates, salicylates, thiazides, oral hypoglycaemic drugs and digitoxin. Bleeding may appear promptly after commencing treatment or develop insidiously after some weeks.

Chemicals, notably benzene and its derivatives, may — from contact at work or in the home — poison the marrow and produce purpuric manifestations. In those exposed to ionizing radiation anorexia, nausea, vomiting and diarrhoea usually precede the fall in platelet count. It is clearly important in all cases of thrombocytopenia to obtain an accurate drug history and to enquire about the use of chemicals at home and work.

Clinical features
In the idiopathic form a history of an upper respiratory infection within the preceding 3 weeks is commonly obtained. Petechiae appear on the limbs, chest and neck and bleeding from the mucous membranes of the nose and mouth is common; in women menorrhagia may be the only prominent symptom. The patient is usually well apart from the tendency to bleed. However, death can rarely result from cerebral haemorrhage; examination of the fundi may reveal retinal haemorrhages in such high-risk cases. Splenomegaly is uncommon in idiopathic thrombocytopenic purpura and its presence should alert one to the possibility of systemic lupus erythematosus, leukaemia or some other malignant disease.

Investigations
A full blood count should enable leukaemia to be excluded in most cases. Anaemia may be due to prolonged bleeding or to marrow damage; the latter is more likely if the polymorph leukocyte count is also low. When the plate-

lets are less than $20 \times 10^9/l$ the risk of a fatal cerebral haemorrhage is high and platelet transfusions should be considered as a temporary measure to buy time.

A marrow biopsy may reveal nothing but is always worth doing to exclude aleukaemic leukaemia, metastases, myelomatosis or myelofibrosis. Occasionally biopsy of an enlarged lymph node may serve the same purpose. Platelet antibodies may be found in the idiopathic form of the disease, whilst if systemic lupus erythematosus is suspected LE cells and DNA antibodies should be looked for.

Haemolytic–uraemic syndrome

This rare disease presents acutely with a microangiopathic haemolytic anaemia, thrombocytopenia and renal failure. It is seen mainly in early childhood but has been reported in older children and adults. In Britain a number of small outbreaks have occurred, suggesting an infective cause. The annual incidence in this country is about 0.3 per 100 000 children under 16 years of age. In most patients the disorder is preceded by a diarrhoeal illness and various organisms including *Campylobacter, Esch. coli, Salmonella, Shigella* and viruses have been isolated from the stools. Pallor is the commonest presenting sign, oliguria or anuria are frequently seen and there may be haematuria, jaundice or a petechial rash.

Disseminated intravascular coagulation can be demonstrated by the presence of thrombocytopenia, coagulation defects and fibrin degradation products in the blood. Most patients recover from their renal failure but some have residual renal impairment and a small proportion die.

Thrombotic thrombocytopenic purpura

This fatal condition is also rare and of unknown aetiology. It presents with fever, thrombocytopenic purpura, haemolytic anaemia, splenic enlargement and fluctuating neurological abnormalities. Only in the terminal stages of the disease are all these features present. It may occur at any age but is seen mainly in young adults. It has some similarities with the haemolytic–uraemic syndrome mentioned above, and disseminated intravascular coagulation is also present in these patients. At autopsy multiple petechial haemorrhages and hyaline thrombi are found in the capillaries and small arterioles.

Hypersplenism (see also Anaemia, p. 225)

An enlarged spleen is associated with many acute and chronic infections, autoimmune disease, congenital metabolic disorders, malignant infiltration and portal hypertension. Thrombocytopenia is not invariable, but when it does occur it may be due to excessive pooling of platelets in the enlarged organ or to their premature destruction. Normally about 30% of the platelets in the circulation are sequestered in the splenic sinusoids, but as the spleen enlarges this proportion may rise to 90%, with a corresponding fall in the peripheral count. This dilutional phenomenon is seen in both infiltrative and congestive splenomegaly and is rarely of much clinical significance, although excessive bleeding may follow trauma or major surgery. A more pronounced thrombocytopenia is, however, seen in some autoimmune disorders where the spleen is enlarged from reticulo–endothelial hyperplasia and the platelets are being actively destroyed. This is probably the case in Felty's syndrome, in which rheumatoid arthritis is accompanied by a severe neutropenia and thrombocytopenic purpura.

COAGULATION DEFECT

Coagulation defects may be inherited or acquired. Haemophilia is the best known of the congenital forms but there are others which are too rare to merit any discussion here. Acquired defects are commoner and result from a lack of vitamin K, impaired synthesis of coagulation factors in the liver or their excessive consumption as a result of intravascular clotting.

Hereditary

Aetiology
Haemophilia is the commonest and most severe of the congenital coagulation disorders. It is due to a variable deficiency of factor VIII. The disease is almost entirely confined to males but is transmitted by apparently normal females. Despite its congenital nature no family history can be traced in about 30% of cases, suggesting a high incidence of sporadic mutation. There are about 3000–4000 males with this condition in the UK.

Christmas disease, which is due to the absence of factor IX, is much rarer than haemophilia but cannot be distinguished from it clinically; the mode of inheritance is the same in that it is confined to males. *Von Willebrand's disease* is also rare and is inherited as an autosomal dominant trait. Unlike the other two it affects both sexes equally. The abnormal bleeding in this disorder is associated with defective platelet aggregation as well as a lowered factor VIII and factor VIII-related antigen level. An acquired form of Von Willebrand's disease is occasionally found in association with systemic lupus erythematosus, autoimmune thyroiditis and lymphoid malignancies.

Clinical features
All haemophiliacs bleed excessively during surgery and after injury, but only those with very low factor VIII levels are severely handicapped by the disease. Even then the condition is rarely evident until the boy begins to walk. Haemarthroses, particularly of the knee joints, are the commonest complication and can lead to crippling deformities if whole plasma or factor VIII concentrates are not given immediately. Haemorrhages into muscle are also common and may produce permanent contractures if the bleeding is allowed to continue. Alimentary bleeding is uncommon and intracranial

haemorrhage is rare. Although haematuria is frequent in adult haemophiliacs it is rarely seen in childhood. Excessive bleeding following injury, surgery or dental extraction may be the first indication of the presence of Von Willebrand's disease in either sex.

Investigations

The platelet count, plasma fibrinogen level and prothrombin time will be normal but the partial thromboplastin time is prolonged in all the hereditary disorders. Specific assays of the individual clotting factors will be necessary to make a definitive diagnosis. In haemophilia the factor VIII concentration may range from 0–50% of normal levels, depending upon the severity of the disease.

Neonatal haemorrhage

Haemorrhagic disease of the newborn is caused by lack of vitamin K. It is virtually confined to breast-fed babies and can be prevented by a single oral dose of 1 mg of vitamin K at birth. Even supplementary feeds with formula milk may provide enough of this essential substance. Bleeding from one or more sites usually appears between 5 and 10 days after delivery. This may take the form of haemorrhage from the umbilicus, a blood-stained nasal discharge or bruising on the trunk or limbs. Fits, loss of consciousness and even death may result from intracranial haemorrhage. The prothrombin time will be prolonged but a normal blood count, including platelets, will enable disseminated intravascular coagulation to be excluded from the differential diagnosis.

Malabsorption (see also Loss of weight, p. 265)

Absorption of the fat-soluble vitamin K is inevitably impaired in diseases which cause steatorrhoea. These include gluten enteropathy, Crohn's disease, cholestatic liver disease and biliary tract obstruction. In a severely jaundiced patient a prolonged prothrombin time with consequent bleeding may also be due to failure by the liver to synthesise some of the clotting factors. In this situation the parenteral administration of vitamin K will not restore the prothrombin time to normal.

Drugs

Gross depletion of vitamin-K-dependent clotting factors has been reported as an occasional complication of intensive antibiotic therapy. Several cases have now been described after major surgery following the administration of third-generation cephalosporins and latamoxef. All these patients had prolonged prothrombin times but nothing else to suggest disseminated intravascular coagulation. Clinically significant bleeding from an abdominal wound occurred in one case within a week of starting therapy.

In every patient the coagulation defect was corrected within 2–3 days by vitamin K. Whether this disorder is due to the elimination of vitamin-K-producing bacteria in the gut by antibiotics which are excreted in the bile, or by some toxic effect on the liver is not clear. The former seems a little unlikely in view of the rapidity with which the condition develops and the lack of evidence that intestinal bacteria are an important source of vitamin K in man.

Anticoagulants

Heparin greatly enhances the inhibiting effect of antithrombin III, which is one of the naturally-occurring inhibitors of the coagulation process. It is given intravenously or subcutaneously and its anticoagulant effect is measured by the prolongation of the partial thromboplastin time; an effective dose will maintain this between 60 and 90 seconds. In excessive amounts heparin will cause oozing from wounds and venepuncture sites but this usually ceases within hours of stopping the drug.

Overdosage with oral anticoagulants is more serious — these drugs produce a delayed reduction in the vitamin K dependent clotting factors. Both phenindione and warfarin interfere with the metabolism of vitamin K in the liver, but the effect of warfarin lasts longer. It will be several days before the prothrombin time reaches its peak after a loading dose or returns to normal after stopping treatment.

Easy bruising and menorrhagia can occur even with therapeutic doses. Loin pain and haematuria are the commonest manifestations of overdosage but massive haematomas in the subcutaneous tissues may follow minor trauma in the elderly. Treatment is hazardous unless the prothrombin time is monitored at least once a fortnight and the dose adjusted to keep it within the therapeutic range; this is usually two to four times that of the control.

The addition of other drugs such as antibiotics or allopurinol may potentiate their action by inhibition of the liver enzymes which inactivate the anticoagulants; this may cause dangerous bleeding. If this happens a fresh whole blood transfusion will return the prothrombin time to normal fairly rapidly but vitamin K, even when given intravenously, will take many hours to do so.

Excessive bleeding is occasionally due to the presence of naturally-occurring anticoagulants which are not normally present in the blood. An inhibitor of factor VIII has been found in some haemophiliac patients following repeated blood transfusions, and other inhibitors of coagulation have been described in systemic lupus erythematosus.

Disseminated intravascular coagulation

The defibrination syndrome, as it was originally called, is now widely recognised as an acute and potentially lethal complication of many clinical situations. These include antepartum haemorrhage, eclampsia, mismatched blood transfusions, septicaemia, severe viral infections, extensive burns, snake bites, cardiothoracic surgery and malignant disease, particularly of the prostate. The onset is usually abrupt with depletion of the coagulation factors and thrombocytopenia following widespread intravascular clotting in the microcirculation. Why this should happen is still obscure but the most likely explanation is that substances are released from damaged red cells or platelets in these situations which trigger off the coagulation mechanisms. Bleeding manifestations are usually more obvious than any due to the thrombotic process.

The condition should be suspected in any patient who develops excessive bleeding or bruising for no apparent reason during the course of a serious illness or following surgery. The prothrombin and partial thromboplastin times are both prolonged and the plasma fibrinogen level usually falls to less than 1.5 g/l (150 mg/dl). Fibrin degradation products will be present in the blood and should be looked for. Thrombocytopenia is usual and occasionally evidence of intravascular haemolysis will be found.

CHAPTER 18
Anaemia

SYNOPSIS OF CAUSES★

CHRONIC BLOOD LOSS
Gastrointestinal diseases; Intestinal parasites; **Menorrhagia; Uterine neoplasm.**

DEFECTIVE BLOOD PRODUCTION
LACK OF ESSENTIAL FACTORS
Erythropoietin; **Thyroid; Iron; Vitamin B$_{12}$**; Pernicious anaemia; **Folic acid.**

MARROW DEPRESSION
Drugs; Poisons; **Radiation; Infections; Connective tissue disorders; Neoplasia; Leukaemia; Myelomatosis**; Myelofibrosis; Thalassaemia.

BLOOD DESTRUCTION
Hereditary spherocytosis; Sickle-cell anaemia; Hereditary enzyme deficiencies; Infections; **Rhesus disease**; Poisons; **Auto-immune disorders**; Hypersplenism.

★ Bold type is used for causes more commonly found in Europe and North America.

PHYSIOLOGY

Before the causes of anaemia are discussed it is necessary to outline the physiology of blood formation.

The haemocytoblast, derived from reticulo–endothelial cells in the bone marrow, is the progenitor of erythrocytes, leukocytes and platelets. In erythropoiesis, and under the stimulus of erythropoietin and other essential factors, maturation occurs successively into pro-erythroblast, normoblast, reticulocyte and normal red blood corpuscle. The process may be retarded or even arrested by a deficiency of one of these essential factors, or by the action of toxic agents on the marrow. Both may affect the production of leukocytes and platelets as well as erythrocytes.

The mature red cell is a flexible non-nucleated biconcave disc uniquely designed to transport oxygen from the lungs to the tissues by virtue of its shape and haemoglobin content. Each haemoglobin molecule is made up of two pairs of polypeptide chains and four haem groups. The oxygen is

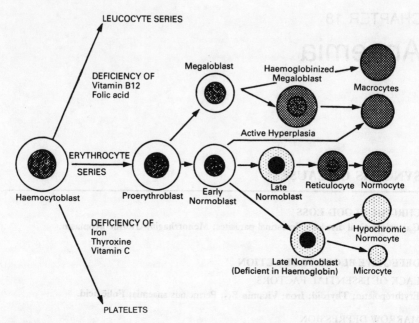

FIGURE 11

reversibly bound to the iron-containing haem complexes and exchanged for carbon dioxide in the capillaries.

Haemoglobin is not a single substance but minor variations in its molecular structure do not affect its biological properties. Fetal haemoglobin is normally replaced by adult haemoglobin during the first few months of life.

The lifespan of the red cell is about 120 days and the number of cells at any one time is fairly constant. There is in consequence a balance of some precision between the influx of new cells into the circulation and the destruction of ageing erythrocytes by macrophages of the reticulo–endothelial system, which takes place mainly in the spleen. This balance may be upset by excessive production, as in polycythaemia, or by a reduction in their number as a result of blood loss, impaired erythropoiesis or their premature demise.

Anaemia can be regarded as a reduction in the oxygen-carrying capacity of the blood. It is considered to be present when the haemoglobin level is below the lower limit of the normal range. This is generally accepted as being 13–14 g/dl in men and 11.5–12.0 g/dl in women.

ESSENTIAL FACTORS

These substances promote the differentiation, proliferation and maturation of the red cell precursors in the marrow. Some are natural secretions of the body, such as erythropoietin and the thyroid hormones, whilst others are normal constituents of the diet. The latter include iron and vitamins, notably vitamin B_{12} and folic acid.

Erythropoietin

This hormone is a glycoprotein which is mainly secreted by the kidneys; in man about 10% appears to come from the liver. It is thought to combine with receptors on the red cell precursors, thereby stimulating their proliferation and maturation.

The oxygen content of the arterial blood is the major factor in regulating erythropoiesis, acting indirectly on the kidneys to control the output of erythropoietin. Its production is increased by testosterone — which may explain the higher red cell count and haemoglobin levels in men — and by hypoxia due to anaemia, cardiopulmonary disease or living at high altitudes.

The secondary polycythemia associated with hypernephromas, renal cysts and hepatic cancer is probably caused by an increased secretion of this hormone. On the other hand, lack of erythropoietin contributes to the anaemia of chronic renal failure.

Thyroid hormones

Thyroxine or triiodothyronine must be accounted as an essential factor for their deficiency in hypothyroidism sometimes gives rise to a normocytic normochromic anaemia curable only by their administration.

Iron

Iron is quantitatively the most important trace element in man and is an essential component of the haemoglobin molecule. It is present in meats, especially kidney and liver, egg yolk, green vegetables and fruit. The average daily intake on a Western diet is 10–20 mg, but under normal conditions only 1–2 mg are absorbed. This takes place mainly in the proximal jejunum after ferric iron has been changed to the ferrous form in the stomach by reducing agents such as ascorbic acid in the diet. Increased amounts are absorbed in iron deficiency and in the haemolytic anaemias.

About 1 mg of iron is normally lost daily in erythrocytes and epithelial cells from the alimentary and renal tracts, and in desquamated skin. In men this is replaced from the diet, but in women of reproductive age the blood lost during each menstrual period is equivalent to a further daily loss of at least 1 mg. The balance in the menstruating female is therefore precarious and pregnancy puts a further strain upon the iron stores; by the end of the third trimester about 0.5 g will have been transferred to the fetus.

In the growing child and adolescent the iron requirement is greater than in the adult male and is similar to that of the premenopausal woman.

The adult human body contains 4–5 g of iron, of which two-thirds is present in the haemoglobin of the circulating red cells. About 1 g is stored in the tissues as ferritin or the much more insoluble haemosiderin. Although the latter has a high iron content it can only be slowly mobilised when required. A low serum ferritin concentration, determined by radioimmune assay, is now considered to be a reliable measure of depleted iron stores. Approximately 0.5 g is contained in myoglobin and the cytochromes involved in intracellular oxidation, but this is not available for erythropoiesis.

A small amount of iron, bound to the glycoprotein transferrin, is transported in the serum. The serum iron concentration ranges from 14–29 μmol/l (80–160 μg/dl) but this is only about one-third of the total iron-binding capacity of the serum, which is a measure of the serum transferrin. Thus about two-thirds of the serum transferrin is normally unsaturated.

Vitamin B$_{12}$

Cyanocobalamin is found in most animal foods, especially muscle, liver and kidney. To a lesser extent it is present in milk, cheese and eggs. In the stomach it binds to a carrier protein called intrinsic factor which is secreted, along with hydrochloric acid, by the gastric parietal cells. The bound vitamin B$_{12}$ is absorbed in the ileum where it parts company with intrinsic factor and is transported, attached to another protein, to the liver. Here it is stored for distribution to the marrow as required.

A daily intake of 2 μg is normally sufficient, but even this amount is absent from the diet of strict vegetarians. With so minute a requirement the effects of deprivation only give rise to anaemia after several years.

Vitamin B$_{12}$ is a co-enzyme in a number of chemical reactions leading to DNA synthesis. It is intimately involved in folate metabolism and a lack of one or other of these vitamins leads to the abnormal production of megaloblasts in the marrow. In the nervous system vitamin B$_{12}$ is necessary for the formation of myelin sheaths and its deficiency may cause a peripheral neuritis or subacute combined degeneration of the spinal cord. These neurological manifestations can occur independently of those due to interference with erythropoiesis and are not always accompanied by a megaloblastic anaemia.

Folic acid

Folates are widely distributed in food of both animal and vegetable origin but are destroyed by cooking and exposure to light. This water-soluble vitamin is absorbed from the duodenum and upper jejunum and stored in the liver; the normal daily requirement is about 200 μg. Its role in erythropoiesis is not fully understood but it appears to be essential for the synthesis of DNA.

Folic acid deficiency, resulting from inadequate intake, malabsorption, increased demand or treatment with folate antagonists, produces megaloblastic changes in the red cell precursors identical to those seen in vitamin B$_{12}$ deficiency.

DIAGNOSTIC APPROACH

Except in gross cases anaemia is rarely diagnosed on appearance alone. It is often discovered on a routine blood count in patients who complain of readily-induced fatigue, shortness of breath, abdominal pain, diarrhoea or abnormal uterine bleeding. Mild degrees of anaemia may, however, exist without giving rise to any signs or symptoms. That this is often the case in the elderly was shown by one series of nearly 500 apparently healthy individuals over the age of 65 in whom a haemoglobin level of less than 12 g/dl was found in 7.5% of the men and 20% of the women. In the majority this was due to iron deficiency caused by gastrointestinal blood loss.

The nature of the anaemia must be established as soon as possible in order to narrow down the search for a possible cause. Fortunately the widespread use of electronic cell counters has greatly facilitated this task. In addition to providing an accurate estimate of the total red cell count they will also measure the mean cell size and haemoglobin content.

A microcytic, hypochromic picture is usually evidence of iron deficiency, of which the commonest cause is chronic blood loss from the alimentary tract or uterus. The patient should be questioned closely about any gastrointestinal symptoms or menorrhagia. No history is complete without a record of any drug therapy for many compounds, particularly anti-inflammatory drugs, produce gastric erosions and occult bleeding. A low serum ferritin level will confirm a diagnosis of iron deficiency and will differentiate this condition from other, less common, causes of a microcytic hypochromic picture such as the sideroblastic anaemias associated with pyridoxine deficiency, alcoholism, lead poisoning, drugs, autoimmune disorders, myelomatosis and thalassaemia.

A macrocytic anaemia is seen in vitamin B_{12} deficiency and folate deficiency, and megaloblastic changes will be found in the bone marrow, provided that neither of these vitamins has been given beforehand. Serum B_{12} and folic acid levels will differentiate between these two disorders. A Schilling test will distinguish between malabsorption of vitamin B_{12} due to ileal disease and malabsorption caused by lack of intrinsic factor.

Pernicious anaemia should be suspected in anyone over the age of 40 with a macrocytic anaemia who has evidence of other autoimmune disorders such as hypothyroidism, diabetes or vitiligo, or a family history of any of these conditions. Macrocytosis can, however, occur without megaloblastic changes in the marrow as a consequence of alcoholism, cytotoxic therapy, haemolysis, neoplasia or recent haemorrhage.

A normocytic, normochromic picture is seen immediately after acute blood loss and in hypothyroidism, marrow depression, chronic infections, connective-tissue diseases, leukaemia and the haemolytic anaemias. The age of the patient, ethnic origin, history of previous illnesses, accompanying symptoms and physical examination will often provide clues to the underlying cause.

Blood films are rarely required in the investigation of most cases of anaemia but may show morphological changes in the red cells as a result of iron deficiency, megaloblastosis, fragmentation in the circulation, hereditary spherocytosis or sickle-cell disease. If malaria is suspected a thick film should be made to demonstrate the parasites.

A full white count is often helpful and should be done routinely. The presence of numerous white cell precursors is virtually diagnostic of leukaemia but may occasionally be due to a leukaemoid reaction to metastases in the marrow, miliary tuberculosis or a viral infection. Platelet counts should be reserved for those cases where there is evidence of abnormal bleeding or easy bruising. Thrombocytopenia is usually associated with leukaemia, drug-induced damage to the marrow or autoimmune disease.

Reticulocyte counts are seldom indicated but will be raised in haemolytic disorders and after recent haemorrhage; a rise in the reticulocyte count will follow the administration of vitamin B_{12} or folic acid to a patient with a megaloblastic marrow. Further investigations will inevitably depend upon the type of anaemia and its possible causes. In this chapter they are classified according to whether they result in chronic blood loss, defective blood production or premature destruction of the red cells.

CHRONIC BLOOD LOSS

The causes of acute blood loss have been described in the preceding chapters. Even when blood loss is severe the blood is likely to be restored to normal within a few weeks. This is not the case, however, if the bleeding continues or recurs.

The main limiting factor in replacing the lost red cells is the amount of iron available for erythropoiesis. As the body iron stores are used up the mean corpuscular haemoglobin falls before there is any appreciable reduction in cell numbers. Later the typical picture of a microcytic, hypochromic anaemia develops with the appearance of anisocytosis, poikilocytosis and target cells in the blood film.

Low levels of serum iron and saturated iron-binding capacity are not reliable indications of iron depletion — they are also seen in illnesses due to infection, malignancy, renal disease and connective-tissue disorders. On the other hand, a serum ferritin level of less than 15 μg/l is said to be an infallible guide to iron deficiency in adults.

The great majority of all cases of anaemia are due to alimentary haemorrhage or menorrhagia and clearly these causes should be the first to be eliminated. Antepartum and postpartum haemorrhage are not discussed here as in practice they are promptly treated at the time. Epistaxis, haemoptysis and haematuria are rare causes and will not be considered further; anaemia in these patients is often due to other factors.

Gastrointestinal diseases

These include such diverse conditions as oesophagitis, gastric erosions, peptic ulceration, intestinal parasites, Crohn's disease, diverticulitis, ulcerative colitis, angiodysplasia of the colon and neoplasms of the alimentary tract. Gastric erosions are a common and unsuspected cause of silent bleeding in the elderly arthritic patient taking non-steroidal anti-inflammatory drugs for pain relief. Peptic ulceration of the stomach or duodenum is probably the commonest cause both of alimentary haemorrhage and of the consequent anaemia; indigestion is not necessarily a prominent symptom and may even be denied.

Inflammatory bowel disease usually presents with abdominal pain or diarrhoea but cancer of the colon frequently causes chronic blood loss without abdominal symptoms. In rectal cancer bleeding is usually obvious though often mistakenly attributed to haemorrhoids; most of these growths are within reach of the examining finger. It is often claimed that haemorrhoids are a common cause of iron-deficiency anaemia but this is not borne out by experience; the danger lies in accepting piles as an adequate explanation and overlooking a much more serious lesion higher up the alimentary canal.

Investigations

If gastrointestinal haemorrhage is suspected further investigations will be necessary to confirm this and to establish the cause. When the bleeding is small the stools may be normal in appearance and chemical tests will be necessary to detect the presence of blood. At least three faecal specimens should be tested, but negative results do not exclude a gastrointestinal lesion as the bleeding may be intermittent. If doubt persists, the search for occult blood should be repeated. The most sensitive tests will detect a loss of as little as 5 ml a day but false-positive results may be found unless meat is temporarily excluded from the diet.

In many centres fibreoptic endoscopy has replaced the traditional barium meal as the initial investigation of the upper gastrointestinal tract. In skilled hands most of the stomach and duodenum can be visualised and uncommon causes of blood loss such as a cancer of the pancreas may be detected by intubation of the ampulla of Vater. When endoscopic facilities are not available the barium meal is still the main diagnostic tool in defining lesions in the oesophagus, stomach and duodenum. Small bowel meals are of limited value in detecting abnormalities in this radiological no-man's-land; even quite extensive Crohn's disease may be missed.

When the history points to the large bowel, proctosigmoidoscopy must be carried out before requesting a barium enema since the latter will not reveal lesions in the rectum. Colonoscopy now enables practically the whole of the large bowel to be seen and photographed.

When the source of bleeding has not been discovered by other means laparotomy may be inevitable.

Intestinal parasites

Infestation of the proximal small bowel by the hookworm *Ancylostoma duodenale* or *Necator americanus* is considered to be one of the commonest causes of anaemia from blood loss in Africa, the Far East, the West Indies and South America. Both species attach themselves to the intestinal mucosa and ingest blood. The female produces over 2000 eggs a day and the diagnosis is made by finding ova in the stools.

Infection by the liver fluke *Schistosoma mansoni* or *S. japonica* is endemic in Africa, Asia, the Middle East, South America and some Caribbean islands. Invasion of the colon results in chronic blood loss. The parasites migrate to the liver in the portal vein and produce portal hypertension; massive haemorrhage from oesophageal varices is a not uncommon cause of death. Both these conditions are rare in the UK but may be seen in immigrants or visitors from these countries.

Menorrhagia

Iron deficiency due to blood loss at the menstrual periods is very common. In 1983 the World Health Organisation reported that 230 of the 464 million women in developing countries suffered from anaemia due to deficiency of iron or folate or both. In five surveys carried out in the UK no less than 25% of women of childbearing age were found to be anaemic.

The menstrual periods normally start between the eleventh and sixteenth year of life and last between 2 and 7 days. Having become established they continue monthly, unless interrupted by pregnancy or disease, until the menopause, which takes place in most women between 45 and 50 years of age. The regular monthly cycle depends upon ovulation occurring and the consequent secretion of progesterone during the luteal phase. Anovulatory cycles are irregular and may be heavier, because of the unopposed action of oestrogen on the endometrium. That menorrhagia is present in a given case should be suspected if the woman admits to heavy periods.

Intra-uterine contraceptive devices frequently cause excessive or prolonged menstruation and intermenstrual spotting is not uncommon. Other local causes of menorrhagia are leiomyomata of the uterus and endometriosis. General causes include hypothyroidism, corticosteroid therapy and less commonly haemorrhagic disease, particularly thrombocytopenia. Excessive haemorrhage may occur during anticoagulant therapy and in some women taking contraceptive pills with a high oestrogen content. Menorrhagia has also been observed during treatment with spironolactone.

In metropathia haemorrhagica the bleeding is characteristically painless, profuse, prolonged and irregular. Failure of ovulation leads to endometrial hyperplasia from the unopposed action of oestrogens on the endometrium. It is most commonly seen towards the end of the reproductive period of life.

The investigation of abnormal uterine bleeding falls within the province of the gynaecologist to whom such cases should be referred.

Uterine neoplasm

Postmenopausal and intermenstrual bleeding demand thorough investigation as they are frequently due to cancer of the cervix or of the body of the uterus. Reference to a gynaecologist must be made without delay. Cervical cytology, curettage and biopsy will be required.

A rare cause of intermenstrual bleeding is excessive oestrogen secretion by an ovarian neoplasm; in order of frequency this is likely to be a granulosa-cell tumour, adrenal rest tumour or an ovarian cyst.

DEFECTIVE BLOOD PRODUCTION

Erythropoiesis may be impaired by a deficiency of essential factors, inherited abnormalities in the structure of haemoglobin, or depression of bone-marrow activity by toxic chemicals or systemic disease.

LACK OF ESSENTIAL FACTORS

Anaemia from this cause may be due to a reduction in the secretion of hormones which normally stimulate erythropoiesis, or from failure of the dietary factors to reach the marrow as a result of malabsorption or an inadequate intake.

Erythropoietin deficiency

The normocytic, normochromic anaemia of chronic renal failure is due to a combination of impaired production and persistent mild haemolysis. The retention of toxic substances in the blood is thought to be partly responsible for this, since uraemic serum has been shown to damage normal red cells and to inhibit the proliferation of red cell precursors in the marrow. The anaemia is however refractory to removal of these substances by haemodialysis so that this cannot be the only explanation. It is likely that the destruction of erythropoietin-producing tissue in chronic renal disease deprives the marrow of its major stimulus to blood formation.

Thyroid deficiency (see also Obesity, p. 291)

A mild, normocytic, normochromic anaemia is a common feature of untreated hypothyroidism. It is curable only by the administration of thyroxine or triiodothyronine. The macrocytic anaemia which is present in some hypothyroid individuals is due to an accompanying pernicious anaemia and will respond to vitamin B_{12} injections. Circulating antibodies to both thyroid constituents and gastric parietal cells may be found in the blood.

Iron deficiency

Chronic blood loss accounts for the great majority of cases of anaemia due to lack of iron. However, 'iron-deficiency anaemia' reported by the laboratory is apt to be equated with nutritional deficiency. As a result of this common error iron therapy is commenced without looking for a possible source of bleeding. Dietary deficiency is seldom the only cause of an iron-deficiency anaemia in the developed countries, but certain age groups are particularly vulnerable. Premature or underweight infants have reduced iron stores and grow more rapidly than the normal child; iron-deficiency anaemia is therefore common in the first few months of life unless their diet is fortified with iron from the beginning. In infancy the haemoglobin level is normally only 11–12 g/dl, but iron deficiency is usually avoided by the early introduction of mixed feeding.

In adolescence the growth spurt calls for an increase in the daily requirement of iron and anaemia is sometimes seen in teenagers and otherwise healthy recruits to the armed forces. In pregnancy about 500 mg of iron is transferred from the maternal iron stores to the fetus. This transfer should be tolerated without affecting the mother provided that iron stores have not been depleted by previous pregnancies, menorrhagia, gastrointestinal blood loss, dietary deficiency or malabsorption. The routine administration of oral iron during pregnancy has done much to reduce the incidence of anaemia from this cause.

Iron-deficiency anaemia is not uncommon in old age. Although in some instances this may be due to an impoverished diet it is far more likely to be due to occult bleeding from the alimentary tract.

Finally, the iron intake may be adequate but malabsorption often follows partial gastrectomy and occurs in gluten enteropathy, tropical sprue and Crohn's disease. Failure of the serum iron concentration to rise significantly 3 hours after an oral dose of iron and ascorbic acid provides objective evidence of malabsorption in these patients.

Vitamin B₁₂ deficiency

Megaloblastic anaemia is caused by defective DNA synthesis in the red-cell precursors and is almost invariably due to lack of vitamin B_{12} or folic acid. Since the production of leukocytes and platelets is also affected the anaemia may be accompanied by leukopenia, thrombocytopenia or the presence of hypersegmented polymorphonuclear leukocytes in the circulation. A raised mean corpuscular volume (MCV) of more than 95 fl in an anaemic patient is often the first indication of megaloblastic changes in the marrow. The diagnosis must however be confirmed by marrow biopsy, as macrocytosis associated with a normal marrow is seen in many other situations. These include alcoholism, cytotoxic therapy, haemolytic states, neoplasia and recent haemorrhage.

Vitamin B_{12} is produced by bacterial synthesis and is absent in plants. Dietary deficiency is therefore sometimes seen in strict vegetarians, whose only supply is from bacterial contamination of their food. In Scandinavian countries megaloblastic anaemia was once common from infestation of the upper intestine by *Diphyllobothrium latum*, a fish tapeworm which takes up vitamin B_{12} and thus deprives the host of adequate supplies. A similar mechanism may account for the deficiency which is sometimes seen in the blind loop syndrome.

The main cause of vitamin B_{12} deficiency, however, is malabsorption as a result of ileal disease or lack of intrinsic factor from the stomach. The former may be due to gluten enteropathy, Crohn's disease, tropical sprue, tuberculosis, lymphoma, scleroderma or ileal resection. The latter is a rare complication of partial or total gastrectomy, and can be avoided by prophylactic treatment. However, it is more commonly due to pernicious anaemia.

Pernicious anaemia

Aetiology

In this disease the gastric mucosa is destroyed by a chronic inflammatory process with failure of production of hydrochloric acid and intrinsic factor. This lack of intrinsic factor results in an inability to bind and absorb vitamin B_{12} in the ileum. That the underlying cause is an autoimmune disorder is suggested by the nature of the gastric lesion, the presence of circulating parietal cell antibodies and the association of pernicious anaemia with Hashimoto's thyroiditis, diabetes mellitus or Addison's disease in the same individual. Heredity is important — about one-third of the patients are found to have a relative with the same disease.

Pernicious anaemia has an overall incidence in Northern Europe of about 1–2 per thousand of the population, but is much commoner than this in old age. It rarely presents before the age of 40 except in those with a family history. As with most autoimmune disorders it appears to be commoner in women. The anaemia may be accompanied by peripheral neuritis or subacute combined degeneration of the spinal cord, and gastric carcinoma is four to five times more frequent in patients with this disease than in the rest of the population.

Clinical features

The onset is insidious and, apart from a sore tongue and paraesthesiae, which may precede the blood changes by many months, the symptoms are usually those of lassitude and breathlessness. Impairment of taste is often noticed but rarely mentioned. Occasionally, however, the neurological symptoms are more prominent and the patient may present with mental confusion, numbness of glove and stocking distribution in the limbs and difficulty in walking.

Examination may show little more than a smooth tongue, but if the anaemia is severe the characteristic lemon-yellow pallor of the skin may be observed, particularly in daylight. When neurological changes are present the knee and ankle reflexes are absent or increased according to whether the peripheral nerves or cord are affected; the plantar responses may be extensor and impairment of sensation may be present in the lower limbs.

Investigations

The blood count will confirm the presence of anaemia and the MCV will be greater than 95 fl unless there is a co-existing iron deficiency or thalassaemia trait. The reticulocyte count is often normal but will show a striking rise by the fourth or fifth day after giving vitamin B_{12} — the lower the initial haemoglobin level the greater the rise. A marrow biopsy should be carried out as soon as possible, and before any treatment is given, because a single dose of B_{12} or folic acid will return erythropoiesis to normal within 24 hours. This will show an increase in the number of megalocytes and megaloblasts with occasional giant metamyelocytes. Blood should be taken on admission for serum B_{12} assay and antibody studies; the finding of antibodies to gastric parietal cells or intrinsic factor will support the diagnosis but more importantly the presence of thyroid antibodies should draw attention to the possibility of hypothyroidism developing later.

A Schilling test will demonstrate malabsorption of the vitamin. It is particularly useful when the prior administration of B_{12} or folic acid has corrected the blood and marrow abnormalities. In this procedure an oral dose of radioactively labelled vitamin B_{12} is given and its excretion measured in a 24-hour urine collection. It is essential to give a large intramuscular dose of 1000 μg of unlabelled vitamin B_{12} immediately before the test in order to saturate the liver stores; this has the added advantage of commencing treatment whilst awaiting the results. By giving the radioactive B_{12} with and without intrinsic factor is is possible to differentiate between pernicious anaemia and malabsorption due to small bowel disease. Normally more than 10% of the radioactivity is excreted in the urine within 24 hours; in pernicious anaemia the figure will be less than 5%.

When gastric symptoms are present a barium meal or endoscopy should be done to exclude a gastric neoplasm. Both procedures will show the atrophic gastric mucosa which is a characteristic feature of this disease.

Folic acid deficiency

Although folic acid is widely distributed in food of animal or vegetable origin dietary deficiency is common in the developing countries and not unknown in the UK, particularly in alcoholics and in elderly people living on inadequate diets. Folic acid requirements are increased during growth and in pregnancy, haemolytic disorders and malignant disease. The absorption of this vitamin may be impaired in gluten enteropathy, tropical sprue, extensive Crohn's disease and following the prolonged administration of anticonvulsant drugs. Impaired folate metabolism is an inevitable consequence of the administration of folic acid antagonists such as methotrexate in the treatment of malignant disease.

Macrocytic anaemia is seen in less than 2% of pregnant women in Britain and is due in the great majority of cases to folic acid deficiency. It results mainly from increased fetal demands and the incidence is higher in multigravidae and twin pregnancies. Its occurrence has fallen following the widespread practice of giving folic acid along with iron to pregnant women. In tropical countries vitamin B_{12} deficiency may contribute to the anaemia.

A blood count will reveal the presence of a macrocytic anaemia but a marrow biopsy will be necessary to confirm that this is due to megaloblastosis. In folate deficiency the serum folate level will be less than 3 μg/l. Unfortunately, some patients have low serum vitamin B_{12} levels as well, which may cause some confusion. These will, however, return to normal within 2 weeks of giving folate alone.

Further investigations will depend upon the most probable cause. If malabsorption is present a small bowel meal may show the typical appearances of Crohn's disease or gluten enteropathy, although the latter should always be confirmed by jejunal biopsy using a Crosby capsule.

MARROW DEPRESSION

Damage to the stem cells or sinusoidal capillaries can lead to failure of erythropoiesis despite an adequate supply of the essential factors. This may also affect the maturation of the platelets and leukocytes so that the anaemia which results is often accompanied by thrombocytopenia, agranulocytosis or both of these potentially lethal disorders.

Aplasia, or complete arrest, is fortunately rare and usually fatal within a matter of weeks. As a rule marrow biopsy shows 'islands' of surviving cells and the condition is one of hypoplasia which may eventually recover completely. A hypoplastic marrow is quite common in anorexia nervosa and may result in leukopenia or thrombocytopenia; it is rarely severe enough to cause anaemia.

Pancytopenia may present acutely with prostration, headache, nausea, sweating, rigors and high fever. The blood picture is one of a severe normocytic, normochromic anaemia, though occasional macrocytes may be seen; the reticulocyte count will not be raised. Bruising and bleeding from mucous membranes are due to the low platelet count, and agranulocytosis will cause ulceration in the mouth. Unless infection is countered by strict isolation and antibiotics the patient will perish from septicaemia.

Transfusions of blood and platelets will temporarily correct some of these deficiencies and buy time, but even if the marrow recovers it may be months before the blood count returns to normal.

Known causes include drugs and other toxic chemicals, ionising radiation and viral infections; in many cases, however, the cause remains obscure.

The anaemia associated with chronic infections, connective tissue disorders, renal failure and malignancy is often due to a combination of marrow depression and increased haemolysis, too few red cells being produced to balance the increased rate of destruction. A hypochromic anaemia is not always due to iron deficiency and other causes should be sought if it fails to respond to iron. Normal or elevated serum iron and ferritin levels should arouse suspicion.

The presence in the marrow of red-cell precursors containing iron granules arranged in a ring around the nucleus is diagnostic of sideroblastic anaemia which may be due to alcohol, drugs, lead poisoning and neoplasia. It may also be caused by hereditary defects in the synthesis of the alpha- and betaglobin chains in the haemoglobin molecule. These disorders are relatively common in Africa, the Mediterranean littoral, the Middle East and Asia and are known collectively as the *thalassaemias*.

Drugs

Therapeutic agents are being increasingly recognised as an important cause of marrow damage. Drug-induced hypoplastic anaemia is less common than agranulocytosis or thrombocytopenia but may persist long after withdrawal of the drug.

Toxic effects are almost inevitable when cytotoxic drugs are used, but idiosyncratic reactions to other medication are impossible to predict in advance. Symptoms are unrelated to dose or duration and may appear at once or after weeks or even months of treatment. A full drug history is essential in any anaemia in which the cause is not immediately apparent, and a textbook on adverse drug reactions should be consulted.

Drugs which are known to cause aplastic anaemia include carbimazole, chloramphenicol, chlorpropamine, gold salts, indomethacin, oxphenylbu-tazone, phenylbutazone, phenytoin, potassium perchlorate, tolbutamide and trimethoprim. In addition, many other drugs besides those mentioned above can cause thrombocytopenia or agranulocytosis without producing much damage to the red-cell precursors. These include such well-known compounds as carbamazepine, dapsone, meprobamate, phenothiazines, rifampicin, semisynthetic penicillins, sulphonamides, spironolactone and the thiazide diuretics.

Poisons

In industry, preventive measures have greatly reduced the incidence of anaemia from toxic chemicals. Benzene derivatives are, however, present in many household products such as paint removers, cleansing fluids, adhesives, insecticides and hair dyes. The risk of exposure in chemical plants, laboratories, dry-cleaning establishments and laundries must not be forgotten.

Ionising radiation

The bone marrow is highly sensitive to such radiation but its susceptibility varies greatly in different individuals. Exposure may be from external sources such as the gamma and neutron radiation from atomic explosions and nuclear energy plants, or from X-rays used in diagnosis or therapy. Depression of marrow activity is common in patients receiving extensive radiotherapy and may call for cessation of treatment. Internal sources include radioactive isotopes given therapeutically or accidentally ingested or inhaled. A potential hazard is the contamination of food and water supplies by the release of radioactive material from nuclear energy plants.

Infections

Many infections are accompanied by a moderate fall in the haemoglobin level. A mild normocytic or slightly hypochromic anaemia is often associated with a low serum iron, which is due to a defect in the release of iron from the storage sites in the reticulo–endothelial system. A refractory anaemia with a hypocellular marrow is recognised as an occasional complication of viral infections such as rubella, influenza, mumps, hepatitis and infectious mononucleosis. Chronic miliary tuberculosis sometimes involves the marrow and produces a pancytopenia.

Connective tissue disorders (see also Fever, p. 324)

Anaemia is common in all of these chronic inflammatory diseases and is usually normocytic and normochromic; occasionally it may be sideroblastic in type. In rheumatoid arthritis alimentary blood loss from the prolonged use of non-steroidal anti-inflammatory drugs will accentuate the anaemia by producing iron deficiency. The anaemia of lupus erythematosus may be accompanied by leukopenia and a low platelet count, and in some cases an inhibitor of erythropoietin has been demonstrated. In cranial arteritis and polymyalgia rheumatica leukocytosis is often present, whilst an eosinophilia is not uncommon in polyarteritis nodosa. The ESR is usually elevated in all these disorders.

Neoplasia

The pathogenesis of anaemia in the various forms of malignancy is complex. In the alimentary tract blood loss may be largely responsible. Growths elsewhere can produce antigens which result in immune-mediated suppression of erythropoiesis or reduced red-cell survival. Alternatively, they may invade the marrow, producing a leuko–erythroblastic anaemia which is characterised by a raised white cell count and the presence of immature leukocytes and nucleated red cells in the peripheral blood.

Leukaemia

Aetiology
Leukaemia is caused by the gross proliferation of primitive lymphoid or myeloid cells which infiltrate the marrow, blood and other tissues. The replacement of normal marrow by these primitive blast cells leads to anaemia, neutropenia and thrombocytopenia. In many animals the disease can be transmitted by viruses but a viral origin has not been established in man. There is an increased incidence following exposure to ionising radiation from atomic explosions, nuclear energy plants or radiotherapy for ankylosing spondylitis.

Acute lymphatic leukaemia is the commonest type seen in childhood and adolescence; it occurs more frequently in children with Down's syndrome. Acute myeloid leukaemia, on the other hand, is uncommon in childhood and is more often seen in the middle-aged or elderly.

In their chronic forms both types are rare in childhood, have a male preponderance and usually present after the age of 40. An abnormal 'Philadelphia' chromosome is present in the marrow cells in about 80% of adults with chronic myeloid leukaemia. Myelomonocytic and eosinophilic leukaemia are rare. The presence of a persistent, absolute lymphocytosis in the blood, accompanied by an increased percentage of small lymphocytes in the marrow, is supposed to distinguish chronic lymphatic leukaemia from other lymphoproliferative diseases. In practice however there is inevitably some overlap and a similar blood picture is seen in such rarities as Waldenström's macroglobulinaemia, Sézary's syndrome and hairy cell leukaemia.

Clinical features

The acute form is seen most often in young children and presents as a brief febrile illness with pallor, haemorrhages into the skin and alimentary tract, and either pharyngitis or pneumonia. Enlarged lymph nodes may be palpable and the liver and spleen enlarge but may not easily be felt. Bone pain is not uncommon and headache may be due to meningeal infiltration or intracranial haemorrhage.

The chronic form is seen chiefly in middle or later life. The onset is insidious with little beyond a complaint of debility and loss of weight, or dyspnoea due to the anaemia. Occasionally there may be left hypochondriac pain from infarction of an enlarged spleen and this organ, particularly in the myeloid type, may extend below the umbilicus and reach the right iliac fossa. Lymphadenopathy is the more prominent feature in chronic lymphatic leukaemia. Purpura and other haemorrhagic manifestations may be present at diagnosis or appear later.

Investigations

The blood picture is one of a normocytic, normochromic anaemia unless prolonged bleeding has led to iron deficiency. The white cell count varies widely but is often greatly increased and may exceed $100 \times 10^9/l$ (100 000 per mm^3). In myeloid leukaemia it is composed largely of immature cells. The alkaline phosphatase normally present in the cytoplasm of mature neutrophils is absent or low in chronic granulocytic leukaemia. Platelet deficiency is common, especially in the acute forms of the disease, but an initial thrombocythaemia is found in some cases of chronic myeloid leukaemia. The marrow in all cases provides the diagnosis, consisting mainly of primitive blast cells.

Myelomatosis

Aetiology

Multiple myeloma is the commonest form of plasma cell tumour in Britain.

It results from the uncontrolled proliferation of a single clone of B lymphocytes in the marrow, disrupting its normal function and invading the surrounding bone and soft tissues. The monoclonal cells produce a homogenous immunoglobulin which can be detected in the serum by protein electrophoresis.

Solitary plasmacytomas can arise in bone and extra-medullary sites such as lymph nodes, but the disease has usually spread to other parts of the skeleton by the time the diagnosis is confirmed. Other plasma cell neoplasms such as Waldenström's macroglobulinaemia, immune-related amyloidosis and heavy chain disease are rare.

Clinical features
Although myeloma occasionally occurs in young adults it is found mainly in the elderly of both sexes. Back pain, aggravated by movement and relieved by rest, is the commonest presenting symptom. Some loss of weight is usual over the preceding months, and there is an increased risk of severe infections because of the reduced levels of normal immunoglobulins. Infection is the commonest cause of death in this condition.

Hypercalcaemia should be suspected if there is nausea and vomiting, constipation, polydipsia and mental confusion. Acute renal failure from hypercalcaemia or the poisoning of the proximal renal tubular cells by light chains excreted in the urine is another major cause of death in this disease. Spinal cord compression and a peripheral neuropathy, unrelated to pressure on nerve roots, are sometimes seen.

Investigations
A normocytic, normochromic anaemia is common but a sideroblastic picture is found in some patients. Rouleaux formation on the blood films and a raised ESR are due to the high concentration of myeloma protein in the plasma. In most cases a monoclonal band of IgG or IgA can be demonstrated by protein electrophoresis. When this is not present free light chains may be found in the urine by a similar technique, but Bence–Jones proteinuria will not be demonstrated by the routine dipstick tests for protein. Serum immunoelectrophoresis will enable the myeloma protein to be identified and may show reduced levels of the normal immunoglobulins.

Blood should be taken for blood urea, serum creatinine and calcium estimations to assess the degree of renal impairment and to exclude hypercalcaemia. A raised blood urea or serum creatinine level is probably the most important indicator of a poor prognosis.

The diagnostic feature of this disease is a plasmacytosis in the affected tissues and this may be found in a marrow biopsy or in an extramedullary site such as a skin nodule or enlarged lymph node. X-rays of the skeleton may show generalised osteoporosis or discrete osteolytic bone lesions; these are most likely to be seen in the skull, vertebrae or pelvis. Pain arising from a collapsed vertebra in the thoracic or lumbar spine is a common mode of presentation.

Myelofibrosis

This is a rare proliferative disorder related to chronic myeloid leukaemia and polycythaemia vera. Replacement of active marrow by fibrous tissue is progressive and ultimately fatal. Haemopoiesis is taken over by the liver and spleen and these organs are characteristically enlarged.

The condition arises insidiously in middle age with increasing weakness and anaemia. The patient may bleed from the accompanying thrombocytopenia.

The blood picture is typically leuko-erythroblastic with a reduced platelet count. Marrow biopsy is essential for the diagnosis but an aspirate may yield no fragments. A trephine biopsy, preferably from a different site, will show the fibroblastic proliferation and acellular marrow.

Thalassaemia

Aetiology

The thalassaemias are a group of inherited disorders affecting the synthesis of the alpha- or betaglobin chains in the haemoglobin molecule. As a result, the production of red cells is impaired, with consequent anaemia.

The thalassaemias are named after the specific globin involved. Alpha-thalassaemia is common in the Far East and parts of Africa but is rarely seen in the UK. Beta-thalassaemia, however, is encountered in immigrants from Cyprus, Greece, Italy, India, Pakistan and South-East Asia. The heterozygous form, or *thalassaemia minor*, is very common in these populations. If the genetic defect is acquired from both parents then the resulting anaemia will be much more severe and the term *thalassaemia major* is used. Occasionally, thalassaemia is associated with the production of an abnormal haemoglobin as well, which further complicates the picture.

Clinical features

Thalassaemia minor is well tolerated and may be symptomless, being discovered on a routine blood count. The anaemia is apt to worsen during pregnancy.

Thalassaemia major is a much more serious disorder and presents in the first year of life with pallor, listlessness and failure to thrive. A very low haemoglobin level stimulates erythropoietin production, which leads to gross hypertrophy of the marrow. This, in turn, causes osteoporosis and deformity of the skull from expansion of the marrow spaces. Pathological fractures and hepatosplenomegaly were common before it was discovered that regular blood transfusions from an early age could suppress the clinical manifestations of the disease. Unfortunately this inevitably leads to a vast accumulation of iron in virtually all the organs of the body; the liver, endocrine glands and particularly the heart are most affected. Few sufferers survive adolescence, ultimately dying of cardiac failure.

Investigations

In thalassaemia minor the blood count will show a mild microcytic, hypochromic anaemia with a low mean corpuscular volume and haemoglobin content. A normal serum iron, iron-binding capacity and ferritin level will exclude iron-deficiency as the cause. Haemoglobin electrophoresis will demonstrate an increased percentage of HbA_2 or fetal haemoglobin in beta-thalassaemia, but not in alpha-thalassaemia minor. This technique may also reveal the presence of an abnormal haemoglobin such as HbLepore or HbS.

In thalassaemia major the haemoglobin level may be as little as 3 g/dl and the red cells will exhibit severe microcytosis, hypochromasia and fragmentation. On electrophoresis the normal adult haemoglobin will be largely replaced by fetal haemoglobin and HbA_2.

The presence of thalassaemia minor in both parents is often sufficient to establish the diagnosis. More extensive investigations to determine the exact nature of the genetic defect is outside the scope of most laboratories — if it is at all possible, patients should be referred to an expert in this field.

BLOOD DESTRUCTION

The haemolytic anaemias are caused by the premature destruction of red cells in the reticulo–endothelial system or circulation as a result of inherited defects, megaloblastosis or environmental factors. They are not seen very often in the UK, but their incidence is increasing as a result of immigration from countries where haemoglobinopathies and congenital enzyme deficiencies in the red cells are common. In megaloblastic anaemias some degree of haemolysis is usual and accounts for the raised reticulocyte count and mid hyperbilirubinaemia. These conditions have already been dealt with in the preceding section.

In the acquired form the red cells are originally normal but their cell membranes are disrupted by toxic substances, intracellular organisms or the deposition of antigen–antibody complexes on their surface. In tropical countries invasion of the erythrocytes by malarial parasites is the commonest cause of an acquired haemolytic anaemia, but this is rarely seen in Britain. Occasionally, haemolysis may result from excessive trauma to the red cells during their passage through the circulation. Fragmentation occurs when the red cells are forced through the fibrin threads in the renal capillaries of patients with malignant hypertension, or damaged by turbulence around prosthetic aortic or mitral valves following cardiac surgery.

Haemolysis releases iron and bilirubin. The iron is conserved in the storage depots and anaemia only appears when destruction has outpaced compensatory erythropoiesis. Increased amounts of unconjugated bilirubin will be present in the blood, but this rarely exceeds 70 μmol/l (4 mg/dl). Jaundice, if present, will be mild, but excess urobilinogen will be detected in the urine.

The shortened lifespan can be measured by labelling some of the patient's erythrocytes with radioactive chromium and measuring their rate of disappearance from the circulation. This technique is rarely used in practice, but it has the advantage of identifying the site of destruction; if the spleen is mainly involved splenectomy will reduce the haemolytic process.

In chronic haemolytic disorders the premature destruction of the red cells takes place mainly in the spleen. As a result this organ enlarges and may be palpable.

Intravascular haemolysis is rare in the UK though common in countries where malaria is endemic. In the UK it may be seen in conditions where the erythrocytes are fragmented in the circulation, in autoimmune haemolytic anaemias of the cold antibody type, and in paroxysmal nocturnal haemoglobinuria. This rare disease is due to the proliferation of an abnormal clone of stem cells which produce erythrocytes that are readily lysed by complement. In the majority of cases there is a platelet abnormality as well. These patients present with episodes of thrombosis in unusual sites and haemoglobinuria in the early morning urine.

Haemoglobinuria is the hallmark of intravascular haemolysis and may be mistaken for haematuria unless the urine is examined under the microscope. Increased levels of haemoglobin and methaemoglobin are always present in the plasma, and haemosiderin may be demonstrated in an early morning urine specimen by staining the sediment with Prussian blue.

Some of the more important causes of a haemolytic anaemia are now discussed in detail.

Hereditary spherocytosis

Aetiology
This genetic defect in the shape of the red cell is inherited as an autosomal dominant disorder. It appears to be due to some abnormality of the fibrous proteins in the cell which maintain the normal biconcave appearance of the mature erythrocyte. Spherocytes are less deformable than the normal red cell and this makes them particularly vulnerable to sequestration and destruction in the spleen.

Hereditary spherocytosis may be inherited from either parent or result from spontaneous mutation. It is particularly prevalent in Northern Europe.

Hereditary elliptocytosis is an allied disorder in which the red cells are oval or elliptical in shape; these cells are less liable to premature destruction in the splenic microcirculation and significant haemolysis only occurs in about 10% of cases.

Clinical features
Although this disease can present at any time in life, anaemia is rarely apparent in childhood, increased erythropoiesis compensating for the increased rate of destruction. Sudden 'aplastic' crises may however occur when the overactive marrow is temporarily inhibited by an intercurrent infection; this is particularly likely to happen during the first 6 years of life.

With increasing age the spleen enlarges and eventually the haemolytic process can no longer be compensated for by increased production. The resulting anaemia may be due in part to folate deficiency, since this vitamin is excessively utilised in any chronic haemolytic disorder. The condition is usually discovered by early adult life, but may remain undetected until the development of pigmented gallstones with resulting jaundice and colic draws attention to its presence. Finally, it sometimes presents in the elderly as a result of a lack of folic acid in the diet or the natural decline in erythropoiesis which occurs in old age.

The history may reveal evidence of a similar disorder in another member of the family or of previous episodes of unexplained anaemia or jaundice. An 'aplastic' crisis may present, with a sudden fall in the haemoglobin concentration sufficient to cause cardiac failure. In the older child and adult the spleen is usually palpable, and chronic ulceration of the ankles is seen in about 15% of cases.

Investigations
The blood film will show the characteristic spherocytes and a negative Coombs test will usually distinguish this condition from autoimmune haemolytic anaemia of the warm antibody type. Whenever possible the parents should also be investigated in order to establish the hereditary nature of the disease. Splenectomy is often valuable in restoring the haemoglobin level to normal.

Sickle-cell anaemia

Aetiology
This congenital haemolytic disorder is due to the inheritance of a gene which produces an abnormal betaglobin chain in adult haemoglobin. It is mainly confined to the inhabitants of Central Africa and their descendants who have emigrated to other parts of the world. In the United States about 10% of Blacks carry the gene. The sickle-cell trait is also found to a lesser extent in the inhabitants of Greece, Turkey and the Middle East.

In the heterozygous state both normal adult and sickle haemoglobin are generated, but the latter is not present in sufficient amounts in the red cells for sickling to occur except in conditions of extreme hypoxia. When both parents are carriers of the trait the affected individual will produce no adult haemoglobin and most of the haemoglobin in the red cells will be abnormal.

The sickling phenomenon only occurs when the sickle haemoglobin is deoxygenated and the molecules aggregate together to form an intracellular gel. This stretches and deforms the membrane of the red cell to produce the characteristic sickle or holly-leaf shape. The sickle cell is more rigid than normal and is sequestered and destroyed more rapidly in the spleen; moreover, sickling causes occlusion of the smaller blood vessels and infarction of the tissues beyond the block. This is facilitated by a low oxygen tension, stasis, dehydration and metabolic acidosis. In some patients the situation is further complicated by the presence of other haemoglobinopathies such as thalassaemia and haemoglobin-C disease.

Clinical features
The sickle-cell carrier is usually healthy, but should avoid such activities

as deep-sea diving or flying in unpressurised aircraft at high altitudes where the reduced oxygen tension causes sickling to occur. In the homozygous individual the story is very different. The disease usually appears towards the end of the first year of life when the marrow stops producing fetal haemoglobin. A moderate haemolytic anaemia develops which may be exacerbated by intercurrent infections, folate deficiency or any of the factors mentioned above which increase sickling. Acute obstruction of the blood supply to various tissues, notably the skeleton, often accompanies the fall in haemoglobin level. This leads to the sudden onset of excruciating pain in the back, chest or extremities which may last for many hours.

When organs other than the bones are affected infarction may cause cerebrovascular accidents, priapism, hepatitis, abdominal pain or gross haematuria. Chronic vascular complications from repeated occlusion of the blood vessels include refractory leg ulcers, renal failure, blindness and possibly the increased susceptibility to infection in these patients from progressive infarction of the spleen. Children with this disease are particularly liable to die from overwhelming pneumococcal infections. The increased production of bilirubin leads to the formation of pigmented gallstones, and cholelithiasis is very common in the survivors.

Investigations

The blood count will reveal the severity of the anaemia and blood films will usually show target cells and the characteristic sickle-shaped erythrocytes. The diagnosis is confirmed by sickling and solubility tests and by the demonstration of sickle haemoglobin on electrophoresis; in the homozygous state about 90% of the haemoglobin will be in this form.

Hereditary enzyme deficiencies

An inherited deficiency of certain enzymes in the red cell may lead to its premature destruction. Lack of the enzymes involved in the anaerobic pathway of glycolysis can cause a haemolytic anaemia but this is fortunately rare. The enzyme most affected is pyruvate kinase, but few laboratories possess the facilities to carry out the necessary investigations. Much commoner are congenital deficiencies in the enzymes involved in the hexose monophosphate shunt which normally consumes about 10% of the glucose metabolised by the red cell.

Deficiency of glucose-6-phosphate dehydrogenase is very common in blacks and has been found in about 10% of Black American males. It is inherited as a sex-linked trait, the gene coding for this enzyme being located on the X-chromosome. It is also widespread among White and Oriental populations and is particularly prevalent in Greeks, Sardinians, Chinese and Thais.

The red cell survival is nearly normal in most of these individuals unless they are exposed to oxidant drugs such as antimalarials, phenacetin, sulphonamides and nitrofurantoin. Naphthalene in moth balls is another oxidant chemical which may be ingested by affected infants.

Favism is a severe form of this disorder produced in Mediterranean races by eating broad beans. It may be fatal.

There is a lag of 2–3 days after ingesting the drug before gross haemolysis appears. During this crisis the haemoglobin level will fall precipitately and the urine will be coloured red. Heinz bodies may be present in blood smears and many of the red cells will have pieces missing from their cytoplasm. Fortunately the crisis is limited in its duration and most patients recover. Occasionally a typical haemolytic episode may be triggered off by a bacterial or viral infection, or by diabetic keto-acidosis.

Infections

The role of infections in exacerbating the anaemia of hereditary haemolytic disorders has already been discussed. Some organisms, however, cause haemolysis by a direct effect upon the circulating red cells. Malaria is the prime example of this but some bacteria such as *Bartonella bacilliformis* may also invade the red cell, whilst others produce enzymes which damage the cell membrane. The most dramatic example of this is the haemolysis produced by the clostridial organisms which cause gas gangrene.

Free haemoglobin and methaemoglobin will be found in the plasma and haemoglobinuria will be present. The colour of the urine in blackwater fever is due to altered haemoglobin and is an indication of the severity of the malarial infection.

Rhesus disease

A severe haemolytic anaemia may present at birth as a result of the passage across the placenta of maternal antibodies which are lethal to the infant's red cells. This situation usually arises in Rh-negative women who give birth to Rh-positive infants. The first child is rarely affected, because immunisation of the mother normally takes place at delivery, when Rh-positive cells from the fetus cross the placenta. A woman may, rarely, have been immunised previously by a transfusion with Rh-positive blood or an abortion.

In subsequent pregnancies the antibodies will be present early in pregnancy and the fetus may be severely affected in utero; about 15% will be stillborn. The survivors may suffer severe brain damage from the high serum levels of unconjugated bilirubin that follow severe haemolysis in the first few days of life.

In the past, treatment by exchange transfusion was the only effective method of removing this excess bilirubin and reducing the subsequent morbidity. The incidence of this disease in Britain has fallen dramatically, however, since it has become routine practice to give anti-D gammaglobulin to non-immunised Rh-negative women immediately after delivery of a Rh-positive child. This removes the fetal cells by lysis and prevents immunisation of the mother.

Poisons

Certain chemicals can destroy normal red cells if present in high enough concentration in the blood. In industry this may result from exposure to arsenic in the form of arsine gas, lead, copper, sodium and potassium chlorate. The raised copper levels in Wilson's disease sometimes cause haemolysis and account for the haemolytic anaemia which is occasionally seen in this disorder.

The role of oxidant drugs in precipitating a haemolytic crisis in patients with glucose-6-phosphate dehydrogenase deficiency in their red cells has already been referred to under congenital enzyme deficiencies. Other drugs produce an autoimmune type of haemolytic anaemia and are discussed in the following section.

Autoimmune disorders

Aetiology

In these disorders the erythrocytes become coated with antibody and the cells are damaged by the interaction of antigens with this antibody, presumably as a result of activation of the complement system. Loss of cell membrane, fragmentation and spherocyte formation occur and the injured cells are rapidly removed by the reticulo–endothelial tissues, particularly the spleen. When the damage is extensive there will be intravascular haemolysis with consequent haemoglobinuria.

In warm antibody autoimmune haemolytic anaemia the immune reaction develops at body temperature and the antibodies are usually of the IgG class. In at least half of the patients with this type there is some underlying disorder such as Hodgkin's disease, chronic lymphatic leukaemia, systemic lupus erythematosus or an ovarian neoplasm.

In cold antibody autoimmune haemolytic anaemia the immune reaction takes place at lower temperatures and haemolytic episodes are precipitated by cooling; thus they are more likely to occur in winter. This type is associated with certain infections, particularly those caused by *Mycoplasma pneumoniae* and viruses, and presents as an acute haemolytic anaemia some 2–3 weeks after the onset of the initial illness; syphilis was once a common cause. A more chronic form appears in the elderly which may be associated with some underlying malignancy. The cold agglutinins which are present in high titres in this type are usually IgM antibodies.

In drug-induced autoimmune haemolytic anaemia the drug is thought to act as a hapten and to evoke the production of IgG or less commonly IgM antibodies. With carbromal and methyldopa the haemolytic reaction is slow in onset and intravascular haemolysis is uncommon. A more dramatic reaction with severe haemolysis and haemoglobinuria may follow an intravenous penicillin infusion of more than 20 million units a day, or the administration of quinine, quinidine and stibophen.

Clinical features

These are very variable and will depend on the severity of the haemolytic process, the type of antibody and the nature of any underlying disease. In mild cases there may be little to find apart from the anaemia, slight icterus and splenomegaly. During acute haemolytic episodes there will be increasing lassitude, cramps, backache and haemoglobinuria. Raynaud's phenomenon and diffuse mottling of the skin after cooling are seen in elderly patients with cold antibodies. A recent respiratory illness will raise the possibility of a *Mycoplasma* or viral infection. A full drug history should be taken to exclude any known drug cause.

Investigations

The anaemia is usually normocytic and normochromic, but a few macrocytes and nucleated red cells may be seen on a blood film; the presence of numerous spherocytes would indicate that the anaemia is of the warm antibody type. A marked but transient leukocytosis may be seen during haemolytic crises, accompanied by a rise in the reticulocyte count. The direct Coombs' test is usually positive. There will be a modest rise in the serum bilirubin level, depending on the degree of haemolysis. The urine should be examined for the presence of urobilinogen, haemoglobin and haemosiderin.

In the cold antibody type the cold agglutinin titre will be elevated and there is likely to be an increase in the IgM fraction on plasma immuno-electrophoresis; a mono spot test for infectious mononucleosis should be done and serum taken for mycoplasma and viral antibodies. Serological tests for syphilis should be requested if this diagnosis is suspected.

In the warm antibody type it is necessary to establish whether or not there is some underlying disease. LE cells and DNA antibodies should be looked for with systemic lupus erythematosus in mind, and lymph node or marrow biopsy may help establishing the diagnosis of a lymphoproliferative disorder such as Hodgkin's disease.

Hypersplenism

This is not a clinical entity but it is seen in a number of chronic disorders in which the spleen is enlarged. It appears occasionally in portal hypertension, in rheumatoid arthritis as Felty's syndrome, in chronic lymphatic leukaemia, sarcoidosis and systemic lupus erythematosus.

It is thought that a heightened activity of the spleen's normal function of sequestrating effete red blood cells worsens an existing anaemia by increased haemolysis. That this may be so is confirmed by a rise in the haemoglobin level after splenectomy.

CHAPTER 19
Cough

SYNOPSIS OF CAUSES*

RESPIRATORY TRACT

Laryngotracheitis; **Whooping cough**; **Laryngitis**; Laryngeal neoplasm; **Bronchitis**; Bronchiectasis; **Asthma**; **Bronchial neoplasm**.

LUNGS

Pneumonia; Lung Abscess; **Tuberculosis**; **Fibrosis**; Embolism; **Cardiac failure**.

* Bold type is used for causes more commonly found in Europe and North America.

PHYSIOLOGY

Coughing is a defensive mechanism designed to protect the airways from the harmful effects of inhaled noxious substances and to clear them of retained secretions. The act of coughing may be voluntary but is more commonly the result of a reflex response to stimulation of irritant receptors in the nose, oropharynx, larynx, trachea or bronchi. In inflammatory lung disease and pulmonary fibrosis or oedema the cough reflex is activated by stretch receptors in the distal airways and interstitial tissues. Depending on which receptors are stimulated the impulses travel to the coughing centre in the midbrain by afferent fibres of the trigeminal, glossopharyngeal, superior laryngeal or vagus nerves.

The cough reflex begins with a deep inspiration, closure of the glottis, relaxation of the diaphragm and tensing of the muscles of respiration. The intrathoracic pressure builds up and, when the glottis suddenly opens again, a forced expiration expels the compressed air, carrying with it any solid or liquid contents.

DIAGNOSTIC APPROACH

Healthy individuals seldom cough unless exposed to noxious fumes or a dusty environment. A persistent cough is abnormal and enquiry should be made about its character, duration and any accompanying symptoms. An acute non-productive cough, particularly if it is associated with a sore throat or nasal discharge, is likely to be due to an upper respiratory infection. In pneumonia the cough may be dry at first but most cases will eventually produce some purulent sputum; fever and general malaise are usually apparent from the onset. Paroxysms of coughing ending in the high-pitched sound of inspiratory stridor due to laryngeal spasm is virtually diagnostic of whooping cough, a disease which is almost entirely confined to children in the first 5 years of life.

A chronic, non-productive cough occurs in asthma and diffuse pulmonary fibrosis. In both disorders it is associated with dyspnoea, particularly on exertion, and there may be a history of exposure to known allergens or industrial dust. The presence of other diseases such as rheumatoid arthritis, lupus erythematosus or systemic sclerosis should remind one of the possibility of cryptogenic fibrosing alveolitis.

A dry cough accompanied by hoarseness in a middle-aged adult is commonly due to chronic laryngitis from excessive smoking or overuse of the voice. The occupation of the patient may be relevant here for the latter is an occupational hazard of auctioneers, actors, politicians and singers in particular. Hoarseness persisting for more than a month should be investigated further, for it may be due to a laryngeal carcinoma or to involvement of the recurrent laryngeal nerve by a bronchial neoplasm.

Sputum production is always pathological — the healthy individual swallows the normal secretions of the respiratory tract. Purulent sputum is yellow or green in colour and is evidence of continuing infection in the bronchial tree or alveoli. Examination of the chest and plain X-rays will usually enable its source to be identified, but sputum culture cannot always be relied upon to isolate the offending organism.

A chronic productive cough is seen in chronic bronchitis, bronchiectasis, pulmonary tuberculosis and neoplasms of the bronchus. Chronic bronchitis occurs mainly in cigarette smokers and those who work in dusty occupations; the sputum is white or mucoid in appearance in the absence of acute infection. In bronchiectasis large volumes of purulent sputum are coughed up, particularly on rising in the morning. In the elderly bronchitic the possibility of tuberculosis or an underlying neoplasm should always be considered and blood in the sputum, however slight, should never be assumed to come from an inflamed bronchus until these other disorders have been excluded.

The timing of a cough may throw some light on its probable cause. A persistent cough at night is commonly due to obstructive airways disease but a paroxysm of coughing in an elderly patient which wakes them from sleep may also herald the onset of pulmonary oedema; the distinction between late-onset asthma and left ventricular failure can sometimes be very difficult unless the attack is actually witnessed by the doctor.

Associated symptoms such as fever and sweating would point to infection and loss of weight would suggest tuberculosis or neoplasm. When dyspnoea is the major complaint reference should be made to the causes listed in the following chapter.

The extent of the physical examination will obviously depend upon the age of the patient, the history and the likely pathology. Examination of the chest may reveal signs of consolidation, a pleural rub, scattered rhonchi or localised crepitations at the bases.

Finger clubbing is an important sign and should be looked for. Common pulmonary causes include bronchiectasis, bronchial neoplasm, tuberculosis, lung abscess and fibrosing alveolitis. The rare dominant hereditary form should be suspected if the clubbing is gross and has been present for many years; enquiry should be made about clubbing in other members of the family.

Investigations

Whenever possible the sputum should be examined and, if purulent, sent to the laboratory for culture. Acute upper respiratory infections are usually self-limiting and transient in nature so that further investigations are rarely necessary. A chest X-ray will only be called for if there is evidence of lung involvement. It should, however, be emphasised that any cough lasting a month or more justifies a chest X-ray, particularly if there is a history of cigarette smoking or haemoptysis.

Laryngoscopy may be necessary if there is accompanying hoarseness, and bronchoscopy is always indicated if there is any suspicion of a bronchial neoplasm. In skilled hands a fibreoptic bronchoscope can be passed safely down the bronchial tree using a local analgesic and mild sedation.

Lung function tests may be helpful in patients with chronic airways obstruction or suspected pulmonary fibrosis.

CAUSES IN THE RESPIRATORY TRACT

Upper respiratory infections are for the most part viral in origin. They are the commonest of all diseases in Britain and account for about half the time lost from work or school. Antral infection following a cold may result in postnasal discharge with persisting cough, particularly at night. Acute viral and streptococcal infections of the pharynx often give rise to a dry cough but this is overshadowed by sore throat and fever. In influenza cough is dry at first but becomes productive as the infection spreads down the respiratory tract; if pneumonia develops the sputum may become blood-stained.

Laryngotracheitis (croup)

This common disorder of childhood is usually associated with viral infections of the upper respiratory tract; occasionally it is caused by staphylococcal or streptococcal infections. It mainly affects children under the age of 3, but it can occur in older children. After a few days of upper respiratory symptoms and fever the child's condition worsens with the development of a harsh barking cough and stridor.

Croup may resolve spontaneously within a week or two, but increasing dyspnoea and cyanosis are ominous signs and require admission to hospital. Nasotracheal intubation and even tracheotomy may be necessary to relieve the obstruction to the airways. X-rays of the chest may show narrowing of the trachea, while lateral X-rays of the neck may reveal a ballooned hypopharynx or infraglottic narrowing.

Whooping cough

Aetiology

Whooping cough is caused by an acute infection of the respiratory tract by *Bordetella pertussis*. It has an incubation period of 7–10 days. Being highly infectious it may appear at any age but the great majority of cases occur before the age of 5. Although it no longer carries a high mortality, symptoms can persist for months despite eradication of the organism with antibiotics. The severity of the disease and the mortality is highest in infants, and milder in vaccinated individuals. Publicity about the adverse neurological complications of vaccination has reduced the uptake of vaccination in Britain in recent years. As a result there have been several major epidemics in this country in the past decade.

Clinical features

This disease commences with a mild catarrhal illness and it is only after a week or two that the characteristic whoop appears. This consists of a rapid series of explosive coughs ending with the expulsion of a little thick phlegm, and followed by the high pitched sound of inspiratory stridor due to laryngeal spasm. Vomiting, cyanosis and apnoea may accompany these bouts of coughing. The whoop may be absent in young infants and previously vaccinated individuals.

The symptoms, which are probably caused by bacterial toxins, may persist for months and recur with any subsequent upper respiratory infection. During an attack the child is often frightened and distressed, the face is congested, epistaxis is common and scattered rhonchi may be audible in the lungs. Between attacks the child may feel quite well. Patients are infectious during the prodromal and early paroxysmal stages. Complications include bronchopneumonia, otitis media and bronchiectasis.

Investigations

The diagnosis can be confirmed by isolating *B. pertussis* from nasopharyngeal swabs on Bordet–Gengou medium, but positive cultures are only obtained in about 30% of cases. Ideally, the swab should be taken immediately after a paroxysm. A white count may show an absolute lymphocytosis, which will support the diagnosis. Agglutination tests for rising antibody titres to this organism are rarely helpful and are seldom done. A chest X-ray is indicated if the possibility of lung involvement exists.

Laryngitis

Chronic laryngitis may be due to oral sepsis and chronic sinusitis, but it is more often caused by excessive cigarette smoking or occupational over-use of the voice as in auctioneers, actors, politicians and singers. Persistent hoarseness and dry cough are present. Tuberculous laryngitis is very rare in the UK. It results from spread of infection from the lungs and may be readily overlooked in the absence of a chest X-ray.

Laryngeal neoplasm

Carcinoma of the larynx is seen in late middle life and is commoner in men. Cough and hoarseness persisting for more than a month in this age group should arouse suspicion and the patient should be referred to an ENT surgeon for laryngoscopy.

Acute bronchitis

Acute bronchitis occurs as an extension of an upper respiratory infection or an exacerbation of the chronic form. It is commoner in winter and spring than in the summer months. It may be accompanied by tracheitis in which there is soreness, increased by coughing, over the trachea and upper sternum. Tightness of the chest is accompanied by an irritating and productive cough. The sputum is at first scanty and viscid and may be streaked with blood but soon becomes mucopurulent and greater in amount. The patient is usually febrile and rhonchi will be audible on auscultation. In uncomplicated bronchitis no radiological changes will be seen.

Chronic bronchitis

Aetiology

Chronic exposure to bronchial irritants results in stimulation of the mucus-secreting cells, reduction in ciliary activity, impaired resistance to infection and spasm of the smooth muscle in the bronchial wall. The factors chiefly responsible are recurrent respiratory infections, atmospheric pollution by smoke and sulphur dioxide, dusty occupations and cigarette smoking. There is a clear association between heavy smoking and the incidence of the disease. Death ultimately results from heart failure due to pulmonary hypertension.

Clinical features

The chief symptom is a persistent cough with the expectoration of mucoid or mucopurulent sputum. Dyspnoea may be denied but the capacity for exertion is progressively impaired. With the development of emphysema this becomes more prominent than the cough except during acute exacer-bations. On examination the chest may appear barrel-shaped and respiratory movements are poor. Rhonchi will be audible throughout the lung fields and may be accompanied by wheezing. In an advanced case cyanosis and finger clubbing are present.

Investigations
Chest X-rays may be normal or show evidence of pulmonary fibrosis or cardiac enlargement. When emphysema is present the lung fields are unduly translucent, especially at the periphery where lung markings are absent. If tuberculosis is a possibility the sputum must be cultured for acid-fast bacilli.

In hospital arterial blood gas analysis will determine the degree of hypoxia and CO_2 retention and help in assessing the effect of treatment. Lung function tests will provide a measure of the severity of the airways obstruction.

Bronchiectasis

Aetiology
Permanent dilatation of the bronchial walls results from a combination of obstruction and infection. It usually involves the lower lobes, but upper lobe bronchiectasis may be caused by apical tuberculosis and bronchopulmonary aspergillosis. Histologically there is disorganisation and destruction of the subepithelial tissues with plasma cell infiltration of the thickened bronchial walls.

Bronchiectasis may complicate any serious respiratory infection in childhood, cystic fibrosis, Kartagener's syndrome, pulmonary tuberculosis and aspergillosis. It is also sometimes seen in patients with hypogammaglobulinaemia, rheumatoid arthritis and systemic lupus erythematosus, in whom an immunological deficiency may lead to failure of the antimicrobial defences to repel repeated infection.

Clinical features
A persistent cough with profuse mucopurulent sputum are characteristic of this disorder. The sputum is more abundant in the early morning and may more than fill the proverbial eggcup. Its production may be provoked by changes of posture on rising. Spread of infection around the infected bronchioles may give rise to episodes of bronchopneumonia and pleurisy. Haemoptysis is common and sometimes massive. Systemic features are rare but include failure to grow, loss of weight, cerebral abscess and secondary amyloidosis. During acute exacerbations coarse crepitations will be heard over the bronchiectatic areas and may be mistaken for a pleural rub. Finger clubbing is common.

Investigations
Chest X-rays are rarely helpful as the only changes likely to be seen are some crowding of the lung markings at the bases. Bronchography, involving the injection of a radio-opaque material into the bronchial tree, may be

necessary to confirm the diagnosis and to determine the extent of the condition. If apical disease is evident on chest X-ray the sputum should be sent for culture with tuberculosis and aspergillosis in mind.

Asthma (see also Dyspnoea, p. 240)

A dry persistent cough of no obvious cause for more than a month suggests the presence of asthma. It can occur at any age and the cough is often most troublesome at night. Many asthma patients are unaware that they have severe airways obstruction at rest, even when the FEV_1 is less than half the predicted value. In a series of 100 patients with asthma studied in an English general practice only 20% were initially recognised to have this disorder. 57% gave a history of a recurrent or nocturnal cough; the diagnosis was based on peak flow readings using a miniature Wright peak flow meter.

Asthma is a very common disease in children. In North Tyneside 11% of a sample of 7-year-old children had asthma, and in another study in Cumbria the prevalence in children under 16 years of age was 15.6%. There appears to be a reluctance on the part of both doctors and parents to use the term 'asthma', even when coughing is accompanied by obvious wheezing and dyspnoea on exertion.

Bronchial neoplasm

Aetiology

Cigarette smoking is the most important cause of lung cancer. It has been stated that 95% of cases are found in cigarette smokers and that the death rate in those who smoke more than 20 cigarettes a day is 40 times that of non-smokers. The risk of developing this disease is increased still further

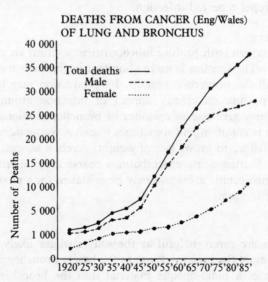

DEATHS FROM CANCER (Eng/Wales)
OF LUNG AND BRONCHUS

FIGURE 12

in those who inhale the smoke and have been smoking for more than 20 years. Of approximately 140 000 deaths from cancer of all causes in England and Wales each year this avoidable disease accounts for more than 35 000 cases, of whom the majority are men.

It is less certain, but likely, that the polluted atmosphere of towns and cities also has an influence on the production of lung cancer, and the role of industrial hazards, such as exposure to asbestos and radioactive chemicals, is well documented.

There are four main types of bronchial neoplasm. The commonest of these are squamous-cell and oat-cell carcinomas, which make up the great majority of growths in cigarette smokers. In non-smokers the predominant tumour is an adenocarcinoma which usually originates in the periphery of the lung and may grow to a considerable size before producing symptoms.

Clinical features
Lung cancer is uncommon before the age of 40 and the peak incidence in men occurs around the age of 65. By the time the tumour is discovered it has probably been present for several years. As the slender hope of cure rests upon the earliest possible diagnosis the various presentations are now detailed; they may be local, systemic or metastatic.

Local symptoms include cough, haemoptysis, dyspnoea and chest pain. Of these, cough is the commonest presenting symptom and may be associated with an influenza-like illness or pneumonia due to infection beyond the occluded bronchus. Any 'unresolved' pneumonia, particularly in a cigarette smoker, should be regarded with grave suspicion. Haemoptysis is rarely severe and may only amount to a little blood-tinged sputum. Dyspnoea on exertion is seen in about half the patients and is often out of proportion to the changes on a chest X-ray. Chest pain was the presenting symptom in one third of a series of 4000 cases; it may be nothing more than a diffuse aching in the chest wall on the side of the growth, or pleuritic in character from an obstructed pneumonia or invasion of the pleura. Unilateral wheezing is occasionally found from narrowing of a bronchus by the tumour.

Systemic manifestations include anorexia, debility, loss of weight, neuromyopathies, thrombophlebitis migrans, hypertrophic pulmonary osteoarthropathy and endocrine disorders due to ectopic hormone production. Oat-cell carcinomas may secrete ACTH, leading to gross adrenocortical over-activity, or cause the inappropriate secretion of ADH. Hypercalcaemia is found in about 6% of all patients with lung cancers and may be due to ectopic hormone production by the primary tumour, or to a local effect of metastases in bone.

Metastatic symptoms may arise from deposits in the liver, brain or bone. Thus the disease may present with a tender enlarged liver, epilepsy of late onset or spontaneous fractures. Intrathoracic spread may cause a recurrent laryngeal nerve palsy, superior vena caval obstruction, unilateral Horner's syndrome, brachial neuritis, pericarditis or chest pain from deposits in the ribs.

Findings in the lungs may be absent until, with increasing stenosis, wheezing becomes audible and stenosis or effusion develops. Finger clubbing and enlargement of the lymph nodes, particularly in the neck, appear late in the disease. Hepatic enlargement should be sought and thrombophlebitis in the limbs is sometimes an early sign.

Investigations

A chest X-ray commonly provides the first evidence but in one series half the cases showed no abnormality within 6 months of death. The films may reveal a round shadow in the periphery of the lung, collapse or consolidation of a lobe or segment, an increase in the hilar or mediastinal shadows or a pleural effusion. A necrotic squamous cell carcinoma may be indistinguishable from a lung abscess. Bronchoscopy will enable bronchial brushings to be taken for cytology and biopsy of the tumour itself if it can be seen through the bronchoscope.

In the absence of a positive identification it may be necessary to proceed to a scalene node or liver biopsy, to confirm the diagnosis and determine the cell type. The cell type will have some influence on the management of the case. Bone, brain and liver scans are sometimes called for to establish the presence of metastases.

CAUSES IN THE LUNGS

In lung disease the cough reflex may be provoked by stimulation of the irritant receptors in the larger bronchi, by retained secretions or distension of the stretch receptors situated in the distal airways and interstitial tissues of the lung.

Pneumonia (see also Fever, p. 317)

An unproductive cough is common at the onset of both lobar and bronchopneumonia. In the former it may be painful, from inflammation of the pleura, and is soon accompanied by much purulent sputum, which may be bloodstained. Pleural involvement is unusual in bronchopneumonia, so the cough is usually painless in this type. Bronchopneumonia is seen mainly in the elderly and in patients with pre-existing pulmonary disease. The nature and amount of sputum will vary with the infecting agent: It is usually purulent in bacterial infections but may be scanty or even absent in pneumonia due to non-bacterial organisms.

Abscess

This may result from aspiration of infected matter or necrosis in a bronchial carcinoma. More frequently however it is a complication of a suppurative pneumonia, due as a rule to *Klebsiella* or staphylococcal infection. It should be suspected if the pneumonia fails to respond to appropriate antibiotic therapy and coughing is precipitated by a change in posture. The production of large amounts of foul-smelling pus suggests a secondary infection with anaerobic organisms.

The diagnosis can only be made by chest X-ray, which shows one or more cavities on the film. Bronchoscopy will be necessary to exclude a bronchial neoplasm or the presence of a foreign body. It has the further advantage of permitting drainage of the abscess and collecting pus which is not contaminated by organisms in the upper respiratory tract.

Tuberculosis (see also Fever, p. 325)

Cough, mucoid sputum and sometimes haemoptysis are usually accompanied by general symptoms such as fever, night sweats, malaise and loss of weight. On the other hand the disease may be indolent, with cough as the only prominent symptom. Apical shadowing is usually evident on chest X-ray and cavitation may be seen. Tubercle bacilli may be found in the sputum or grown on Löwenstein–Jensen cultures.

Fibrosis

Diffuse fibrosis in the interstitial tissues of the lungs has many causes. Occupational hazards include prolonged exposure to coal dust, silica, asbestos and the thermophilic *Actinomycetes* in mouldy hay responsible for farmer's lung. It may occur occasionally as a side-effect of drugs such as nitrofurantoin and busulphan or follow ionising radiation. It is seen in sarcoidosis and in cryptogenic fibrosing alveolitis which may be associated with the connective tissue diseases. All these conditions give rise to a persistent cough, but since dyspnoea is the most striking symptom they are considered in more detail in the following chapter.

Embolism (see also Thoracic pain, p. 30)

Cough is a minor feature of this condition being overshadowed by pleuritic pain, shortness of breath and bloody sputum.

Cardiac failure

In left ventricular failure the paroxysmal dyspnoea of 'cardiac' asthma results from pulmonary oedema. It occurs characteristically at night and is accompanied by cough and frothy blood-tinged sputum. Wheezing is not uncommon. There is often a history of valvular or ischaemic heart disease, or of pre-existing hypertension.

CHAPTER 20
Dyspnoea

SYNOPSIS OF CAUSES*

RESPIRATORY
Laryngeal obstruction; Epiglottitis; **Asthma; Bronchitis; Emphysema; Neoplasm; Pneumonia; Pneumothorax; Pleural effusion; Adult respiratory distress syndrome; Pneumoconiosis**; Extrinsic & cryptogenic fibrosing alveolitis; Sarcoidosis.

CARDIOVASCULAR
Heart failure; Ischaemia; Myocardial infarction; Valvular disease; Congenital heart disease; Pericarditis; **Pulmonary embolism**.

GENERAL
Drugs; **Hyperthyroidism**; Addison's disease; Renal failure; Anxiety state.

* Bold type is used for causes more commonly found in Europe and North America.

PHYSIOLOGY

The purpose of respiration is to supply oxygen to and remove carbon dioxide from the blood. This exchange is effected in the alveoli and the rhythmic activity of breathing is maintained by the respiratory centre in the midbrain. It is sensitive to variations in the blood levels of these gases and to the rise in hydrogen ion concentration which occurs in metabolic acidosis.

Dyspnoea or breathlessness may be defined as an uncomfortable aware-ness of the act of breathing irrespective of its rate or depth. It normally accompanies effort and only becomes significant when the exertion has not previously caused it in the individual concerned. It may be brought on by an increased demand for oxygen or failure of some part of the respira-tory apparatus to deliver it.

Increased demand accounts for the breathlessness associated with exer-cise, anaemia, hyperthyroidism and lack of oxygen at high altitudes. That caused by faulty performance may be due to neuromuscular disorders such as poliomyelitis affecting the respiratory muscles, obstruction to the air flow in the bronchial tree, abnormal stiffness of the lungs or impaired gas exchange in the alveoli. No single mechanism or pathway is responsible for this sensation. The signals which give rise to it probably originate in stretch receptors in the chest wall and lungs and are carried to the brain in afferent fibres of both somatic and autonomic nerves. In some patients fatigue of the respiratory muscles may play a part.

The degree of breathlessness does not always reflect the gravity of the illness. Thus the hyperventilation caused by metabolic acidosis in diabetes and renal failure is not necessarily accompanied by any complaint of dyspnoea, provided that the patient's lungs are healthy. Similarly, some asthmatics develop tolerance to their airways obstruction and are unaware of the severity of their condition.

Although respiration is a rhythmic involuntary process it is highly subject to voluntary control and the play of emotion. Patients with anxiety states often complain of dyspnoea, and frequent sighing may be described by them as breathlessness.

DIAGNOSTIC APPROACH

This will vary with the mode of onset and age of the patient. Sudden breathlessness may result from a spontaneous pneumothorax, pulmonary embolus, myocardial infarction, rapidly forming pleural effusion or obstruction by a foreign body in the air passages. Paroxysmal bouts of dyspnoea are usually due to asthma and may be precipitated by an upper respiratory infection, exertion, emotional upsets or exposure to a potential allergen. In both children and adults it may be accompanied by a troublesome cough, particularly at night. Progressive dyspnoea, at first only on exertion, is commonly due to chronic bronchitis and emphysema, diffuse pulmonary fibrosis or ischaemic heart disease.

In childhood acute respiratory infections and asthma are the commonest causes, but an inhaled foreign body is always a possibility in the very young. Extrinsic asthma should be suspected in any child with a wheezy bronchitis which does not respond to adequate antibiotic treatment. Cyanosis and clubbing of the fingers would point to a congenital cardiac disorder such as Fallot's tetralogy.

When taking a history in adults it is very important to enquire about previous illnesses, drugs recently taken, smoking habits, hobbies and occupations. A sudden onset with chest pain in a healthy young man is probably caused by a spontaneous pneumothorax, but similar symptoms in a woman on the contraceptive pill or during the last trimester of pregnancy are more likely to be due to pulmonary embolism. The inhalation of fumes or dust at work in susceptible individuals may provoke attacks of occupational asthma or the insidious pulmonary fibrosis of extrinsic fibrosing alveolitis. Farm workers and bird fanciers are obvious victims but many others work in environments where exposure to industrial dusts is commonplace. Miners, stonemasons, foundrymen, sandblasters and those who work with asbestos in one form or another are liable to develop pneumoconiosis, and massive fibrosis may occur long after they have moved to safer occupations.

Cigarette smoking may exacerbate these dust diseases, quite apart from its role in causing chronic bronchitis and emphysema.

With advancing age, cardiovascular causes assume increasing importance. A history of rheumatic fever in childhood would point to mitral or aortic valvular disease, while a sudden onset with chest pain is likely to be due to myocardial ischaemia or pulmonary embolism. Breathlessness on exertion may first manifest itself by difficulty in climbing stairs or going up an incline. Orthopnoea, that is to say dyspnoea at rest, is seen in severe cardiac failure and chronic respiratory disease and by the time this occurs the patient is usually cyanosed and seriously disabled. The effect of anaemia, hypertension and thyroid disorders in precipitating heart failure in the elderly should not be forgotten.

Associated symptoms must be noted, because they often point to the most probable cause. Chest pain, as a rule, is prominent in myocardial infarction, pulmonary embolism, pleurisy and pneumothorax. Cough, haemoptysis and fever may be present in both respiratory and cardiac disorders. In chronic heart failure there may be upper abdominal discomfort from congestion of the liver along with swelling of the legs. Palpitations, sweating and tremor of the outstretched hands are not uncommon in anxiety states but the presence of a goitre or a history of thyroid disease in the patient or close relative should suggest hyperthyroidism, which can have an insidious onset in the elderly. Loss of weight is usually indicative of a serious underlying disorder — and gross obesity in itself may sufficiently account for some dyspnoea on exertion.

The extent of the physical examination will obviously depend upon the circumstances but should always involve a thorough examination of the chest and the cardiovascular system. Clubbing of the fingers is seen in congenital heart disease, bacterial endocarditis, bronchiectasis, bronchial carcinoma, tuberculosis and disorders which give rise to progressive pulmonary fibrosis.

Investigations
The history and physical examination should have provided a lead as to which physiological system is involved — in most cases the respiratory or cardiovascular system. A preliminary blood count will exclude severe anaemia as a cause and leukocytosis will point to infection.

An electrocardiogram is essential if dyspnoea is thought to be of cardiac origin. This may need to be repeated if the initial trace is equivocal, particularly if the patient is thought to have had a recent myocardial infarction. It may, however, be completely normal following a quite massive pulmonary embolus. A chest X-ray will reveal an increase in cardiac size or any alteration in its outline.

In acute respiratory disorders a chest X-ray is rarely indicated unless there is some indication of lung involvement. It is, however, essential if the dyspnoea is of long standing. Sputum, when present, must be examined and cultured before any antibiotic therapy is started. If tuberculosis is suspected acid-fast bacilli should be looked for in the sputum or laryngeal swab and Löwenstein–Jensen cultures requested on at least three early morning specimens.

Bronchoscopy will be indicated in the case of a suspected inhaled foreign body or bronchial neoplasm. In an obscure case of pulmonary fibrosis or pleural effusion it may be necessary to proceed to lung or pleural biopsy in order to establish a diagnosis. Occasionally an enlarged lymph node in the supraclavicular fossa may provide histological evidence of tuberculosis, neoplasm or sarcoidosis.

Lung-function studies are of considerable value in diagnosing some respiratory disorders and in evaluating their response to treatment. A simple bedside spirometer, such as the vitalograph, may be used to estimate the vital capacity and forced expiratory volume in one second (FEV_1). Normally 70–80% of the vital capacity should be expelled smoothly and rapidly in this time interval. In obstructive airways disease the FEV_1 is usually less than 70% of the vital capacity and may be as little as 40%. It is thus a measure of the degree of obstruction to expiration.

Another useful means of assessing respiratory function, particularly in general practice, is the Wright peak flowmeter, which measures the maximum expiratory flow rate at the beginning of expiration; the results correlate closely with the FEV_1. Measurement of the transfer factor for carbon monoxide, a non-invasive method of determining the overall efficiency of gas exchange in the lungs, can only be carried out in a pulmonary function laboratory. Arterial blood gas analysis in experienced hands will provide direct evidence of inadequate alveolar ventilation; a raised P_aCO_2 is indicative of carbon dioxide retention whilst a low P_aO_2 is a measure of the degree of hypoxia.

Finally, when presented with an obscure case of dyspnoea the possibility of a metabolic disorder such as thyrotoxicosis, Addison's disease or uraemia should not be forgotten and appropriate investigations should be undertaken.

RESPIRATORY CAUSES

These may obstruct the flow of gases in the air passages, interfere with their exchange in the alveoli or cause splinting and loss of elasticity in the lungs. Breathlessness may result from stimulation of the stretch receptors in the thorax or from the direct effect of hypoxia and CO_2 retention on the respiratory centre.

Laryngeal obstruction

A foreign body is the commonest cause of acute obstruction of the larynx. In one series of 292 cases it was found that 265 occurred in children, most of them under the age of 2. In 124 children the object turned out to be a peanut. In the 27 adults the chief causes were small bones and tooth plates.

Complete obstruction without prompt removal or tracheotomy is rapidly fatal. Partial obstruction is much more common and presents with urgent cough, stridor, choking and violent inspiratory effort.

Obstruction may also occur in acute laryngotracheitis, epiglottitis and the rarely seen laryngeal diphtheria. Oedema of the larynx, along with bronchospasm, may be part of an anaphylactic reaction to insect stings, drugs or foreign sera. Sudden spasm in tetanus is a rare cause, but paralysis of both vocal cords may occur in motor neurone disease or as a complication of poliomyelitis. Obstruction due to an invasive thyroid cancer is self-evident but may require tracheotomy for relief.

A large foreign body passing through the larynx is likely to occlude the right main or lower bronchus, which are nearly in line with the trachea. Acute dyspnoea follows and collapse of the lung occurs. The inhalation of vomit in the anaesthetised patient or coma from other causes may also result in massive collapse, but the patient is not in a position to complain of breathlessness! Bronchoscopy will determine the site and probable nature of the occlusion.

Acute epiglottitis

This potentially fatal disorder of childhood is caused by *Haemophilus influenzae* infection, and is seen in children under 3 years of age. Unlike acute laryngotracheitis there is no cough, but the child is obviously ill, with a high fever, dyspnoea and stridor. The disorder can be recognised by the posture of the patient — the child sits with neck extended, unable to breathe properly and drooling secretions from the mouth.

This is a medical emergency and acute respiratory obstruction may be precipitated by examination of the throat or attempts to take lateral X-rays of the neck. The cherry-red epiglottitis will be visible on direct laryngoscopy when the child is being intubated under general anaesthesia in the theatre; immediate tracheotomy may be necessary if there is any difficulty in passing an endotracheal tube. Recovery usually begins within hours of starting appropriate antibiotic therapy.

Asthma

Aetiology

The airways obstruction in asthma is due to a variable combination of bronchospasm, inflammation of the bronchial walls and plugging of the distal air passages by intraluminal secretions and epithelial debris. Although many different mechanisms have been invoked to explain these changes they probably all act ultimately by causing the release of chemical mediators such as histamine and leukotrienes from the mast cells in the lung.

In extrinsic asthma the degranulation of the mast cells is provoked by the inhalation of a wide variety of common allergens. These include house dust and the house dust mite, pollens, dander from household pets and horses, feathers, *Aspergillus fumigatus* and other moulds. Occasionally, patients are found to be allergic to milk, egg or fish proteins ingested as food. Drugs are a rare cause, with the exception of aspirin and other non-steroidal anti-inflammatory drugs.

Extrinsic asthma usually presents in childhood in atopic individuals and is frequently associated with other allergic manifestations such as eczema, rhinitis and hay fever in the patient or other members of the family. It is commoner in boys and may remit spontaneously at puberty.

Occupational asthma is a form of extrinsic asthma provoked by exposure to dust or fumes at work. Over 200 agents have been identified as causing it in susceptible subjects. These include substances such as di-isocyanates, platinum salts, formaldehyde, epoxy-resin curing agents, antibiotics, biological detergents, colophony used in solder flux, grain and wood dusts. Occupational asthma may occur as a result of irritation of the bronchi in an individual with a pre-existing tendency to bronchial hyperreactivity or result from a specific sensitisation to a particular substance. The symptoms may remit completely if exposure ceases but this is by no means invariable.

When no external stimulant can be identified the term 'intrinsic asthma' is used to describe the condition. This begins in adult life and sometimes follows viral or bacterial infections of the respiratory tract. It is often called 'late-onset' asthma and may present for the first time in the elderly without any previous history of respiratory disease.

Clinical features
The acute attack is sudden in onset and may be triggered off by respiratory infections, inhalation of acrid fumes or smoke, exercise, emotional disturbances and the administration of beta-blocking drugs such as propranolol. It frequently occurs at night and a persistent non-productive cough may waken the patient from sleep. In older children and adults this is usually accompanied by wheezing and a sense of impending suffocation. The average attack lasts an hour or two, unless relieved earlier by bronchodilator drugs, and ends with the expectoration of a small quantity of thick, tenacious sputum. Exercise-induced asthma characteristically begins a few minutes after the activity has ceased.

If the attack lasts many hours the patient becomes increasingly breathless as the terminal bronchioles become blocked by plugs of inspissated mucus. Such an episode can cause death within a few hours unless the obstruction is relieved by vigorous physiotherapy, bronchodilators, rehydration and parenteral corticosteroids. About 1500 sufferers still die annually in Britain through failure of both patients and doctors to appreciate the severity of an attack and to take appropriate measures to bring it to an end.

During an acute bout the patient will be sitting upright or leaning forward in order to make maximum use of the accessory muscles of respiration. Expiration will be prolonged and wheezing may be audible. On auscultation widespread sibilant rhonchi will be heard throughout the lungs. Cyanosis is uncommon except in status asthmaticus when the obstruction may be so severe that the breath sounds are inaudible. Tachycardia, pulsus paradoxus, indrawing of the intercostal spaces during inspiration and physical or mental exhaustion justify admission to hospital.

In some asthmatics, particularly those with the extrinsic type, there may be no symptoms or signs between paroxysms. Others are less fortunate and remain in a state of chronic airways obstruction which is exacerbated by exertion, heavy meals or psychological stress. Such individuals are often labelled as suffering from 'wheezy' bronchitis, for there is a reluctance amongst patients and doctors to accept the diagnosis of asthma and the need for specific treatment.

Investigation
Eosinophilia in the blood or sputum may be helpful in differentiating asthma from bronchitis; it is not confined to those with the extrinsic form. If the sputum looks purulent it should be cultured both for bacteria and moulds. Skin-prick tests will be positive to one or more of the common allergens in atopic individuals. Negative skin tests are common in non-atopic patients and are invariable in those with intrinsic asthma.

In an uncomplicated case chest X-rays will be normal or merely show some hyperinflation of the lungs. If this appearance persists between attacks it indicates some degree of chronic airways obstruction. In allergic bronchopulmonary aspergillosis transient lung shadows may be seen, particularly in the upper lobes.

Objective measurements of lung function can be obtained by using a Wright peak flow meter or portable spirometer. Serial recordings are very useful in assessing the degree of airways obstruction and its response to treatment with bronchodilator drugs and corticosteroids. In severe attacks the measurement of arterial blood gases may be necessary to determine the degree of hypoxaemia and CO_2 retention, particularly if mechanical ventilation is thought necessary.

Bronchitis (see also Cough, p. 230)

The dyspnoea of bronchitis is due to narrowing of the airways by swelling and thickening of the bronchial wall and the presence of retained secretions, commonly accompanied by some degree of bronchial spasm. In chronic bronchitis these changes may eventually lead to emphysema, pulmonary hypertension and cardiac failure.

Emphysema

Aetiology
Pulmonary emphysema may occur as a primary condition but a mixed picture of chronic bronchitis and emphysema is much commoner than the occurrence of either condition alone. It probably results from the destructive effect of proteolytic enzymes such as neutrophil elastase on lung tissue and is much more prevalent in cigarette smokers, particularly those with a homozygous alpha$_1$-antitrypsin deficiency. Destruction of the alveolar walls leads to a reduced number of enlarged air spaces with progressive obliteration of the vascular bed.

Clinical features

In primary emphysema there is but one symptom, dyspnoea, coming at first on exertion and ultimately at rest. In the commoner variety associated with chronic bronchitis this will be accompanied by wheezing and a productive cough. In the early stages there may be little to find apart from occasional rhonchi and diminished breath sounds on auscultation. As the disease progresses there will be gross overinflation of the lungs and laboured breathing may be evident, even at rest. The chest movements will be limited, the breath sounds inaudible and central cyanosis may be present.

Investigations

The blood count is usually normal but a secondary polycythaemia is not uncommon in cyanosed patients; a raised serum bicarbonate level is evidence of CO_2 retention. The chest X-ray may be entirely normal to begin with but, as the disease advances, will show overinflation of the lungs, flattening of the diaphragms and attenuation of the vessels at the periphery. Large bullae may be seen, particularly at the bases. Spirometry will record a diminution of vital capacity and FEV_1. A low transfer factor for carbon monoxide will confirm the impaired exchange of gases in the lungs, but this cannot be measured accurately if the vital capacity is less than one litre. Arterial blood gas analysis may be necessary to determine the degree of hypoxia and to study the effect of treatment.

Neoplasm (see also Cough, p. 232)

Whilst cough and discomfort in the chest are usually the earliest symptoms of a bronchial carcinoma it should be realised that dyspnoea may be present long before complete occlusion of the bronchus takes place. This may be due to infection distal to the growth or to a pleural effusion. Occasionally lung metastases from breast, kidney or prostate may present with increasing breathlessness on exertion in an otherwise symptomless patient.

Pneumonia (see also Fever, p. 317)

Dyspnoea is a characteristic feature of all pneumonias; its severity depends upon the amount of lung involved. It is usually present at rest and may be increased on exertion for some weeks following recovery. In the elderly the onset may be insidious and without fever. There may be no symptoms for a long time in pulmonary tuberculosis but dyspnoea is sometimes out of proportion to the physical signs.

Pneumothorax (see also Thoracic pain, p. 31)

The sudden onset of breathlessness in this disorder is usually overshadowed by severe chest pain. It is seen mainly in healthy young men and the diagnosis is usually obvious from examining the chest, and confirmed by

X-ray. It can however occur from rupture of a bulla in an emphysematous patient and should always be considered if there is a sudden worsening in their condition.

Pleural effusion

Aetiology
The commonest cause of a pleural effusion, which is often bilateral, is congestive cardiac failure. Other conditions which give rise to a transudate are ascites, usually associated with cirrhosis of the liver, and the nephrotic syndrome. Exudates are most frequently produced by inflammation or malignancy. They are usually unilateral and may complicate pneumonia, tuberculosis, subphrenic abscess, pulmonary embolism or systemic lupus erythematosus. Alternatively, they may result from invasion of the pleura by dissemination of lymphoproliferative disorders or metastases from such neoplasms as breast, bronchial, ovarian or prostatic carcinomas. Frank blood in the pleural fluid may result from trauma or the presence of a mesothelioma.

Clinical features
Dyspnoea is the prominent symptom, though in some cases it may be preceded by pleuritic pain. On examination there will be diminished or absent movement on the affected side with dullness to percussion and reduced or absent vocal fremitus. Breath sounds will be absent on auscultation and aegophony will indicate the upper level of the effusion. Accompanying signs and symptoms will depend upon the causal condition.

Investigations
Chest X-rays will confirm the presence of fluid and indicate the site for aspiration. Removal of the fluid may help in diagnosis or be done to relieve the breathlessness. Transudates have a total protein content of less than 30 grams per litre and a low white cell count, whilst exudates have a higher protein content and may be frankly purulent. If tuberculosis is suspected a specimen should be sent for Löwenstein–Jensen culture; acid-fast bacilli are rarely seen in the pleural fluid. In an obscure case only pleural biopsy may provide the diagnosis.

Adult respiratory distress syndrome

This is the commonest and most serious respiratory complication in severely ill or injured patients. The aetiology of 'shock lung' is unknown but it results in pulmonary capillary damage and increased capillary permeability. If the patient survives the profound hypoxaemia they may end up with widespread pulmonary fibrosis. The mortality rate is over 50% despite respiratory support with intermittent positive pressure respiration. Chest X-rays will show diffuse bilateral infiltrates. Recovery depends upon the prompt treatment of the underlying cause; in some cases there is evidence of fat embolism, disseminated intravascular coagulation or aspiration pneumonitis.

Pneumoconioses

The term 'pneumoconiosis' is confined to lung disease resulting from the inhalation of inorganic dust. Only small particles are likely to reach the alveoli, where they are engulfed by macrophages in an attempt to remove them. The release of chemicals by the damaged macrophage is thought to provoke the fibrous reaction which may eventually lead to massive pulmonary fibrosis.

The commonest of these conditions in Britain is caused by exposure to coal dust, but the clinical course of *coalworker's pneumoconiosis* is very varied. In many miners it produces few symptoms, even after years of exposure, its presence being detected radiologically by the appearance of numerous small nodular opacities 2–5 mm in diameter in the lungs. Dyspnoea on exertion in many of these cases of so-called 'simple' pneumoconiosis is probably due to other causes such as chronic bronchitis associated with cigarette smoking.

In a minority the lesions increase in size and may occupy as much as one-third of the area of the lungs. These patients become progressively more short of breath as the result of massive pulmonary fibrosis and consequent emphysema. This is more likely to occur if the coal dust contains a high proportion of silica.

Caplan's syndrome is an unusual form of massive fibrosis which occurs in individuals with rheumatoid arthritis or a positive rheumatoid factor; the fibrotic lesions in these patients often cavitate and have the histological appearance of rheumatoid nodules.

Silicosis may develop in foundrymen, tool grinders, stonemasons and sandblasters. The radiological picture is similar to that seen in coalworker's pneumoconiosis but is more likely to progress to massive fibrosis, despite removal from the dusty environment. It has become infrequent in recent years because the hazard has been recognised and precautions have been taken. Pulmonary tuberculosis is a recognised complication of this disease.

Asbestosis is caused by the inhalation of asbestos dust. The substance is widely used in the manufacture of fireproof and insulating material as in ship building, roofing and the lining of clutches and brakes. The inhaled fibres provoke fibrosis in the alveoli and may reach the pleura. The process starts in the lower lobes and spreads diffusely to involve the rest of the lung. Breathlessness on exertion is the most prominent symptom and may be accompanied by a productive cough. Apart from the workers themselves the condition has been reported in close relatives and others living in the vicinity of a mine or factory where asbestos is being processed.

There is an increased risk of bronchial cancer in asbestos workers and their relatives, particularly if they smoke cigarettes, and pleural mesotheliomas develop in a high proportion of those exposed to this dust. Epidemiological studies also reveal an increased incidence of cancers of the stomach, larynx, ovary and breast. Chest X-rays may show a bilateral ground-glass appearance in the lower lobes, streaky reticular shadowing, a honeycomb appearance or a shaggy outline to the heart; calcification of the pleura and pericardium may be seen. Asbestos bodies and fibres in the sputum provide evidence of exposure to this toxic substance.

Extrinsic fibrosing alveolitis

Aetiology

This is a pneumonitis caused by an allergic reaction to a wide variety of allergens in inhaled organic dust. Initially this results in acute inflammation of the alveoli and surrounding interstitial tissue with narrowing and obstruction of the respiratory bronchioles. These changes usually resolve spontaneously provided that there is no further exposure to the allergen.

Repeated exposure however will result in the formation of non-caseating granulomata with consequent pulmonary fibrosis. Common examples of this condition are *farmer's lung*, caused by the inhalation of thermophilic *Actinomycetes* or fungal spores in mouldy hay, and *bird fanciers' lung*, where the antigen is avian protein contained in the 'bloom' on the feathers or in the excreta. It has also been reported in workers exposed to malt in whisky production, mushroom compost, mouldy sugar cane, cork dust, maple bark and grain contaminated by the grain weevil.

Clinical features

This disorder should be suspected in any individual who complains of acute dyspnoea some 4–8 hours after exposure to an organic dust. It is usually accompanied by fever, chills and general malaise and may be mistaken for a viral or *Mycoplasma* pneumonia. In farm workers an acute onset often follows forking hay or other mouldy feedstuffs during the winter months when the cattle are confined indoors. A similar acute illness may be seen in pigeon fanciers exposed to intermittent high concentrations of avian protein when cleaning out the lofts.

Pulmonary fibrosis due to repeated exposure to low doses of the antigen is much more insidious in onset. By the time the patient presents with increasing shortness of breath the condition may be irreversible. The diagnosis is likely to be overlooked unless a detailed account of the patient's occupation and hobbies is obtained. On examination crepitations will be heard in the middle and lower zones of the lungs. Clubbing is uncommon, but cyanosis and signs of heart failure may be present in the advanced case.

Investigations

Chest X-rays may be normal following acute exposure but as the condition progresses nodular shadows, reticular markings and cystic changes appear. Precipitin tests may help to determine the cause. They are positive for *Micropolyspora faeni* in most cases of farmer's lung.

Cryptogenic fibrosing alveolitis

Pulmonary fibrosis in which no causal agent can be identified is seen in late middle-age. It is often associated with other diseases much as rheumatoid arthritis, systemic lupus erythematosus, Sjögren's syndrome, polymyositis, chronic active hepatitis and ulcerative colitis. Circulating immune complexes have been found in some patients and IgG and complement have been demonstrated in lung tissue by immunofluorescence.

Dyspnoea is increasingly easily provoked and may be accompanied by an unproductive cough. Central cyanosis at rest, clubbing of the fingers and toes and congestive cardiac failure are late signs. On auscultation showers of fine inspiratory crepitations will be heard at the bases.

Chest X-rays will usually reveal small irregular opacities or a ground-glass appearance, particularly in the lower lobes. Pulmonary function tests will show a marked reduction in transfer factor, vital capacity and FEV_1. An open-lung biopsy may enable this condition to be distinguished from other causes of pulmonary fibrosis such as sarcoidosis, but this procedure is not without risk. Tests for rheumatoid factor and antinuclear antibodies are positive in many patients, even in the absence of disease outside the chest.

Sarcoidosis

Aetiology

This widespread granulomatous disease of unknown aetiology may affect any organ in the body. It is slightly more common in women, particularly in those of childbearing age, and the majority of cases present before the age of 40. Although no antigen has been identified there is evidence of impaired cellular immunity in some patients and circulating immune complexes have been detected during the acute phase of the illness. The fact that the lungs and intrathoracic lymph nodes are the tissues most commonly involved suggests that the causative agent probably enters the body through the respiratory tract. In a world-wide series of nearly 4000 cases an abnormal chest X-ray was present in 92%; of these, half showed bilateral hilar shadows only without any radiological evidence of pulmonary infiltration.

Sarcoidosis may affect the skin, eyes, skeleton, nervous system and myocardium. Granulomas are frequently present in the liver but rarely cause hepatic dysfunction. Hypercalcaemia is sometimes seen, particularly during the summer months, but hypercalciuria is even commoner and is caused by the enhanced absorption of calcium in the small bowel. Both these abnormalities are probably due to hypersensitivity to vitamin D.

Clinical features

These will obviously depend upon the organs which are affected. Enlarged hilar shadows on a routine chest X-ray are often the first evidence of the disease. Their presence may be associated with an acute onset of malaise, slight fever, erythema nodosum on the shins and a transient arthralgia. There are unlikely to be any respiratory symptoms unless the lungs are involved. Spontaneous recovery is the rule, though the radiological abnormalities may take a year or two to disappear.

The gradual onset of increasing dyspnoea, often without any history of a preceding acute illness, is seen in those with pulmonary infiltration. This may be accompanied by a dry unproductive cough and central cyanosis. Apart from scattered crepitations there will be little to find in the chest. In the later stages finger clubbing may develop. Death may result from respiratory failure, cor pulmonale or a massive haemoptysis from an aspergilloma in the damaged lung. Sarcoidosis of the upper respiratory tract is rare and presents with hoarseness, stridor or dyspnoea; it is usually accompanied by lupus pernio.

Investigations

Chest X-rays commonly show hilar enlargement and this may be accompanied by diffuse miliary nodules or larger, irregular shadows with a more uneven distribution. A Mantoux test is usually negative. The ESR is often elevated when the disease is active, and an increased level of serum angiotensin-converting enzyme is found in about 60% of cases. Pulmonary function studies will show a restrictive defect in ventilatory function with a low transfer factor. Biopsy of liver, lung, lymph node or skin at the site of a Kveim test may show sarcoid tissue. The test itself is positive in about 70% of cases untreated with corticosteroids. Hypercalcaemia should be excluded especially if there is any evidence of renal impairment.

CARDIOVASCULAR CAUSES

The heart is a muscular pump which discharges its contents into the pulmonary and systemic systems against resistance. Failure may be said to have begun when the circulation is no longer adequately maintained and blood accumulates behind the failing ventricle.

Failure of the organ as a whole sometimes occurs acutely in a previously healthy heart as in the myocarditis of rheumatic fever or diphtheria. In most cases, however, it begins on one side or the other of a heart which is already the seat of chronic disease. Failure is commonly precipitated by an extra-cardiac cause such as anaemia, intercurrent infection, hypertension or pulmonary embolism.

Heart failure

In left ventricular failure breathlessness is the earliest symptom to appear. It is due to pulmonary oedema which may be confined to the interstitial tissues. In hypertension, cardiomyopathy and valvular disease the onset of failure may be very gradual. The patient adjusts to its first appearance during some customary exertion by reducing activity; it may be many months before increasing dyspnoea brings him to the doctor.

In contrast to this the onset may be acute as in myocardial infarction or paroxysmal nocturnal dyspnoea. In an attack of 'cardiac asthma' the patient is suddenly awakened by urgent breathlessness and may struggle to the window for more air. Wheezing is often present and some frothy and blood-stained fluid may be coughed up. Pallor, cyanosis and sweating are accompanied by tachycardia and crepitations at the lung bases. The attack usually subsides in an hour or so but can be relieved earlier by the intravenous administration of opiates, aminophylline or diuretics. The use of diuretics carries some risk, in an elderly man with an enlarged prostate, of precipitating acute retention of urine the following morning.

Right ventricular failure is due, most often, to preceding left ventricular failure and its causes. The term *cor pulmonale* refers to right heart failure resulting from pulmonary hypertension due to various lung disorders such as pulmonary embolism, chronic bronchitis, emphysema, fibrosing alveolitis and the pneumoconioses. Excessive retention of salt and water by the kidneys results in oedema of the legs and, in the bedfast patient, over the sacrum. The congested liver is usually palpable and often tender; faint icterus may be present. The rise in peripheral venous pressure is evident in the distended jugular veins. The height of venous pulsations above the manubrium sterni should be measured with the patient reclining at an angle of 45°.

Ischaemia (see also Thoracic pain, p. 32)

With increasing age the blood supply of the myocardium is progressively impaired with consequent hypoxia of the ventricular muscle. This is mainly due to atherosclerosis of the coronary arteries and may be accelerated by the presence of hypertension, diabetes mellitus or hypothyroidism. Rarely it may be due to inflammation of the coronary arteries, as in polyarteritis nodosa, or to a viral myocarditis. The main symptoms are dyspnoea and anginal pain which are induced by exertion. They occur more readily in the presence of anaemia, thyrotoxicosis, hypothyroidism and abnormalities of cardiac rhythm.

Myocardial infarction (see also Thoracic pain, p. 34)

Left ventricular failure accounts for the acute shortness of breath and tightness in the chest which accompany and sometimes overshadow the characteristic chest pain.

In the elderly dyspnoea alone is the presenting symptom in some 30% of cases. Such premonitory symptoms as readily-induced fatigue and shortness of breath may not uncommonly precede the event. Needless to say these are usually elicited in retrospect and may be found to have been present for weeks or even months.

The diagnosis is readily confirmed as a rule by serial ECGs, supported if necessary by serum enzyme estimations.

Valvular disease

Aortic stenosis is usually a sequel of rheumatic fever but may be congenital or atheromatous in origin. With the onset of left ventricular failure dyspnoea appears. Inadequate filling of coronary and cerebral vessels leads to anginal pain and syncopal attacks. A harsh systolic murmur is maximal to the left of the sternum and is often clearly audible at the apex and in the neck.

Mitral stenosis is the commonest sequel of rheumatic myocarditis and is sometimes accompanied by regurgitation. The raised pressure in the left atrium leads to pulmonary hypertension and slowly increasing dyspnoea begins years after the initial attack of rheumatic fever. Cough and haemoptyses are common and a malar flush is characteristic. The heart is not enlarged in the absence of regurgitation, but a diastolic thrill may be felt at the apex and a diastolic murmur follows the opening snap of the mitral valve; these may disappear with the onset of atrial fibrillation.

X-rays will show enlargement of the left atrium and dilatation of the main pulmonary artery will give a straight line appearance to the left border of the heart. Calcification of the mitral valve may be seen on a PA film.

Congenital heart disease

This is a fairly rare cause of dyspnoea; congenital cardiac abnormalities occur in about one in 100 births. When the defects are multiple, as in Fallot's tetralogy, the child is cyanosed and dyspnoeic; without surgical treatment survival to adult life is unlikely.

The forms most likely to be encountered otherwise are patent ductus arteriosus, coarctation of the aorta, pulmonary stenosis and septal defects. In mild cases symptoms may be absent for many years. In others bacterial endocarditis may supervene or evidence of cardiac failure appears as dyspnoea. Surgical treatment is often curative.

Pericarditis (see also Thoracic pain, p. 36)

This may be due to viral infection, myocardial infarction, rheumatic fever, tuberculosis, malignant infiltration, connective tissue disease or renal failure. Pain is the cardinal symptom and dyspnoea is only conspicuous when a pericardial effusion is present.

As the intrapericardial pressure rises ventricular filling is impaired and may lead to cardiac tamponade. This is a life-threatening situation which may end in cardiac arrest unless the pressure is promptly relieved by pericardial aspiration.

The most important physical signs of this condition are a raised jugular venous pressure and a paradoxical arterial pulse which diminishes in volume and may even disappear during inspiration.

Constrictive pericarditis rarely ends in heart failure but breathlessness is common and orthopnoea is present in about 20% of cases. It may result from blunt trauma to the chest, tuberculosis, lymphoproliferative disorders, radiation fibrosis and, very occasionally, mixed connective tissue disease. Patients frequently complain of a feeling of congestion in the head when bending forward. Clinical findings include a raised jugular venous pressure and systolic retraction of the ribs in the left axilla (Broadbent's sign).

Pericardial calcification on a chest X-ray is pathognomonic of this condition but is present in only one third of cases; it is not necessarily due to tuberculosis. An ECG will show low voltage QRS complexes in the chest leads, and paradoxical ventricular septal motion on echocardiography is said to be a constant finding.

Pulmonary embolism (see also Thoracic pain, p. 30)

The sudden onset of dyspnoea in those confined to bed with heart failure or following an operation or childbirth should suggest this diagnosis. It is usually accompanied by pleuritic pain, and evidence of deep venous thrombosis may be present in the calves. Pulmonary embolism should also be remembered in a woman on the contraceptive pill. On the other hand, increasing dyspnoea in an older subject without obvious cause or chest pain may be due to multiple small emboli.

GENERAL CAUSES

These include such diverse conditions as anaemia, living at high altitudes, the effects of certain drugs on pulmonary function, metabolic disorders and psychological factors. Dyspnoea may result from direct stimulation of the respiratory centre, damage to the lungs or cardiac failure. Some of the more important ones are considered below.

Drugs

Mention has already been made of such drugs as aspirin and beta-blockers which produce or exacerbate asthma. Dyspnoea may, however, be evoked by other mechanisms. A wide variety of drugs, notably cytotoxic chemicals, can cause a diffuse interstitial pneumonia and pulmonary fibrosis during treatment. The list grows longer each year and includes amiodarone, bleomycin, busulphan, carbamazepine, cyclophosphamide, gold, nitrofurantoin, penicillamine and sulphonamides. Drugs such as hydralazine, isoniazid, phenytoin and procainamide may produce systemic lupus erythematosus in susceptible individuals. This drug-induced form commonly results in pulmonary involvement. Finally, large amounts of the weedkiller paraquat, when ingested, cause extensive and usually irreversible destruction of the lungs. Lower doses may produce transient pulmonary infiltrates and temporary impairment of lung function without necessarily causing permanent damage.

Hyperthyroidism (see also Loss of weight, p. 281)

The presence of dyspnoea in a thyrotoxic patient points to incipient cardiac failure which may be accompanied by atrial fibrillation. In the elderly lack of eye signs or an obvious goitre may result in this diagnosis being overlooked.

Addison's disease (see also Loss of weight, p. 283)

Shortness of breath after quite modest exertion is a little-recognised symptom of chronic adrenocortical insufficiency. In a personal series of 70 cases of Addison's disease it was present in 55%. Suspicion may be aroused by an abnormally small heart shadow on a chest X-ray taken to exclude other causes. In one of the above cases the diagnosis was delayed for over 2 years because the radiologist's report was disregarded. An ECG may show flattened or inverted T waves in the chest leads which return to normal within 2 or 3 days of starting corticosteroid therapy.

Renal failure

Dyspnoea in terminal renal failure is due to a combination of severe anaemia, pulmonary oedema from the retention of salt and water, and metabolic acidosis.

Anxiety state

The role of the psyche in determining the onset of asthma should not be forgotten.

Neurotic subjects, especially young women, sometimes exhibit episodes of acute hyperventilation which are preceded by a feeling of suffocation and accompanied by a sense of unreality and panic. During an attack they will complain of lightheadedness, dyspnoea, palpitations and paraesthesia in the extremities and around the mouth. Carpopedal spasm may develop if the attack is prolonged. The symptoms are mainly due to hypocapnia and can often be relieved by breathing into a paper bag. Often the sensation gets better rather than worse on exercise.

Epidemics of dizziness, headache, fainting, shivering, pins and needles and hyperventilation leading to tetany have been described. In one of these outbreaks in a girls' school the symptoms were not transient but persisted for days. The previous occurrence of an epidemic of poliomyelitis was thought to have rendered the girls vulnerable to mass hysteria.

CHAPTER 21

Tachycardia

SYNOPSIS OF CAUSES*

SUPRAVENTRICULAR

Sinus tachycardia; Paroxysmal supraventricular tachycardia; Atrial fibrillation; Atrial flutter; Junctional tachycardia.

VENTRICULAR

Ventricular tachycardia; Ventricular fibrillation.

---

* Bold type is used for causes more commonly found in Europe and North America.

PHYSIOLOGY

The action potentials which initiate cardiac contraction normally arise in the sino-atrial node and spread across the atria to reach the atrio-ventricular node, which lies in close proximity to the coronary sinus. The atria and ventricles are electrically insulated from one another by connective tissue and fat and, in most individuals, this node provides the only pathway between them. The conduction velocity within this junctional tissue is much slower than that elsewhere and this delay is reflected in the PR interval on the electrocardiogram.

From the atrio-ventricular node the impulses travel down the bundle of His and into the subendocardial network of Purkinje fibres, where they excite in turn the ventricular muscle in the septum, apex and base of the heart. The pacemaker cells in the sino-atrial node have a faster intrinsic rate of discharge than those elsewhere, so that sinus rhythm is the norm. Catecholamines from the sympathetic nerve endings and adrenal medulla increase the rate, whilst vagal stimulation slows it down.

In healthy adults the resting pulse rate is about 70–80 beats a minute but may be as low as 40 or as high as 90 beats a minute. It tends to be slower in athletic individuals, in whom pulse rates under 50 are not uncommon. In children the resting pulse rate is faster, averaging about 120 beats a minute at birth and slowing gradually during childhood to reach adult levels at puberty.

Tachycardia is a transient or persistent increase in the heart rate above the upper limit of normal; in practice this means one in excess of 90 beats a minute in an adult. It is often much faster than this. Sinus tachycardia is the normal physiological response to such causes as excitement, pain, anger, fear, fever and exercise. It occurs in many diseases, especially those of the heart itself, and is a prominent feature of shock irrespective of the cause.

The ectopic rhythms differ from sinus tachycardia in that the action potentials arise from sites other than the sino-atrial node. For example, impulses which have already passed through the atrio-ventricular node may return to the atria via abnormal pathways to add to the stimuli reaching this junction. In the Wolff–Parkinson–White syndrome there is an anatomically distinct accessory pathway which permits this re-entry. In other cases it is thought that the impulses return along some part of the conducting tract which is physiologically but not anatomically separate from the rest of the tissue.

Ectopic rhythms may also arise from pacemaker cells in the atria, atrio-ventricular node, bundle of His or Purkinje fibres when their intrinsic activity is sufficiently enhanced to exceed the sinus rate. Similarly they may originate from non-specialised cells in the myocardium which generate action potentials in response to injury, hypoxia or electrolyte imbalance. The commonest irregularity is the premature systole produced by an occasional impulse from an ectopic focus in the atria or ventricles; this, however, does not cause tachycardia. Such impulses occur quite frequently in otherwise healthy individuals and may be provoked by caffeine in tea or coffee, alcohol or heavy smoking.

In the middle-aged or elderly, on the other hand, atrial or ventricular ectopic beats may be the first indication of underlying heart disease. They occur in about 80% of patients with myocardial infarction and may precede more serious dysrhythmias.

DIAGNOSTIC APPROACH

Psychogenic and systemic disorders should be considered first for, in the great majority of cases, tachycardia is of extracardiac origin. Nervous tachycardia ordinarily subsides quickly but in the consulting room it may persist in a patient who is outwardly calm and indeed claims to be at ease and unperturbed. This may be due to fear of what may be found at examination, or to repressed anxiety.

Slight exertion in the obese, in sedentary persons who are 'out of condition' and in convalescence may raise the heart rate unduly and should be evaluated accordingly. Sinus tachycardia is a normal accompaniment of raised body temperature and is readily induced in anaemia. Questions should be asked about consumption of tea and coffee, alcohol and tobacco.

A list of all drugs taken should be noted, with particular attention to any psychotropic drugs or sympathomimetics.

A cardiac disorder should be suspected if the patient complains of syncope, anginal pain, breathlessness or swelling of the legs. There may be a history of rheumatic fever in childhood or of previously recorded hypertension. Digitalis toxicity may be the cause of a rapid heart rate in patients already on this drug, particularly if they have been given diuretics as well. In hospital a rise in pulse rate in the first week or two after surgery may be the first indication of deep venous thrombosis and a warning of impending pulmonary embolism.

Palpitations are commonly due to multiple ectopic beats in an anxious individual. However, episodes which begin and end suddenly, and which are associated with a rapid heart rate, may be the only clue to a paroxysmal ectopic rhythm. Attacks vary in duration from a few minutes to many hours and may be precipitated by exertion or occur in bed at night. These patients often present in normal rhythm in the surgery or consulting room.

Examination will determine the rate and regularity or otherwise of the heart beat and will disclose any other evidence of cardiac abnormality. An irregular pulse is commonly due to atrial fibrillation but multiple ectopic beats can mimic this arrhythmia. Anaemia sufficient to produce tachycardia is likely to be obvious from inspection of the conjunctivae and nail beds. Any thyroid enlargement should be noted. Fever, palpable lymph nodes or splenic enlargement will point to a systemic disease.

Investigations will clearly depend upon the history and clinical findings. If an ectopic rhythm seems likely an electrocardiogram is essential to establish its nature. An ECG recorded after exercise may be helpful in eliciting tachycardias provoked by exertion, but this procedure is potentially dangerous if the resting ECG is abnormal and shows evidence of ischaemic changes. In an obscure case of palpitations continuous ambulatory recording of the ECG for 24 hours may be invaluable in demonstrating intermittent ectopic rhythms.

SUPRAVENTRICULAR CAUSES

Sinus tachycardia

The heart rate in sinus tachycardia ranges from 90–180 beats a minute, but rarely exceeds 150 at rest. Although the pulse may vary with emotion, changes of posture and exertion it can be maintained for hours, days or weeks at this elevated level, depending on the underlying cause. Sinus tachycardia, though accompanying many systemic diseases, is ordinarily overshadowed by more specific signs and symptoms. There are, however, a few conditions which merit special consideration.

Sinus tachycardia is a prominent feature of anxiety states, where it may be accompanied by praecordial discomfort, palpitations, tremor of the outstretched hands, sweating, irritability, fatigue and shortness of breath. The fear of heart disease is readily induced and may indeed perpetuate the tachycardia. This group of symptoms first gained recognition during the First World War, when it was regarded as of cardiac origin and called the effort syndrome.

This psychologically-induced tachycardia must be distinguished from tachycardia due to hyperthyroidism, which often presents with similar symptoms. A history of weight loss despite a good appetite, eye signs and a palpable goitre; however slight, should enable this distinction to be made. A normal serum thyroxine level, however, does not exclude thyrotoxicosis — the serum triiodothyronine level is a better guide to thyroid function in these patients.

It is also important to exclude drugs as a possible cause of sinus tachycardia before blaming it on the psyche. These include caffeine and other methylxanthines in tea and coffee, ephedrine and other sympathomimetic drugs used in asthma, atropine and the phenothiazines which have anticholinergic activity, and vasodilators such as prazosin used in the treatment of hypertension. It is astonishing how often these medications are overlooked.

When the pumping action of the heart is impaired by disease the cardiac output can only be maintained if the rate is increased to compensate for the fall in stroke volume. Sinus tachycardia is therefore a prominent feature of both left and right ventricular failure and is commonly seen in myocardial infarction, myocarditis, pericarditis and cardiomyopathy. It is consistently present in major pulmonary embolism.

Sinus tachycardia is readily recognised on an ECG, provided that normal P waves can be identified before each QRS complex. The rate rarely exceeds 150 a minute and the ventricular complexes will be normal in width unless bundle branch block is present. Gradual slowing of the rate may follow pressure on the carotid sinus or eyeball, but for obvious reasons these manoeuvres are rarely carried out in practice unless there is some doubt about the nature of the rhythm.

Paroxysmal supraventricular tachycardia

In this disorder the ectopic impulses are generated in the atria or atrioventricular node. When they arise in the atria the cause is usually digitalis toxicity in a patient with a diseased heart. In this form the atrial rate varies between 140 and 240 a minute but since it is usually accompanied by some degree of atrio-ventricular block not all these impulses will reach the ventricles. When the ectopic focus is in the junctional tissue the impulses gain re-entry to the atria via an accessory pathway which, in patients with the Wolff–Parkinson–White syndrome, is the bundle of Kent. Paroxysmal nodal tachycardia is commonly seen in otherwise healthy children and adults.

The onset and cessation are usually sudden and an attack may last for only a few minutes or persist for several hours. If brief palpitations may be the only symptom, but angina and cardiac failure may develop in patients with heart disease if the attack is prolonged for many hours. It may be followed by a spontaneous diuresis and patients should be asked if they have noticed polyuria afterwards.

The ECG will show a regular tachycardia of between 140 and 240 beats a minute. In atrial tachycardia the P waves will precede the QRS complexes but in nodal rhythm they will be difficult to identify as they may coincide with or follow the ventricular complexes. Failure to slow the rate by carotid sinus massage may help to distinguish this ectopic rhythm from sinus tachycardia if there is any doubt about the tracing.

Atrial fibrillation

This is the commonest of the ectopic tachycardias. The impulses, which may be more than 400 to the minute, bombard the atrio-ventricular node, where many are blocked. The ventricular contractions are completely irregular in rate and strength and vary between 60 and 200 per minute depending upon the degree of block. Atrial fibrillation may alternate with normal rhythm before becoming established.

The commonest causes are mitral valve disease, ischaemic heart disease and hyperthyroidism in the elderly. It is occasionally seen in otherwise healthy individuals but thyrotoxicosis should always be excluded by the appropriate tests before making a diagnosis of 'lone' atrial fibrillation. The pulse is rapid and wholly irregular but, as the beats vary in strength, not all reach the wrist. The heart rate must therefore be determined by auscultation.

No discrete P waves will be seen on the ECG, the atrial activity being represented by irregular deflections known as 'f' waves. The QRS complexes occur at irregular intervals and rarely exceed 160 per minute. The ventricular rate may slow in response to carotid sinus massage.

Atrial flutter

Flutter, like atrial fibrillation, is occasionally seen in apparently healthy individuals but is usually associated with rheumatic heart disease, myocardial infarction or cor pulmonale. The atrial rate is rapid and regular between 220 and 360 per minute. The ventricles cannot respond to such a rate, and in consequence block occurs. In adults this is often a two to one block with a ventricular rate between 130 to 170 beats a minute. With a greater degree of block it may fall to as low as 70 a minute. Clearly the existence of atrial flutter may be overlooked without an ECG.

The onset resembles that of paroxysmal atrial tachycardia but the attacks last longer and may persist for weeks. The pulse rate will depend upon the degree of atrio-ventricular block and may rise or fall suddenly if this alters during the course of the examination. Signs of organic heart disease such as gallop rhythm or congestive failure may be found.

With a high degree of block the condition can be readily diagnosed from the ECG. The regular rapid P waves produce a characteristic saw-tooth appearance which is best seen in standard leads II, III and AVF, with ventricular complexes after every second to fourth P waves. It is more difficult to diagnose with a 2:1 block for the second P wave will be buried in the QRS complex and the tracing will resemble that of paroxysmal supra-ventricular tachycardia. Carotid sinus massage may increase the degree of block and reveal the characteristic appearance on the ECG.

Junctional tachycardia

The pacemaker cells in the atrio-ventricular node normally have an intrinsic rate of discharge of between 40 and 60 impulses a minute. If this is enhanced in conditions such as rheumatic fever, digitalis intoxication or myocardial infarction it may override the sinus rhythm and result in a slowly fluctuating tachycardia which is indistinguishable clinically from sinus tachycardia. An ECG however will show atrio-ventricular dissociation with absence of P wave activity before some of the QRS complexes.

VENTRICULAR CAUSES

Ventricular tachycardia

This may complicate any form of heart disease but is commonly due to myocardial infarction or chronic ischaemia. It may be precipitated by a number of drugs which include digitalis, tricyclic antidepressants, sympatho-mimetic compounds and quinidine. Ventricular tachycardia is said to be present when there is a run of six or more ventricular ectopic beats at a rate of more than 120 beats a minute. This arrhythmia is particularly dangerous because it may progress to ventricular fibrillation unless it is suppressed by anti-arrhythmic drugs or normal sinus rhythm is restored by cardioversion.

The ECG will show a tachycardia with wide QRS complexes ranging from 120 to over 200 a minute. The QRS complex will usually exceed 0.14 second in duration and P waves may be absent from the tracing. A form of ventricular tachycardia known as *torsade de pointes* can be recognised on the ECG by paroxysms of tachycardia in which the QRS axis undulates over runs of 5–20 beats, so that the points of the QRS complexes appear to be twisting around an imaginary iso-electric line; this abnormality may termi-nate spontaneously or go on to ventricular fibrillation.

Ventricular fibrillation

This may follow ventricular tachycardia and is rapidly fatal unless stopped by the use of an electrical defibrillator. Since the patient will be pulseless the diagnosis can only be made by electrocardiography which will show disorganised chaotic activity on the trace. It accounts for the majority of cardiac arrests, occurring within 48 hours of a myocardial infarction, and is the main justification for having specialised coronary care units in every district general hospital.

CHAPTER 22
Loss of weight

SYNOPSIS OF CAUSES*

DEFICIENT INTAKE
Anorexia nervosa; Starvation; Kwashiorkor; Drugs.

MALABSORPTION
Gluten enteropathy; Tropical sprue; Intestinal infections; Blind loop syndrome; **Crohn's disease; Pancreatic disease; Cystic fibrosis**; Lactose intolerance; Drugs; **Operation sequelae**.

ABNORMALITIES OF METABOLISM
Infections; Acquired Immunodeficiency syndrome (AIDS); Rheumatoid arthritis; Neoplasia; Lymphomas; Diabetes mellitus; Hyperthyroidism; Addison's disease.

* Bold type is used for causes more commonly found in Europe and North America.

PHYSIOLOGY

The amount of food habitually consumed varies greatly between one healthy adult and another. This is not explained by differences in build, physical activity or basal metabolic rate. The weight of most adults remains fairly constant without particular attention to diet, but in some any excess is promptly registered on the scales.

There is nevertheless a well recognised tendency to increase in weight in middle age. This may be related to a reduction in physical activity without a corresponding reduction in the intake of food. Loss of weight is common in the elderly and, whilst this is often pathological, it is equally likely to result from lessening of physical activity and of appetite.

Digestion is begun mechanically by mastication and intestinal peristalsis followed by a chemical attack upon the individual constituents of the food. In fat digestion the bile salts emulsify and pancreatic lipase hydrolyses the fat into glycerol and fatty acids. Protein is reduced by pancreatic and intestinal enzymes to polypeptides and amino acids. Carbohydrates are broken down by other enzymes to monosaccharides, of which glucose is the most important.

Absorption follows, taking place through the microvilli of the small intestine whence the products of digestion pass into the blood and lymph vessels. Water, mineral salts and vitamins are also taken up. These include the fat-soluble vitamins A, D and K and the water-soluble vitamins B and C. The B complex includes folic acid and vitamin B_{12} which is mainly absorbed in the lower ileum. Malabsorption may result from incomplete digestion due to lack of enzymes or bile salts, or from damage to the absorptive mechanisms of the intestinal mucosa.

DIAGNOSTIC APPROACH

Loss of weight is common to many illnesses and is not of much diagnostic value on its own. It may be due to inadequate intake, malabsorption or the deranged metabolism associated with chronic inflammation, neoplasia or endocrine disease. The possible causes to consider will obviously differ according to the age and sex of the patient, the ethnic origin and any accompanying symptoms and signs. When taking a history it is necessary to explore the social background and to find out if any drugs are being taken, and for what purpose.

In childhood, *failure to thrive* is perhaps more important than any recent loss of weight. By plotting the child's height and weight on a standard growth chart its growth can be compared with that of healthy children of the same age and sex. A knowledge of its previous height and weight is often valuable in determining whether it is remaining in the same percentile of the population, or is deviating from it. Its performance can also be contrasted with that of other members of the family.

If malnutrition can be excluded the most probable causes in the UK will be allergy to cow's milk, cystic fibrosis, gluten enteropathy or chronic respiratory and renal infections. The combination of repeated respiratory infections and fatty stools in an undersized child will point to cystic fibrosis, which is relatively common and often presents early in life. Lactose intolerance should be considered in children of the immigrant population.

Malignant disease and hyperthyroidism are rare in childhood. Diabetes mellitus is uncommon in this age group but may appear acutely with rapid loss of weight, thirst, polyuria and dehydration. The diagnosis is not difficult provided that the urine is tested routinely. Anorexia nervosa is virtually unknown below the age of 12 and a thorough search should be made for an organic cause in a younger child; in a recent case this turned out to be achalasia of the oesophagus.

Anorexia nervosa is, however, the commonest cause of a poor appetite and consequent loss of weight in adolescent girls and young women in Britain. It will be accompanied by primary or secondary amenorrhoea, depending on the age of onset, unless oral contraceptives are being taken. The diagnosis is usually apparent from the history of dieting or psychological stress and is confirmed by the physical findings. This condition is rare in males, who present with loss of weight and obstinate constipation — numerous fruitless investigations may be carried out before the true nature of their illness is recognised.

In adult life the spectrum widens to include a variety of inflammatory, neoplastic and endocrine disorders; *gluten enteropathy* should still be considered in the differential diagnosis for it may not appear until old age. Loss of weight with painless lymphadenopathy in a young man should remind one of *Hodgkin's disease*, which is now curable with aggressive chemotherapy. *Crohn's disease* and *peptic ulceration* are common in middle life and *malabsorption* may follow partial gastrectomy or intestinal resection. *Alcohol* and *drug abuse* are becoming increasingly common, particularly in the drifting inhabitants of the larger cities, and often lead to malnutrition. Weight loss is a common presenting feature of *AIDS*, which is particularly prevalent in homosexual men and intravenous drug abusers.

Recent loss of weight in a middle-aged adult who has previously enjoyed good health may be due to a gastric or colonic *neoplasm*; dysphagia, vomiting, abdominal pain or diarrhoea will draw attention to the alimentary tract. *Pancreatic insufficiency*, with the exception of cystic fibrosis, is mainly confined to the elderly of both sexes in whom it may be due to chronic inflammation or pancreatic carcinoma; it usually presents with a short history of abdominal pain, steatorrhoea and weight loss. Jaundice will suggest *biliary obstruction* and the causes of this should be considered. In a middle-aged or elderly cigarette smoker the first thing to exclude is a bronchial cancer. Occult neoplasms or drugs may be responsible in old age.

Some underlying systemic disorder will be suspected in the presence of fever, frequency of micturition, arthralgia or respiratory symptoms. The physical examination may reveal finger clubbing, increased pigmentation of the skin, a pleural effusion or enlargement of lymph nodes, liver or spleen. Goitre may be apparent, with prominent eyes, tremors and tachycardia suggesting hyperthyroidism.

Investigations will vary widely depending upon the most probable cause; these will be discussed in the text.

When faced with unexplained weight loss it is sensible to tackle the problem systematically by considering the causes of deficient intake, malabsorption and deranged metabolism separately. In this chapter they are considered in that order.

DEFICIENT INTAKE

Restriction of food consumption may be deliberate, in the following of food fads or 'slimming' cures, or from the anorexia of chronic conditions such as alcoholism, cardiac failure, liver disease, renal impairment or depressive illness. Alternatively, the intake may have been cut down to avoid the post-prandial pain or discomfort of achalasia, oesophagitis, peptic ulceration or mesenteric ischaemia. The weight loss which is common following partial gastrectomy appears early and is largely due to the taking of smaller meals to avoid discomfort and the 'dumping' syndrome. In the UK the most extreme example of voluntary restriction is that seen in anorexia nervosa which is becoming increasingly common, particularly in middle-class adolescent females.

Anorexia nervosa

Aetiology
This condition was first described in England by Sir William Gull in 1874. Since the cause was unknown he believed that the diagnosis could only be made by the exclusion of other wasting diseases. We are still ignorant of the true nature of this malady, which has been variously described as a psychiatric disorder, an endocrine or metabolic disturbance, or a combination of the two. An attractive hypothesis, because it offers hope for effective treatment, is the suggestion that it is primarily due to dopamine overactivity in the hypothalamus which is triggered off by psychological stress or overzealous dieting.

Anorexia nervosa is rare in males and mainly affects adolescent girls and young women between the ages of 12 and 24. It may follow disturbed family or sexual relationships, death of a close relative, unhappiness at school or work, or the stress engendered by forthcoming examinations.

Clinical features
The most prominent symptom is avoidance of carbohydrates, with consequent loss of weight. The term 'avoidance' includes consumption and then riddance by self-induced vomiting or purgation, as well as exclusion from the diet. The weight loss will be greater than 10% of the calculated optimum weight for the patient's age, sex and height as determined from standard tables or growth charts; in many cases it may be as much as 40% of their normal weight.

In females this is accompanied or preceded by amenorrhoea of at least 3 months' duration, unless the patient is taking an oral contraceptive. The diagnosis is more difficult in males, who usually present with loss of weight and obstinate constipation.

The patient is moody, irritable and resentful of her parents' natural concern. She may deny having any symptoms and is often astonishingly energetic despite her cachectic appearance. In a personal series of over 150 cases, about one-third admitted to feeling depressed, and in 40% the illness appeared to have been precipitated by dieting because patients believed themselves to be overweight. 44% of this series confessed to self-induced vomiting, purgative abuse or both. Constipation, fatigue and insomnia were very common and, not surprisingly, many of the worst affected complained of feeling the cold. About one-third described abdominal discomfort after eating and blamed this for their loss of appetite. Other symptoms included headache, giddiness, dry skin, falling hair, nocturia and dyspnoea on exertion.

The full extent of the weight loss can only be appreciated when the patient is undressed. Much of the subcutaneous fat will have disappeared and the body will be thin to the point of emaciation. The back and limbs are often covered by fine downy hair, and acrocyanosis of the extremities is common. The palms and soles of the feet may have an orange or yellow hue, which is due to hypercarotenaemia, and ankle oedema is not uncommon.

Hypotension will be found in about 30% of cases and is often accompanied by bradycardia. Hypothermia is rare and is seen only in grossly emaciated patients. Secondary sexual characteristics are usually well-preserved, but atrophic breasts and scanty pubic or axillary hair are not unusual in chronic anorexics of many years' duration.

Mild forms are common, particularly amongst university students, and many recover without any specific treatment. Even in those more severely affected eventual recovery is the rule, but death can occur from intercurrent infection or suicide. Many, however, are left with abnormal eating habits and quite a number go on to develop bulimia.

Investigations

The haemoglobin level and ESR are usually normal, but leucopenia is common and mild thrombocytopenia is occasionally seen. The bone marrow, on the other hand, often shows marked hypocellularity, fat depletion and the presence of a gelatinous acid mucopolysaccharide material.

On a chest X-ray the heart is characteristically small and vertical in position; the cardiothoracic ratio is reduced, but returns to normal on refeeding. An ECG may show sinus bradycardia, first-degree heart block and reduced or inverted T waves. Non-specific abnormalities are often present on an electroencephalogram, while a CT brain scan may show dilated ventricles and widened sulci.

The fasting plasma glucose level is often at or below the lower limit of the normal range, and may be accompanied by an elevated growth hormone level. The serum carotene level is often elevated, and raised cholesterol levels are found in about 30% of cases. The serum transaminase and bilirubin concentrations are sometimes elevated, whilst hypokalaemia and a modest increase in the blood urea are not uncommon in those who indulge in self-induced vomiting or purgative abuse. Hypocalcaemia, probably due to vitamin D deficiency, is occasionally found but hypomagnesaemia is rare. The serum zinc concentration is sometimes subnormal, but there is no convincing evidence that zinc deficiency is responsible for this disease.

Anorexia nervosa is associated with many abnormalities of endocrine and hypothalamic function. Thermoregulation is often faulty and partial diabetes insipidus is not uncommon in more severe cases. Hypothalamic hypogonadism is the rule, with low serum gonadotrophin and sex hormone levels but normal prolactin concentrations.

Many patients have low serum triiodothyronine (T3) levels, together with low or low normal thyroxine (T4) levels and normal TSH concentrations. This 'low T3 syndrome' is also seen in other wasting conditions and may be accompanied by the prolonged achilles reflex half-relaxation time which is found in hypothyroid patients.

There is an increased secretion of corticotrophin-releasing hormone by the hypothalamus in this disorder which can lead to increased adrenocortical activity; elevated plasma and urinary cortisol levels are found in some patients and revert to normal on refeeding.

Starvation

Inadequate intake of food may be seen in large families because of poverty and bad housekeeping. In old people living alone malnutrition and loss of weight result from straitened means, physical disability, loneliness and apathy leading to anorexia. Deficient or bad teeth may contribute in such cases to the inadequate intake; such a remediable cause is easily overlooked.

The symptoms and signs of malnutrition are non-specific and may amount to no more than unexplained lethargy and muscular weakness. Deficiency of iron or vitamins should be suspected if there is anaemia, angular stomatitis, a smooth tongue, hyperkeratosis of the skin, flattened nails or spontaneous bruising on the trunk or limbs. In the elderly loss of height and a kyphotic spine are commonly due to osteoporosis but osteomalacia should always be considered as an alternative diagnosis in the housebound individual, particularly if there is any evidence of a proximal myopathy.

Wernicke's encephalopathy due to thiamine deficiency is occasionally seen, especially in alcoholics. It usually presents acutely with confusion, delirium, confabulation, ataxia, diplopia and nystagmus.

In the developing and tropical countries, and in prisoners of war, deprivation, especially of protein and vitamins, may be of extreme degree. According to the World Health Organisation protein–calorie malnutrition is the major dietary problem of the world today; it is often accompanied by vitamin and mineral deficiencies. In many developing countries half the children suffer from protein deficiency while some 2% will have kwashiorkor.

Kwashiorkor

This severe deficiency disease is unknown in the UK but is common in Africa and Central America. While basically due to protein starvation there is also deficiency of carbohydrates, fats and vitamins. The picture may be complicated by malaria, dysentery or intestinal parasites. Diarrhoea is a constant feature and is partly due to the profound atrophy of the intestinal mucosa which is seen at autopsy.

Kwashiorkor appears soon after weaning. The infant is miserable and undersized; muscle wasting in the limbs is obscured by oedema, especially of the feet. The dry, pigmented, hyperkeratotic lesions of the skin resemble those of pellagra. The hair is characteristically dry, straight, sparse and easily pulled out; it may become reddish or yellow in colour and sometimes

white from lack of pigment. Acrocyanosis is common and hepatosplenomegaly may be found. The distended belly is due to flaccid abdominal
muscles, ascites or the presence of a malarial spleen.

Drugs

Diminished intake of food may be due to anorexia induced by a wide
variety of medicines. Anorexia caused by digitalis should be well known but
is still overlooked, even in hospital. Most cytotoxic drugs and many antibiotics may be responsible. Whenever possible the current medications
should be stopped for at least 48 hours in order to see if the appetite will
return. It must not be forgotten that drugs once prescribed for obesity may
have continued to be taken long after the target weight has been passed.

MALABSORPTION

If loss of weight has taken place despite an adequate and accustomed intake
of food we must next consider whether it has been digested and absorbed.
The concept of *malabsorption* is valuable, for it enables us to consider
together a score of disorders which have in common a failure to absorb one
or more of the constituents of the diet. This may be due to inherited
abnormalities, structural damage to the small bowel, intestinal infections,
drugs, radiotherapy to the abdomen, and deficiency of bile salts or
pancreatic enzymes. Many of these causes are distinctly uncommon and will
only be referred to briefly. In the UK the commonest causes are gluten
enteropathy, Crohn's disease and pancreatic insufficiency.

It is convenient to consider the clinical features of malabsorption and
such general investigations as may be necessary at the outset. The symptoms and signs seen particularly in the individual disorders will be discussed
in the text, together with any special investigations which may be required.
Malabsorption is likely to give rise to lassitude and loss of weight along with
abdominal discomfort and chronic diarrhoea. Abdominal symptoms may,
however, be minimal and overlooked. Other complaints may arise from the
lack of various constituents in the diet.

Steatorrhoea is frequently present and, when severe, several pale, bulky
ill-smelling stools are passed daily. These characteristically float in the
lavatory pan, adhere to its side and are flushed away with difficulty. In mild
cases, however, the stools may be normal in appearance, particularly if the
patient is on a low-fat diet.

Abdominal pain suggests the presence of an inflammatory or obstructive
lesion such as pancreatitis or Crohn's disease, while jaundice would implicate the liver and biliary tract. Anaemia is commonly due to deficiency of
iron, vitamin B_{12} or folic acid. Other evidence of vitamin deficiency may
be seen in excessive bleeding or bruising from lack of vitamin K. Lack
of vitamin D will lead to osteomalacia with myopathy, bone pains and
fractures.

Investigations

The scope and order of the investigations will depend upon the most likely cause. A full blood count will disclose any anaemia and a microcytic, hypochromic picture is most likely to be due to malabsorption of iron; failure of the serum iron level to rise significantly 3 hours after a dose of oral iron and ascorbic acid will confirm this. A macrocytic picture is probably due to deficiency of vitamin B_{12} or folic acid; marrow biopsy, serum vitamin levels, a Schilling test and the response to their administration will determine which is lacking.

The serum calcium, phosphate and alkaline phosphatase should be estimated for evidence of osteomalacia, but a normal calcium level does not exclude this diagnosis — secondary hyperparathyroidism will tend to keep it in the normal range. X-rays of the chest, spine and pelvis may reveal decalcification and Looser's zones (pseudofractures). In the absence of the latter only a bone biopsy will enable osteomalacia to be distinguished from osteoporosis.

Estimation of the serum bilirubin, liver enzymes and prothrombin time will help to exclude liver or biliary tract disease. Hypokalaemia may result from a combination of inadequate intake of potassium and excessive loss in the stools from chronic diarrhoea. A low serum albumin level is an indirect measure of protein loss.

Steatorrhoea, whether obvious or occult, is present in many cases of malabsorption and inspection of the stools followed by chemical analysis is essential. A butter-fat absorption test may be used for screening purposes but an estimation of faecal fat is the only reliable measure of fat absorption. Normally the quantity excreted over a period of 4 or 5 days does not exceed 18 mmol (5 g) per 24 hours. During this period the diet should contain at least 70 g of fat a day. Not surprisingly, this test is very unpopular with the laboratory staff and should only be requested if the butter-fat test is abnormal, or if there is other strong evidence which points to malabsorption as the cause of weight loss.

Gluten enteropathy

Aetiology

The coeliac disease of children, idiopathic steatorrhoea of adults and non-tropical sprue are now recognised to be the same disorder. The cause lies in an inherited idiosyncrasy to the toxic effects of some constituent of gluten on the intestinal mucosa.

'Gluten' is the name given to a group of proteins present in barley, rye, wheat and oats. It is possible that some other disorders such as tropical sprue, allergy to cow's milk and acute gastro-enteritis in childhood are associated with a temporary sensitivity to this substance.

The damage to the mucosal cells results in loss of the villi in the upper part of the small intestine, thus reducing the area available for the digestion and absorption of food. Whether this is due to the lack of an enzyme responsible for breaking down gluten or to some abnormal immunological reaction to its presence is still uncertain.

There is an association between this disease and dermatitis herpetiformis, and many patients with these bullous skin lesions have an abnormal jejunal mucosa. In both disorders there is a high incidence of the HLA antigens B8 and Dw3. Lymphomas of the small bowel and other malignancies of the alimentary tract are late complications of this life-long disease.

Clinical features

Gluten enteropathy is fairly common in the UK. It may present in early childhood or be discovered for the first time in old age. When it occurs in children there will be irritability, failure to grow, a protuberant belly and steatorrhoea. In milder cases it may not be recognised until adult life but a careful history often reveals episodes of diarrhoea in the past. Loss of weight, anaemia, bone pains from osteomalacia or a tendency to bleed excessively from lack of vitamin K may draw attention to its presence.

Evidence of malabsorption should be sought in all patients with dermatitis herpetiformis because of the known association with this disease, even when there are no symptoms to attract attention to the gastrointestinal tract.

Investigations

A full blood count and routine biochemistry will disclose any anaemia or biochemical evidence of osteomalacia. The stools should be inspected and, if steatorrhoea is suspected, they should be collected for faecal fat estimation. The diagnosis is confirmed by jejunal biopsy, using a Crosby capsule, which will show the characteristic flat, atrophic mucosa. Ideally this procedure should be repeated after some months on a gluten-free diet to demonstrate a morphological improvement following this treatment.

A small bowel meal in this disorder may show intestinal hurry, segmentation, flocculation of barium and dilatation of loops of bowel; in children the most constant sign in gluten enteropathy is a dilated duodenum. Strictures may be due to ulceration of the small intestine or lymphoma, but only laparotomy will enable this distinction to be made.

Tropical sprue

This disease resembles gluten enteropathy but differs from it in occurring in the tropics, in its infective and epidemic character and in its response to folic acid and tetracyclines. It often begins acutely with abdominal discomfort, anorexia, diarrhoea and loss of weight. Glossitis and stomatitis are common. The symptoms may subside on leaving the tropics but anaemia due to vitamin B_{12} or folate deficiency often persists.

The disorder is rare in the UK but is sometimes seen in travellers returning from abroad. The diagnosis is based on the history, absence of intestinal parasites, evidence of malabsorption and subtotal villous atrophy on jejunal biopsy.

Intestinal infections

Giardia lamblia infestation will, when heavy, impede fat absorption and produce steatorrhoea. It has recently been reported in tourists returning from Eastern Europe. The organism will be found in duodenal aspirates and the stools.

Whipple's disease is a rare infection in which glycoprotein is deposited in the macrophages of the small intestine, lymph nodes and other tissues. Electron microscopy has shown that these glycoprotein deposits are made up of unidentified rod-shaped bacilli.

Whipple's disease mainly occurs in middle-aged White men, and the onset of diarrhoea and weight loss is often preceded by a transitory polyarthralgia affecting the larger joints. Fever, lymphadenopathy and increased skin pigmentation should arouse suspicion. Steatorrhoea is nearly always present and a small bowel meal may show thickening of the intestinal wall. Jejunal biopsy will reveal dilated lymphatic spaces and villi distended by swollen macrophages containing glycoprotein. Clinical improvement follows a prolonged course of antibiotics, the one most favoured being tetracycline.

Tuberculous enteritis and tabes mesenterica are now seldom seen in the UK. Widespread involvement of the gut and mesenteric lymph nodes will interfere with absorption. It can be mistaken, even at operation, for Crohn's disease.

Blind loop syndrome

The blind loop syndrome is the name given to malabsorption caused by an overgrowth of the normal bacterial flora in a stagnant loop of bowel. The microorganisms achieve this by competing for vitamins in the food, by releasing enzymes which interfere with the digestive processes or by producing toxins which directly damage the intestinal mucosa. *Escherichia coli* may cause vitamin B_{12} deficiency, whilst anaerobic organisms such as *Bacteroides* species deconjugate bile salts and impair the absorption of fat.

The underlying pathology may be a jejunal diverticulum, a blind loop of duodenum following a partial gastrectomy, intestinal scleroderma or a fistula between adjacent loops of bowel in Crohn's disease. The diagnosis is usually inferred from the history and radiological findings and the response to treatment with broad-spectrum antibiotics.

Crohn's disease (see also Lateral abdominal pain, p. 86)

In regional enteritis steatorrhoea and malabsorption are seen in over half of cases. This may result from very extensive involvement of the small bowel, from widespread resection or from fistula formation with the development of stagnant loops and overgrowth of the normal bacterial flora. In one such patient a fistula between stomach and colon effectively bypassed the whole of the small intestine; this was missed on barium meal and follow-through and was only discovered when a barium enema was carried out.

Pancreatic disease (see also Epigastric pain, p. 58)

Pancreatic insufficiency is a common cause of steatorrhoea, particularly in the elderly. In this age group the onset of diarrhoea is often sudden and rapidly disabling. It may be due to chronic pancreatitis or carcinoma and the nature and duration of the symptoms is very similar in both disorders. Typically there is a short history of 1 or 2 years of diarrhoea, abdominal pain and progressive loss of weight. Epigastric pain, often radiating through to the back, will distinguish pancreatic disease from other causes of malabsorption such as gluten enteropathy and Whipple's disease, which are usually painless. Both benign and malignant disease may destroy enough islet-cells to produce diabetes mellitus.

Haematological abnormalities are often absent and the haemoglobin level rarely falls below 10 g/dl. The liver function tests will be normal unless the bile ducts are obstructed. A glucose tolerance test may show impaired glucose tolerance even when there are no symptoms or signs to suggest diabetes.

Pancreatic calcification on a plain X-ray of the abdomen is seen in about half of cases of chronic pancreatitis. A small bowel meal is seldom helpful and may confuse the situation by showing a jejunal diverticulum.

A jejunal biopsy will exclude gluten enteropathy and Whipple's disease. Endoscopic retrograde cholangio-pancreatography or angiography may help to distinguish between chronic inflammation and carcinoma but this can be extremely difficult, even at laparotomy.

The rare Zollinger–Ellison syndrome is due to the formation of an islet-cell tumour of the pancreas with the resulting excessive secretion of gastrin and hyperchlorhydria. The excess acid inhibits the action of bile and lipase with consequent diarrhoea and steatorrhoea. Weight loss occurs but is overshadowed by the symptoms of peptic ulceration. The diagnosis is confirmed by finding high fasting serum gastrin levels of more than 300 pmol/l (600 ng/l). It is sometimes associated with adenomas or hyperplasia of other endocrine glands.

Cystic fibrosis

Aetiology
This multisystem disease is inherited as an autosomal recessive trait. It is the commonest gene defect in Northern Europe and one in 20 men and women are carriers. It has an incidence in the UK of about one in 2000 live births.

The main abnormality lies in the production of extremely viscid secretions by exocrine tissue in the lungs, liver, pancreas, intestinal tract and testis. Although the sweat glands appear to be normal there is a marked and selective increase in the salt concentration of the sweat, which is of diagnostic value.

Cystic fibrosis is the commonest disorder of the pancreas in childhood. It usually becomes apparent within a few months of life and in the past few sufferers reached adolescence, death resulting from an overwhelming chest infection or cor pulmonale. With the use of antibiotics, physiotherapy and pancreatic extracts many now survive to adult life; a mild case may escape detection until then.

Clinical features

In the neonatal period cystic fibrosis may present as meconium ileus, volvulus or intussusception. In the older child there is failure to grow, despite a good appetite, repeated respiratory infections and steatorrhoea. The distended belly is in marked contrast to the wasted limbs.

Recurrent abdominal pain is not uncommon and patients may present with cirrhosis, cholangitis, gallstones, rectal prolapse or faecal impaction. The excessive loss of salt in the sweat during hot weather can result in dehydration and hypovolaemic shock. In a minority the respiratory involvement is absent. Some 10% develop mild diabetes but a much larger proportion will have impaired glucose tolerance tests. Adult males are sterile from testicular involvement but not necessarily impotent. Nasal polyps are common.

Investigations

The diagnosis is usually based on finding increased sodium concentrations in sweat. In children this is normally less than 70 mmol/l (70 mEq/l). Sweating is stimulated by pilocarpine iontophoresis and at least 100 mg of sweat must be collected on at least two separate occasions. The interpretation of the sweat test, however, can be very difficult because the sodium concentration tends to increase with age and is elevated in some other conditions such as adrenal insufficiency, malnutrition from other causes, ectodermal dysplasia, glycogen storage disease and salt loading. Disturbed liver function tests will draw attention to hepatic dysfunction, and a glucose tolerance test may be abnormal.

Lactose intolerance

In the UK this congenital enzyme deficiency is seen chiefly in Cypriot, Asian and African immigrants, in whom it is common. They appear to have insufficient lactase secreted by the intestinal mucosa to deal with the large amount of milk consumed in this country. The unabsorbed lactose is broken down by bacteria to produce lactic acid and other organic acids which take up water by osmosis with resulting abdominal colic, bloating, diarrhoea and frothy acid stools.

The symptoms often appear a few days after birth and may be mistaken for acute gastroenteritis. In the older child, and occasionally in adults, the intolerance to milk or milk products may be unmasked by intercurrent infection. In the lactose tolerance test a rise of less than 1.1 mmol/l (20 mg/dl) in the blood glucose level after an oral load of 50 g of lactose is very suggestive of this diagnosis, particularly if it is accompanied by symptoms. The only really satisfactory test, however, is the demonstration of lactase deficiency in a mucosal specimen obtained by jejunal biopsy.

Drugs

A few drugs are known to cause steatorrhoea when taken for prolonged periods. Of these the commonest in daily use is phenytoin, and fatty stools should be looked for in all epileptics on this drug who complain of chronic diarrhoea. Phenytoin may also interfere with the absorption and metabolism of folic acid, but osteomalacia in patients on anticonvulsant therapy is more likely to be due to the enzyme-inducing action of these drugs on calciferol metabolism in the liver.

Oral neomycin is another drug which causes steatorrhoea when given to patients with severe liver disease, and other antibiotics such as bacitracin, polymyxin and kanamycin have been implicated.

Colchicine is rarely prescribed nowadays for gout, but cholestyramine binds bile salts in the intestine, thereby reducing fat absorption. The steatorrhoea which results is usually mild and may not lead to much loss of weight. Finally, alcohol in large amounts has a direct toxic effect on the intestinal mucosa but the weight loss in alcoholics has many other causes.

Operation sequelae

Malabsorption with consequent loss of weight is not uncommon after gastric surgery. It may be due to an increased rate of transit through the upper intestine, resulting in inadequate mixing of the food with bile and pancreatic juices, a reduction in hydrogen ion concentration, or the overgrowth of bacteria in a blind loop of duodenum. Total gastrectomy will ultimately lead to vitamin B_{12} deficiency from lack of intrinsic factor. Some increase in faecal fat is usual, even after partial gastrectomy, but rarely causes symptoms. An isolated malabsorption of iron, however, is very common and will present as an iron-deficiency anaemia.

Extensive resection of the small intestine in Crohn's disease, malignancy, mesenteric infarction or a strangulated hernia may cause malabsorption if too little bowel is left; when the ileocaecal valve is also removed the diarrhoea is likely to be even more severe. Resection of the terminal ileum is particularly troublesome for this will interfere with the absorption of bile salts and vitamin B_{12}.

The deliberate short-circuiting of the small intestine in the surgical treatment of gross obesity inevitably leads to malabsorption and the desired loss of weight. Paradoxically, the absorption of oxalates in the large bowel is greatly enhanced by the increased concentrations of bile salts reaching the colon, and the patient's satisfaction with this procedure may be marred by frequent episodes of renal colic and the passage of oxalate stones. Other complications include an increased incidence of gallstones, chronic hepatitis and arthritis.

ABNORMALITIES OF METABOLISM

If the intake of food appears to have been adequate and no evidence of malabsorption is forthcoming it remains to consider whether some derangement of metabolism is responsible for the loss of weight. This may result from inflammatory causes, renal failure, neoplasia or endocrine disease.

Inflammatory causes include a wide variety of chronic non-intestinal infections and the connective-tissue diseases which are discussed in the chapter on Fever — rheumatoid arthritis is mentioned here because loss of weight in this common disorder is more prominent than fever. Some decrease in body weight is usual in malignant disease but this is often accompanied by other symptoms and signs arising from the primary growth which indicate its presence. Of the endocrine diseases only diabetes mellitus, hyperthyroidism and Addison's disease commonly cause weight loss.

Infections

Only those disorders which are likely to be encountered in Europe and North America are mentioned here. In tropical climates such infections as malaria, amoebiasis, schistosomiasis, trypanosomiasis and kala-azar will have to be borne in mind.

Tuberculosis is still endemic in many parts of the world but its incidence in the UK has declined dramatically in recent years. Nevertheless, it should always be considered in the differential diagnosis of unexplained weight loss, especially in the elderly. Chronic miliary tuberculosis, in particular, can be extremely insidious in onset and is often missed.

Subacute bacterial endocarditis is another infection which comes on gradually, with malaise, anorexia, and weight loss. A history of rheumatic fever or cardiac surgery and the presence of cardiac murmurs should bring it to mind; fever may not be noticed by the patient. The same applies to cholangitis, brucellosis and other chronic infections in adults. In children chronic respiratory and renal infections cause failure to thrive.

Many other infections may be responsible for loss of weight in patients whose immunological defences have been suppressed by corticosteroids or other immunosuppressive therapy. This particularly applies to individuals undergoing organ transplants or chemotherapy for malignant disease. The possibility that they have become infected by opportunistic organisms such as *Pneumocystis carinii*, cytomegalovirus or fungi should not be forgotten. Similar infections are responsible for many of the manifestations of the acquired immunodeficiency syndrome, which is described below.

Acquired immunodeficiency syndrome (AIDS)

Aetiology
This worldwide disease, which has already reached epidemic proportions in Africa and North America, is caused by the human immunodeficiency

virus type 1 (HIV-1). This retrovirus was first isolated in France in 1983 and originally called the lymphadenopathy associated virus (LAV) or human T-cell lymphotrophic virus type III (HTLV-III). More recently another retrovirus, HIV type 2, has been isolated from some AIDS cases in France and West Africa.

The importance of the HIV virus lies in the fact that it is mainly transmitted by sexual intercourse and has a symptom-free incubation period of up to 8 years or more before upsetting the natural cellular immunity of the body by destroying the T helper lymphocytes. The invariable consequence of this is that the patient with AIDS dies, often within a year, from an overwhelming infection by one or more pathogenic organisms.

In North America and Europe the main victims so far have been promiscuous male homosexuals and bisexual men, particularly those indulging in anal intercourse, and drug addicts sharing contaminated syringes. Other victims include haemophiliacs treated with infected factor VIII concentrates, patients receiving blood transfusions from an infected donor, and infants infected by placental transfer during pregnancy. In Africa, on the other hand, the virus is spread mainly by heterosexual intercourse and the highest prevalence of HIV antibodies is found mainly in the most sexually active groups, particularly in men who associate with prostitutes.

The HIV virus has been isolated from mononuclear cells in the peripheral blood and from many body fluids. These include plasma, seminal fluid, vaginal secretions, saliva, breast milk, urine and tears. The main vehicles for transmission, however, appear to be blood and semen.

The virus has also been recovered from the cerebrospinal fluid and brains of AIDS patients presenting with presenile dementia, encephalitis, meningitis, myelopathy, radiculopathy or peripheral neuropathy. Kaposi's sarcoma has been reported in about half the homosexual men with AIDS, and a further 5% of cases present with a non-Hodgkin's lymphoma, often of B cell origin. The reason for the development of such tumours is obscure, but it is possible that the immunodeficiency caused by the HIV virus permits infection by another virus which induces these malignant changes.

The introduction of reliable assays for HIV antibodies has revealed the alarming spread of this organism in recent years. In the United States alone about 65 000 people had contracted AIDS by July 1988, of whom nearly half were already dead. About 90% were male homosexuals or bisexual men, and this percentage also applies to the 1600 cases reported in the UK by July 1988. Again, over half the cases have already succumbed to infection.

Because of the long incubation period it is too early to say how many others may be at risk, but it has been estimated that there may be as many as 50 000 carriers of the virus in the UK already. The evidence from Africa suggests that the disease will inevitably spread to the heterosexual population in many countries unless their inhabitants can be persuaded to confine their sexual activity to one faithful partner. Perhaps the only comforting thing about this deadly virus is that it is less infective than the hepatitis B virus; infection is very rare following needle-prick injuries, and there is no evidence of spread by social contact.

Clinical features
There are three phases in the development of this disease; the initial viral infection; the long incubation period and finally the appearance of infections which kill the patient.

The primary viral infection is often symptomless but it can present acutely with fever, headache, sore throat, an erythematous mascular rash, splenomegaly, generalised lymphadenopathy, disturbed liver function, lymphopenia or thrombocytopenia. On clinical grounds it may be indistinguishable from many other transient viral infections and the illness usually subsides spontaneously in a couple of weeks. It may be many months before the HIV antibody tests become positive. Occasionally it can present with puzzling neurological symptoms and signs indicative of an encephalitis, meningitis, myelopathy, radiculopathy or peripheral neuropathy. A history of any homosexual activities, promiscuous sexual behaviour, a recent blood transfusion, intravenous drug abuse, haemophilia, ear-piercing, tattooing, needle-prick injury or acupuncture should arouse suspicion.

During the second phase the HIV infection causes a slow decline of cell-mediated immune function that usually takes several years before it becomes sufficiently impaired to allow secondary organisms to take over. In this symptom-free incubation period the patient is capable of passing on the virus and, apart from some generalised lymphadenopathy, may be apparently healthy. Unless these individuals are tested for HIV antibodies no-one will know that they are carrying the virus.

When the full-blown picture of AIDs finally develops the patient will present with fever, anorexia, malaise, night sweats, chronic diarrhoea and profound loss of weight. If the lungs are involved cough and dyspnoea may be prominent.

In the United States and Europe the commonest secondary invaders are *Pneumocystis carinii*, cytomegalovirus, herpesvirus and *Candida*. In Africa toxoplasmosis, cryptosporidiosis and tuberculosis are also common, but almost any organism can be involved and multiple infections frequently occur. An enteropathic version of AIDs is seen in Uganda which is known as 'slim disease' because of the severe loss of weight and diarrhoea which are the main presenting features. The term 'AIDS-related complex' (ARC) is sometimes applied to patients in whom the disease is less florid and there is doubt about the diagnosis.

A relentless progressive dementia, myelopathy or neuropathy will signal the destruction of nerve cells by the HIV virus, but meningo-encephalitis and focal lesions in the brain may be due to dissemination of non-Hodgkin's lymphoma or invasion by such organisms as *Cryptococcus neoformans*, cytomegalovirus, *Toxoplasma gondii* or Herpesvirus.

Eczema and fungal infections of the skin are common, and immune complex vasculitis and thrombocytopenic purpura have been reported. The most significant skin manifestation, however, is the presence of the multiple vascular nodules of Kaposi's sarcoma which are usually accompanied by deposits in the lymph nodes and gastrointestinal tract. This tumour can also cause a diffuse pneumonitis indistinguishable from lung infections due to cytomegalovirus or *Pneumocystis carinii*. At present there is no cure for AIDs and most patients die within a year or two of the onset of the final phase.

Investigations
During the initial viral illness the blood picture may reveal lymphopenia or thrombocytopenia, and liver function tests may be temporarily disturbed. The HIV antibody tests will be negative and it may be several months before they become positive. A positive test during the incubation period will be the only evidence of infection unless attempts are made to isolate the virus from the blood; this process is difficult and time-consuming and is used only for research purposes. Lymph node biopsy will show only non-specific follicular hyperplasia.

When AIDS finally develops the blood picture may reveal anaemia, leukopenia, lymphopenia or thrombocytopenia. A raised ESR and hyper-gammaglobulinaemia are common findings. The HIV antibody test will be positive in the majority, but negative results are sometimes found in very florid cases and in those infected with the HIV-2 virus.

The routine serological tests for secondary invaders may be negative because of the immunosuppression caused by the virus. Identification will depend upon isolating them from the lungs by bronchopulmonary lavage or lung biopsy, or finding them in blood or stools. Chest X-rays will show the diffuse shadowing associated with a pneumonitis, and CT head scans may demonstrate localised masses or brain atrophy in cases with neuro-logical abnormalities; only a brain biopsy will reveal whether this is due to infection or neoplasm.

Rheumatoid arthritis

Aetiology
This common connective-tissue disorder affects at least a million individuals in the UK with varying degrees of severity. There is no reason to believe that it is less prevalent in other countries. It is seen occasionally in child-hood, as Still's disease, but the onset is more common in the third and fourth decade of life, women being affected about three times as often as men.

The pathological changes in the joints consist of exudation, infiltration of the synovial membrane by lymphocytes and plasma cells, and the prolif-eration of granulation tissue which erodes the articular cartilage and subchondrial bone. The tendons and ligaments are also involved in the inflammatory process.

Extra-articular manifestations are much less common and include subcu-taneous nodules over pressure points, pericarditis, pleural effusions, inter-stitial fibrosis in the lungs and a necrotising arteritis which may be indistinguishable from polyarteritis nodosa. Unusual presentations include Felty's syndrome with lymphadenopathy, enlarged spleen and leukopenia, Sjögren's syndrome — in which involvement of the lachrymal and salivary glands results in conjunctivitis and a dry mouth — and Caplan's syndrome in coal miners, in which rheumatoid nodules in the lungs are associated with pneumoconiosis.

The aetiology is still obscure but there seems little doubt that both genetic and environmental factors are important. Recent research suggests that environmental factors initiate the arthritis but genetic factors determine whether the particular individual will subsequently develop autoimmunity and chronic disease. In one study of patients with transient joint pains many were found to have circulating immune complexes in their blood, but a high incidence of the tissue antigen HLA-DR4 was found only in those who went on to develop rheumatoid arthritis and auto-antibodies to IgG.

Clinical features

In all but a minority (in which the disorder begins acutely) debility, malaise and readily-induced fatigue appear early. These are accompanied by loss of weight, evanescent aches and pains in the muscles and joints with stiffness worst on waking. This may continue for weeks or months before joint swelling appears.

On examination slight fever is common, accompanied by sinus tachycardia. The small joints of the hands and wrists and the knee joints are usually affected first. Wasting of muscle and swelling of the joints gives a spindle-shaped appearance to the fingers. Involvement of tendon sheaths with resulting rupture leads to deformities and the ulnar deviation of the fingers which is commonly found. When the wrists are involved there may be an accompanying carpal tunnel syndrome. Palmar erythema is often seen, whilst subcutaneous nodules are sometimes palpable over the ulna and other bones.

Investigations

A mild normocytic, normochromic anaemia is common but it may be hypochromic as a result of alimentary blood loss from analgesic therapy. The ESR is moderately raised depending upon the activity of the disease. Leukopenia is present in Felty's syndrome. Tests for autoantibodies to IgG (rheumatoid factor) are positive in a high proportion but are not specific for this disease, being also positive in 20–30% of cases of systemic lupus erythematosus.

The earliest radiological change in the joints is localised osteoporosis; later the joint spaces are reduced and erosions seen. Chest X-rays may occasionally disclose a pleural effusion or signs of diffuse interstitial fibrosis.

Neoplasia

As any hope of cure by surgery or other therapy depends upon early diagnosis our dominant concern is for the first evidence of neoplasia. Unfortunately loss of weight is often only apparent when the growth has spread beyond the confines of the affected organ. Malignant disease accounts for about 20% of all deaths each year in England and Wales. The comparative frequency of neoplasms in different sites is shown in the following table. Of the 139 822 deaths in 1985 the four main causes were carcinomas of bronchus, breast, stomach and colon.

Cancer deaths — England and Wales 1985

Malignant neoplasms of	Number	% all neoplasms
Trachea, bronchus and lung	35 792	25.6
Female breast	13 513	9.7
Colon	11 287	8.1
Stomach	9 971	7.1
Lymphatic and haematopoietic tissue other than leukaemia	9 038	6.5
Prostate	6 628	4.7
Pancreas	6 077	4.4
Rectum	6 040	4.3
Bladder	4 669	3.3
Oesophagus	4 570	3.3
Ovary	3 843	2.8
Leukaemia	3 698	2.6
Uterus and cervix	3 492	2.5
Kidney	2 186	1.6
Other sites not identified	19 020	13.6
All malignant neoplasms	139 822	100.0

The clinical manifestations of malignant disease result from local involvement, metastases or systemic disturbances which include loss of weight. Symptoms and signs arising from the primary growth have been discussed elsewhere in this book and will not be considered further.

Metastases
Metastases often remain silent for a long time and, in the case of breast and bowel cancer, this may be several years after the primary has been discovered and removed. Sometimes, however, they provide the first evidence of disease. The various sites in which they may appear are now considered. The lymph nodes adjacent to the growth enlarge first. In breast cancer they are felt in the axilla. Cervical adenopathy is found in carcinoma of the thyroid, in postcricoid neoplasms and in the lymphomas. In the mediastinum hilar enlargement seen on a chest X-ray may be the first evidence of a bronchial tumour or of Hodgkin's disease.

The liver is the site of secondary deposits in three-quarters of patients dying of cancer, and hepatic enlargement is a common finding. In the lungs, secondary deposits are commonly silent, being found on X-ray as circular or 'cannonball' shadows, but pleural metastases may cause large pleural effusions and consequent shortness of breath.

Metastases in the brain are not uncommon and may be single or multiple.

According to their situation and size they may remain silent or cause headache, vertigo, vomiting, impaired vision, fits, ataxia or palsies. These ominous symptoms may be accompanied by presenile dementia and raised intracranial pressure.

Deposits in bone can cause pain from invasion of the periosteum or vertebral collapse and pathological fractures may occur elsewhere in the skeleton. Infiltration of the bone marrow may produce a leuko-erythroblastic anaemia or thrombocytopenia. Initial bone X-rays are often negative but eventually changes in texture become apparent. Bone scans often reveal suspicious areas before the lesions are visible on plain X-rays. In the skin small nodules occasionally provide the first clue to malignancy elsewhere.

Systemic effects

Toxic effects arising from the tumour include lassitude, fever and loss of weight, which is the subject of this chapter. It is often seen, particularly in the terminal stages, and may be due in part to loss of appetite. Naturally, anorexia and weight loss are to be expected in carcinoma of the oesophagus and stomach. Anaemia is most likely in alimentary cancer from haemorrhage, but it may be due to metastases in the marrow from other sites.

A non-metastatic neuropathy sometimes occurs, particularly with bronchial carcinoma and the lymphomas. It may take the form of a sensory or motor polyneuritis with muscle wasting, ataxia and loss of reflexes. It is probably an immune-mediated disorder associated with the release of some antigen by the tumour tissue.

Finally, the association of certain metabolic disturbances with some neoplasms is well known. Although they are uncommon it is important to bear them in mind, because such patients present with weight loss, apathy and mental changes. They appear to be due to the production by these growths of polypeptide hormones. They include hypercalcaemia, which may be associated with bony secondaries, the inappropriate secretion of antidiuretic hormone and the ectopic ACTH syndrome. Bronchial neoplasms are the chief offenders but other tumours have occasionally been incriminated.

Investigations

These will be directed by the symptoms and signs to whatever organ or system falls under suspicion. A routine blood count will reveal the presence of anaemia and the grossly raised white cell count of leukaemia. The ESR is likely to be elevated in most forms of malignant disease.

A chest X-ray may show hilar enlargement, a pleural effusion or the presence of primary or secondary growth. Ultrasonography and computed tomography are now widely used in the detection of neoplasms in most organs of the body, but are likely to be displaced by the technique of nuclear magnetic resonance when this equipment becomes more generally available.

Finally, if a tumour or enlarged lymph node is visible or accessible biopsy will provide histological proof of the diagnosis.

Lymphomas

Aetiology
Hodgkin's disease is the commonest of all the solid tumours of the lymphoid system. It is rare in childhood and is seen most often in young men. *Non-Hodgkin's lymphoma* is commoner in the middle-aged and elderly of both sexes, but is sometimes seen in younger patients with AIDS. The disease is usually widely disseminated by the time the diagnosis is made.

Clinical features
Painless enlargement of lymph nodes, particularly those in the neck and axillae, is often the first manifestation of Hodgkin's disease and may precede other signs and symptoms by months or even years. Involvement of lymph nodes in the mediastinum or abdomen is common but will not be detected on clinical examination. Later there will be night sweats, fever, generalised pruritus and loss of weight. Alcohol-induced bone pain may have been noticed by the patient.

Anaemia is common and may be due to haemolysis, hypersplenism or marrow infiltration. Neurological complications include spinal cord compression from extradural deposits, leuko-encephalopathy and peripheral neuropathy.

Superimposed infection may be due to impaired cellular immunity, hypogammaglobulinaemia or neutropenia from marrow infiltration. Herpes zoster is common in Britain, particularly in patients undergoing treatment, and opportunistic infections such as cryptococcal meningitis or *Pneumocystis carinii* pneumonia may prove fatal. Lymphosarcoma and reticulum cell sarcoma may present in a similar way to Hodgkin's disease, but their course is usually much more rapid.

On examination the characteristic smooth, freely mobile lymph nodes occurring in groups and not adherent to the overlying skin should be looked for. The liver and spleen are usually palpable in the later stages. The skin is often sallow and hyperpigmentation is sometimes present. A pleural effusion may be found.

Investigations
Some degree of anaemia is usually present; an elevated reticulocyte count and a positive Coomb's test will suggest haemolysis and the level of serum unconjugated bilirubin may be increased. A normal white count will exclude leukaemia, but a marked eosinophilia is not uncommon. The ESR is usually high, but reduced immunoglobulins may be found on serum electrophoresis. If AIDS is suspected from the history a blood sample should be taken for HIV antibodies, taking care to avoid needle stick injury.

A chest X-ray may show enlarged hilar shadows, diffuse pulmonary infiltration, or a pleural effusion. A biopsy, usually of a superficial lymph node, will provide the diagnosis in many cases and will exclude other causes of lymphadenopathy such as tuberculosis, sarcoidosis and toxoplasmosis.

Liver and bone scans using radioactive isotopes, lymphangiography and even exploratory laparotomy may be necessary to establish the anatomical extent of the disease. These procedures are likely to be replaced by the non-invasive techniques of computed tomography or nuclear magnetic resonance when this equipment becomes more widely available.

Diabetes mellitus (see also Obesity, p. 290)

Aetiology

Diabetes is not a single disease but a complex metabolic disorder caused by a number of conditions which result in lack of sufficient insulin at cellular level. This deficiency may be due to destruction of the islet cells of the pancreas, to inactivation of this hormone in the circulation or to increased resistance to its action in the tissues. In some individuals more than one of these mechanisms may be operating at the same time. Lack of insulin leads to hyperglycaemia, particularly after a carbohydrate meal. Glycosuria appears when the blood glucose levels exceed the renal threshold for this sugar.

Many surveys have shown that diabetes is the commonest endocrine disorder in the UK, affecting between 1 and 2% of the indigenous popu-lation. Its prevalence amongst Indian immigrants to this country is even greater and may reach 10–15% of the elderly Asian population. Most cases arise spontaneously but there is often a family history of this disease and it may be precipitated by infection, surgery, pregnancy or the adminis-tration of such drugs as corticosteroids, the oestrogen-containing contra-ceptive pill or thiazide diuretics. It may follow an overt attack of pancreatitis or surgical removal of that organ, and it is a recognised complication of acromegaly and Cushing's syndrome.

Patients are classified as type I or type II diabetics depending upon whether or not they need insulin therapy to survive.

Type I, or 'juvenile' diabetes as it was previously called, usually appears in childhood or young adult life, but it can present at any age. These patients are insulin-independent from the start and require insulin therapy for the rest of their lives. This type is now thought to be an autoimmune disease for circulating islet cell antibodies have been detected in the blood several years before the onset of symptoms. In one series they were found in 75% of cases at the time of diagnosis. The underlying pathology is a progressive destruction of the islet cells by chronic inflammation which eventually leads to insulin deficiency and carbohydrate intolerance. Not surprisingly, this type of diabetes is sometimes preceded or followed by other autoimmune disorders such as thyroiditis, pernicious anaemia, Addison's disease or rheumatoid arthritis. The initial stimulus which trig-gers off the inflammatory process is still unknown, but the most likely sequence of events is a subclinical viral pancreatitis followed by deposition of immune complexes in the damaged tissues.

Type I diabetes is a familial condition but precisely what is passed on is still a mystery. There is however a high prevalence of the HLA antigens DR3 and DR4 in insulin-dependent diabetics compared to the normal population, and the inheritance of both these antigens appears to confer a greater genetic susceptibility to this disease than does the possession of either antigen alone.

Type II, or 'maturity-onset' diabetes, has a different aetiology. In these non-insulin-dependent patients the main problem seems to lie in an increased resistance to the action of insulin in the tissues. This type is rarely seen before the age of 30 and its incidence rises with increasing age. Although non-insulin-dependent diabetes may present with loss of weight it is more commonly found in those who are overweight. It is therefore dealt with in more detail in the chapter on Obesity.

Clinical features
In type I diabetes an acute onset is common, particularly in children. It presents with thirst, polyuria, frequency of micturition, blurred vision and loss of weight. If the condition is not recognised immediately these symptoms will be followed by vomiting, dehydration, confusion and even coma. Epigastric pain is not uncommon. In adults the onset may be much more insidious and weeks or months may pass before they seek advice. This particularly applies to those with non-insulin-dependent diabetes. In elderly women pruritus vulvae may be the presenting symptom.

On examination there may be little to find apart from a dry tongue, inelastic skin and obvious loss of flesh. Drowsiness, slow deep respirations and the smell of acetone or nail varnish in the breath are evidence of severe keto-acidosis and insulin must be given without delay.

Investigations
The urine will usually contain both glucose and ketones in abundance, but the latter may be absent in the older patient with type II diabetes. A random blood glucose level of more than 10 mmol/l (180 mg/dl) will confirm the diagnosis. A glucose tolerance test is unnecessary as a rule and is a burden to both patient and pathologist. The blood urea, serum creatinine and electrolytes should be estimated as a guide to the degree of dehydration and electrolyte depletion. Several hundred millimoles of sodium and potassium may have been lost in the urine if keto-acidosis is present.

A polymorphonuclear leukocytosis is often found in diabetic keto-acidosis and does not necessarily indicate bacterial infection. Nevertheless, since diabetes is frequently exacerbated by infection it is probably wise to take a throat swab and chest X-ray, and to send a urine specimen to the laboratory for microscopy and culture.

Hyperthyroidism

Aetiology
Thyrotoxicosis occurs mainly in females and is rare in childhood, the peak incidence being seen in the third and fourth decades. The term 'Graves disease' is still used to describe the syndrome of hyperthyroidism, goitre

and eye signs; these common features are sometimes accompanied by pretibial 'myxoedema', vitiligo, thyroid acropathy and myasthenia gravis. The diffuse enlargement of the thyroid gland in this disorder is due to the production of thyroid-stimulating antibodies which interact with TSH receptors and cause the increased secretion of triiodothyronine (T_3) and thyroxine (T_4). Other autoantibodies are probably responsible for the exophthalmos and other non-thyroidal manifestations of this disease. The passage of these antibodies across the placenta from a thyrotoxic mother to her unborn child is a rare cause of transient neonatal hyperthyroidism.

In older patients thyrotoxicosis is often due to the excessive secretion of thyroid hormones by an autonomous nodule in a multinodular goitre; eye signs will be absent in these cases. The administration of iodine to goitrous individuals in areas of iodine deficiency sometimes results in hyperthyroidism, the correction of the deficiency unmasking the presence of an autonomous adenoma or Graves disease. Finally, an overactive thyroid is occasionally due to the excess production of thyroid-stimulating substances by a pituitary adenoma, bronchogenic carcinoma or trophoblastic tumour.

Clinical features
The symptoms result from a raised metabolic rate and sympathetic over-activity. Exhaustion and debility are often the first symptoms. Loss of weight is usual and may be severe, despite a good appetite. Palpitations, excessive sweating, dyspnoea on exertion and occasionally diarrhoea are prominent. The patient is often restless and irritable, psychoneurosis is common and insanity may occur.

On examination the prominent eyes, flushed excitable appearance, moist skin and the rapid heart, often fibrillating at the menopause, are characteristic. The thyroid gland is usually visible and as a rule palpably enlarged, but rarely the enlarged portion lies behind the sternum; it may then be felt filling up the suprasternal notch. A bruit is heard over the gland in about 60% of cases. Tremors of the extended hands are fine, regular and rapid and are increased by excitement or movement.

Upper lid retraction and 'lid lag' are the commonest ocular manifestations. Exophthalmos may affect only one eye at first; in severe cases paresis of the external ocular muscles will cause diplopia. Finger clubbing, Addisonian-like pigmentation, vitiligo, splenic enlargement and pretibial 'myxoedema' are found occasionally in Graves disease.

Investigations
The diagnosis should always be confirmed by hormone assay before treatment is started. The introduction of radioimmunoassays for the thyroid hormones have made most other thyroid function tests obsolete. A raised serum thyroxine level is usually sufficient to establish the diagnosis except in women on the contraceptive pill and during pregnancy; here an elevated level may be due to the increase in thyroxine-binding globulin which is provoked by oestrogens. A thyroxine-binding globulin estimation will enable a correction to be made for this increased binding and should be

requested at the same time as the thyroxine estimation. Serum triiodothyronine estimations are often of value in confirming hyperthyroidism in cases of T_3-toxicosis with normal serum thyroxine levels. Thyroglobulin and microsomal antibodies should be looked for in the serum for they are of some prognostic value; patients with high titres are more likely to develop hypothyroidism after thyroid surgery or radio-iodine therapy.

Addison's disease

Aetiology

Both adrenal glands must be largely destroyed before the signs and symptoms of this uncommon disease appear. Tuberculosis still accounts for at least 30% of cases in Britain. In the majority of cases, however, the chronic inflammatory process which destroys the adrenals appears to be of an autoimmune nature — circulating adrenal antibodies are commonly found. This form is seen more often in women and may be preceded or followed by other autoimmune disorders such as Hashimoto's thyroiditis, pernicious anaemia, vitiligo, ovarian failure or diabetes mellitus. There is a high incidence of HLA antigens A1 and B8 in these patients. Rare causes include amyloidosis, metastases and, in endemic areas of the world, mycotic infections.

The clinical manifestations of this disease are due to lack of mineralocorticoids and cortisol (hydrocortisone). The hyperpigmentation is caused by excess corticotrophin secreted by the pituitary gland in response to the falling cortisol level in the blood.

Clinical features

The onset is usually insidious and is characterised by increasing lassitude and pigmentation over many months. In some cases there is a history of these complaints for several years before a relatively mild stress precipitates an adrenal crisis. Anorexia and weight loss are almost invariable though the latter rarely exceeds 6 kg. They may be accompanied by episodes of nausea and vomiting. Abdominal pain is less common and may be mistaken for that of a peptic ulcer, cholecystitis or inflamed appendix.

Postural hypotension may cause blurring of vision, giddy spells or fainting attacks. Other symptoms include dyspnoea on quite modest exertion, palpitations and muscle cramps from salt depletion. Mental confusion or hysterical behaviour often herald an impending adrenal crisis which may present with abdominal pain, nausea, vomiting, headache and drowsiness; unexplained fever is not uncommon and is usually accompanied by a rapid pulse and falling blood pressure.

On examination the pigmentation is most marked on the exposed parts of the body but may be seen in the axillae, scars, the palmar creases, over bony prominences and in areas where friction from clothing occurs. It varies in intensity from a light tan to a dirty brown or black colour. Buccal pigmentation was present in 50% of a personal series of 71 cases. The blood pressure is usually low and the systolic pressure may fall below 100 mmHg on standing. A normal blood pressure does not however exclude this condition for the patient may have been hypertensive beforehand.

Investigations

The blood picture is usually normal, but the ESR is sometimes elevated and a relative lymphocytosis has been reported. The characteristic changes in the serum are a low sodium level, hyperkalaemia, a metabolic acidosis and a raised blood urea. Although these abnormalities are invariably present to some degree during an adrenal crisis, they may be absent in the more chronic case.

When tuberculosis is responsible X-rays may show lesions in the lungs and speckled calcification in the adrenals. A small, thin cardiac shadow is typically seen in this disorder and may be commented upon by the radiologist.

Low plasma and urinary corticosteroid levels support the diagnosis, but normal levels may be found for the adrenal remnants are being maximally stimulated by endogenous corticotrophin. A certain diagnosis can only be made if these levels fail to rise significantly after adequate stimulation of the adrenals with injections of animal or synthetic ACTH.

Raised morning plasma ACTH levels will be found in the untreated patient and circulating adrenal antibodies may be detected in those cases due to auto-immune disease. These investigations are outside the scope of most hospital laboratories but fortunately the diagnosis does not depend upon the results of such esoteric tests.

CHAPTER 23
Obesity

SYNOPSIS OF CAUSES*

NON-ENDOCRINE
Idiopathic; **Drugs**; Head injury; Intracranial tumours; Encephalitis.

ENDOCRINE
Diabetes mellitus; **Hypothyroidism**; Cushing's syndrome; **Stein-Leventhal syndrome**; Hypopituitarism; Hypogonadism.

* Bold type is used for causes more commonly found in Europe and North America.

PHYSIOLOGY

Carbohydrates account for at least half the calorie content of most diets. In the alimentary tract they are broken down to monosaccharides, mainly in the form of glucose. This sugar is readily absorbed and passes to the liver where a small proportion is converted into glycogen. The remainder enters the general circulation where it is either burnt as fuel or converted into free fatty acids and glycerol which are stored as neutral fat. Insulin, secreted by the islet cells of the pancreas, is necessary to enable these metabolic processes to take place.

The output of this hormone is largely governed by the blood glucose level. When this rises after food more insulin is released and this, in turn, lowers the level by increasing the utilisation of this sugar in the tissues. In healthy individuals this process ensures that the blood glucose does not normally exceed 9 mmol/l (160 mg/100 ml) after a meal and returns to fasting levels within 2 hours.

Glucose is an essential fuel for brain cells and provides a ready source of energy for other tissues, particularly during exercise when energy requirements are high. In the fasting state free fatty acids, mainly derived from the breakdown of neutral fat in the adipose tissue, are an alternative and more economical fuel. During prolonged starvation and in insulin-deficient diabetics they are the major source of energy but have the disadvantage that their oxidation results in the production of ketones.

The fat depots constitute an active metabolic organ whose main function is to store surplus fat and carbohydrate ingested at meals and to provide a continuous flow of energy to the tissues in the form of free fatty acids. The amount of fat in the body is determined by the balance between these two processes; when intake consistently exceeds energy output the adipose organ will increase in size.

Energy expenditure in man is determined by the sum of the basal metabolic rate, the energy used up in physical activity, and dietary-induced thermogenesis. The first two normally account for about 80% of the total but many studies have failed to show significant differences between lean and fat individuals, except in hypothyroid subjects in whom the basal metabolic rate is abnormally low.

In cafeteria-fed rats, allowed an unlimited intake of their favourite foods, the difference in energy expenditure between thin and obese animals appears to be determined by their capacity to burn excess fatty acids in the mitochondria of their brown fat. This specialised tissue forms only about 1% of their body weight but is now thought to be the site of dietary-induced thermogenesis in these rodents. It is tempting to assume that a similar mechanism operates in man and that a congenital or acquired defect in brown adipose tissue may account for some people growing fat and others remaining thin, despite very similar patterns of food intake and activity. This hypothesis is far from proven but there is evidence that dietary-induced thermogenesis is reduced in patients with idiopathic obesity.

This cannot however be the only factor which determines the size of the adipose organ in man. Insulin is clearly necessary for the conversion of glucose to fat but other hormones such as oestrogens and cortisol also promote its synthesis. The average fat content of women, expressed as a percentage of total body weight, is almost twice that of men of the same age. Impaired glucose tolerance and a tendency to put on weight is not uncommon in women taking the contraceptive pill and in patients of both sexes on corticosteroid therapy.

Little is known about the physiological mechanisms which control the mobilisation of fat. Growth hormone is probably involved, for it is lipolytic in the intact animal and its secretion rises when the blood glucose level is low, at a time when more free fatty acids are required as alternative fuel. There is some evidence, however, that the pituitary secretes at least one other polypeptide hormone, beta-lipotrophin, which also causes the breakdown of neutral fat. The hypothalamus controls the output of most anterior pituitary hormones by secreting specific releasing factors into the portal system of veins which link the median eminence and the pituitary gland. The ventro–medial nuclei may ultimately control the secretion of these lipolytic hormones, since destruction of this area in animals leads to overeating and gross obesity.

Finally, the size of the adipose organ is influenced by the activity of the thyroid gland which controls the basal metabolic rate. In hyperthyroidism energy output is increased and loss of weight is usual despite a good appetite; the reverse is seen in hypothyroidism. The energy requirements of an individual will vary enormously according to age and physical activity; the calorie content of a diet sufficient to maintain a normal weight in youth may be inappropriately high in middle age. Even in the presence of overt endocrine disease obesity can only occur if the carbohydrate intake exceeds the capacity of the body to dispose of it in the metabolic fires.

The range of weight among human beings is surprisingly wide. Cases are recorded with some authenticity that are almost beyond belief. The heaviest known human was Robert Earl Hughes of Indiana USA who weighed 92 kg (14½ stone) when 6 years old and progressively increased in size to reach 486 kg (76 stone) when he died of renal failure at the age of 32. Fortunately such corpulence is extremely rare.

DIAGNOSTIC APPROACH

Obesity is common in countries where carbohydrate foods are cheap and readily available. It has been defined as an increase of more than 20% over the optimal weight for height, age and sex but few doctors will have life insurance tables or growth charts readily to hand. In practice the condition is usually fairly obvious although the full extent of the problem may not be apparent until the patient is weighed and undressed.

In infancy and childhood endocrine disorders are rare. Bottle feeding, a diet of fish and chips and the excessive consumption of sweets are more probable causes of obesity. Sexual maturation is often delayed, but stunting of growth must be taken seriously for it is likely to be due to juvenile hypothyroidism, hypopituitarism or Cushing's syndrome.

In young adults obesity is commonly associated with a sedentary occupation, lack of exercise, the excessive consumption of alcohol, frequent pregnancies or the contraceptive pill. Overeating is an occupational hazard of chefs and housewives. Hypogonadism in the male is rare and readily diagnosed by the lack of secondary sexual characteristics. In the female hypothyroidism and Cushing's syndrome are uncommon causes; obesity, hirsutism and irregular periods are more likely to be associated with polycystic ovaries than with adrenocortical overactivity.

In the middle-aged and elderly adiposity is mainly due to a life-long indulgence in high carbohydrate diets, but diabetes mellitus is not uncommon and hypothyroidism is often missed. The decline in physical activity by middle age may be partly responsible for the increased incidence at this time of life.

There is rarely time for a full dietary history and in any case obese patients often underestimate their carbohydrate intake. A few pointed questions will quickly establish that many are still taking sugar in tea or coffee, eat potatoes with their main meals and have been unable to stick to reducing diets in the past. It is useful to get some idea of when the patient first became overweight. This may date from a head injury, change of occupation, marriage, pregnancy or starting on the contraceptive pill. With hypothyroidism in mind inquiry should be made of cold intolerance, undue fatigue, headaches, constipation and changes in the texture of the skin and hair. Irregular or absent periods, hirsutism in the female or infrequent shaving in the male are all very suggestive of an underlying endocrine cause. A family history of diabetes or thyroid disease may be significant, but obesity in other members of the family is commonly due to a shared habit of overeating.

Examination of the undressed patient is essential to reveal the full extent of the adiposity and its distribution. Truncal obesity with relatively thin arms and legs is seen only in severe Cushing's syndrome, along with a rounded face and the characteristic broad red or purple striae on the lower abdomen, thighs and upper arms. Thin red or white striae are less significant, being seen in anyone who has put on weight rapidly. The skin may be coarse and dry in hypothyroidism or thin and readily lifted off the underlying fat in Cushing's syndrome. The amount and distribution of body hair should be noted and, if abnormal, the external genitalia must be inspected. Loss of the outer third of the eyebrows is common in the elderly and does not necessarily mean that they are suffering from thyroid deficiency.

Examination of the central nervous system may reveal the peripheral neuropathy of diabetes or the characteristic slow relaxation of the tendon reflexes seen in hypothyroidism. The fundi should be routinely examined for any evidence of retinopathy, and the visual fields tested by confrontation to pick up any temporal field loss due to damage to the optic chiasma from an enlarging pituitary tumour. Finally the blood pressure should be taken, bearing in mind that using a normal-sized cuff on a fat arm may result in falsely high readings. A post-prandial urine specimen should be tested routinely for the presence of glucose, but further investigations are rarely justified unless the history or physical examination produce some evidence which points to an endocrine cause.

NON-ENDOCRINE CAUSES

In the synopsis the classification is somewhat artificial, since even the non-endocrine causes of obesity may operate through hormonal mechanisms. Nevertheless, this division does enable the major endocrine disorders to be described separately.

Idiopathic obesity

Most obese subjects fall into this category. It is seen in infants fed on modified cow's milk, in schoolchildren brought up on unrestricted carbohydrate diets and in adults of all ages, particularly women after repeated pregnancies. The only common factor appears to be an excessive intake of carbohydrates over a long period which presumably exceeded the energy requirements of that individual.

While overeating with consequent hyperinsulinaemia may account for most cases of moderate obesity, the suspicion remains that some more fundamental disorder of fat metabolism must be responsible for the grosser forms of adiposity which are seen. A congenital or acquired defect in dietary-induced thermogenesis might well explain a life-long tendency to put on weight and an apparent inability to get rid of it despite repeated attempts at dieting.

When the total body weight exceeds 100 kg (16 stone) more than half the body is composed of fat. This represents about 400 000 kcal of stored energy, theoretically equivalent to 4–5 months supply of food! Attempts at dieting may be defeated by reactive hypoglycaemia between meals.

Obese children do not necessarily grow into fat adults, despite assertions to the contrary. The incidence of diabetes mellitus, heart disease, hypertension, gallstones, hiatal hernia and osteoarthritis is much higher in the obese than in the normal population.

Drugs

Obesity often results from treatment with corticosteroids, oestrogens, progestins and drugs used in psychiatric disorders. It is a common side-effect of therapy with chlorpromazine, haloperidol, pimozide and thioridazine and has encouraged their use in anorexia nervosa. Manic-depressives given lithium salts tend to put on weight and may develop a goitre; the serum thyroxine and TSH levels should be checked at intervals in these patients for evidence of iatrogenic hypothyroidism.

Head injury

An alarming increase in weight occasionally follows severe head injuries. The patient has usually been unconscious for many hours after a fall from a horse or a road traffic accident. Damage to the hypothalamus may be responsible, since transient diabetes insipidus, menstrual irregularities and reversal of the normal circadian rhythm of water and electrolyte excretion have been seen in some cases.

Intracranial tumours

Hypothalamic damage, with consequent overeating and gross obesity, may be due to an astrocytoma of the midbrain, suprasellar tumour or meningioma compressing the hypothalamus from above. Because of their rarity, slow growth and paucity of physical signs they may be missed for years. Loss of vision in the temporal fields from pressure on the optic chiasma may eventually draw attention to their presence.

Encephalitis

Obesity is a rare complication of viral encephalitis and cerebral sarcoidosis.

It may be accompanied by disturbances of sleep and temperature control, suggesting a hypothalamic cause.

ENDOCRINE CAUSES

Maturity-onset diabetes and hypothyroidism are amongst the commonest causes of obesity in middle life. Their earlier recognition would avoid a great deal of unnecessary and prolonged ill-health.

Diabetes mellitus (see also Loss of weight, p. 280)

Aetiology

Type II, or 'maturity-onset' diabetes, is multifactorial in origin and is often associated with obesity rather than loss of weight. In these non-insulin-dependent diabetics the fasting blood glucose level may be normal but hyperglycaemia and consequent glycosuria appear after a carbohydrate meal.

Type II diabetes is rare before the age of 30 and increases in incidence with advancing age. In the UK it is thought to affect at least 3% of the indigenous population over the age of 65. Its prevalence in Indian immigrants to this country is at least three times greater than this, and in one survey carried out in the Midlands 20% in this age group were affected. The reason for this striking racial difference is unknown, but hereditary factors must play a part.

There is good evidence that some non-insulin-dependent diabetics actually secrete more insulin than normal following a carbohydrate meal, presumably in response to the high postprandial blood glucose levels. This paradox can only be explained by an inherited or acquired resistance in these patients to the normal action of insulin on the uptake of glucose by the tissues. Many mechanisms have been suggested which include the production of an abnormal insulin molecule which fails to lock on to the insulin receptors on the cell membranes; defects in the receptors themselves or in the post-receptor pathways; or the presence of circulating insulin antagonists which may inactivate the hormone in the circulation or block its action at cellular level. In some patients more than one of these mechanisms may be operating at the same time. The exposure of the adipose tissues to increased concentrations of glucose and insulin over a prolonged period of time will encourage lipogenesis and may account for the obesity which is so often seen in non-insulin-dependent diabetes.

Naturally-occurring insulin antagonists are normally present in the blood and include adrenaline, cortisol and growth hormone. Insulin antagonism probably explains the carbohydrate intolerance seen in acromegaly and Cushing's syndrome. Recently, antibodies to human insulin have been demonstrated in the blood of some untreated diabetics and in other, non-diabetic patients with autoimmune diseases. By inactivating insulin in the circulation they may contribute to the lack of this hormone at cellular level.

Obese diabetics rarely require insulin unless they are stressed by surgery, myocardial infarction or severe infections. Strict adherence to a low carbohydrate diet is essential to lower the postprandial blood glucose levels.

Clinical features

Many patients with type II diabetes will have been overweight for many years. There may be a history of diabetes in the family, of large babies in multiparous females or of frequent urinary or skin infections. Pruritus vulvae is common and is almost always due to monilial infection. Thirst and polyuria are minimal and may not be complained of by the patient.

The long-term vascular complications may first bring the patient to the doctor. Atherosclerosis is common in diabetics and occurs at an earlier age than in the normal population. Thus they may present in middle age with hypertension, myocardial infarction, strokes or ischaemic legs. Failing vision from diabetic retinopathy, progressive renal failure, perforating ulcers of the feet and local gangrene of one or more toes are due to small vessel disease. A peripheral neuropathy mainly affecting the lower limbs will cause pain, paraesthesiae and eventually loss of all sensation in the feet. Isolated cranial nerve palsies are sometimes seen and other ocular complications include cataracts and glaucoma.

Investigations

Glycosuria may be found only in a postprandial specimen; ketones are usually absent. Proteinuria, however slight, is indicative of renal damage. A urine specimen should be sent for microscopy and culture. Swabs from leg ulcers are likely to grow *Staph. aureus*. Blood for glucose estimation should be taken about one hour after a meal; a level of more than 10 mmol/l (180 mg/dl) will confirm the diagnosis. A full glucose tolerance test is rarely necessary except in border-line cases. A glycosylated haemoglobin estimation above the normal range for the laboratory will also confirm the diagnosis and provides a base-line for determining the effect of treatment.

Hypothyroidism

Aetiology

In infancy hypothyroidism is due to the faulty development of the gland or, in a few cases, to inherited enzyme deficiencies which impair the production of thyroxine (T_4) and triiodothyronine (T_3). Endemic cretinism, due to maternal iodine deficiency, has long disappeared from Europe and North America but still occurs in some mountainous regions of the world such as the Andes and the Himalayas. Mass screening has shown that the incidence of neonatal hypothyroidism in the UK is approximately 1 in 4000 live births. Early diagnosis and treatment is essential to prevent the irreversible brain damage of the untreated cretin.

Thyroid deficiency arising later in childhood may be due to developmental abnormalities of the gland or to the early appearance of autoimmune thyroiditis. Children with Down's syndrome are particularly at risk. In adolescent girls an enlarging goitre is often the first and only sign of a failing thyroid.

Most cases of primary hypothyroidism in adult life are probably due to the production of thyroid microsomal antibodies which eventually destroy the hormone-secreting cells. In a few cases other autoantibodies have been found which either inactivate the hormones in the circulation or block the thyroid response to thyroid-stimulating hormone (TSH) by combining with the TSH receptors. This disorder is much commoner in females and particularly prevalent in middle-aged and elderly women. It is one of the commonest endocrine diseases in Britain, affecting at least 2% of the adult population.

Hypothyroidism with goitre may be induced by a variety of drugs which interfere with hormone synthesis. These include the thioureas and imazoles used in the treatment of hyperthyroidism, para-aminosalicylic acid, cobalt, lithium salts, phenylbutazone, resorcinol in ointments applied to varicose ulcers and the excessive intake of iodine or organic iodine compounds.

The incidence of hypothyroidism following subtotal thyroidectomy for thyrotoxicosis may be as high as 40% at 10 years, a similar incidence to that seen after treatment with radioactive iodine. Secondary hypothyroidism is uncommon but may follow destruction of the pituitary gland by tumour, surgery or infarction accompanying severe postpartum haemorrhage (Sheehan's syndrome). It may then be associated with hypogonadism and secondary adrenal failure.

Clinical features
Obesity, cold intolerance, constipation and a gradual slowing down in mental and physical activity are the cardinal features of hypothyroidism at any age, but may not be apparent in the first few weeks of life. Prolonged neonatal jaundice is sometimes the earliest manifestation of congenital hypothyroidism. Only later will the characteristic features of the cretin become apparent. These include the flattening of the bridge of the nose, the half-open mouth with thickening of the lips and tongue, the protuberant abdomen and umbilical hernia, and the pale cool skin. These placid infants are content to lie quietly for long periods of time showing little interest in their surroundings. The longer the delay in diagnosis the more likely that they will be left with permanent cerebral impairment.

In older children and adults the onset is often very insidious and easily missed. The most frequent presenting symptoms are the non-specific ones of tiredness, lack of energy and weight gain. The tiredness is characteristically present throughout the day and there may be difficulty in waking and a tendency to fall asleep after meals. Inability to cope with normal physical and mental activities may be mistakenly ascribed to depression. In the rare case of juvenile myxoedema this lack of energy and inability to concentrate will result in a deteriorating performance at school. Without regular checks of height and weight the inevitable stunting of growth may be missed for several years. In plump young women the disorder may present with infertility and scanty periods.

In middle age thyroid deficiency begins to affect the heart and central nervous system. Thus it may present with angina, congestive cardiac failure, myocardial infarction, depression, cerebellar ataxia or the carpal tunnel syndrome. Angina pectoris in a middle-aged overweight woman should always bring this diagnosis to mind, particularly if there is no other pathology such as diabetes, valvular heart disease or previously recorded hypertension to account for it. A complaint of dry skin, falling hair, cold intolerance, constipation, menstrual disturbances or increasing deafness may be elicited on direct questioning, but these symptoms are not invariably present. A family history of thyroid disease or other autoimmune disorders should be inquired for, and previous treatment with thyroid surgery or radioactive iodine is obviously relevant; obscure aching in the muscles may precede the more familiar symptoms in these patients.

In the elderly slowness of thought and speech, a poor memory, somnolence, deafness, an unsteady gait and faecal impaction are far too often attributed to advancing senility. Untreated, they become demented or fall victim to hypothermia during the winter months.

Physical examination may be unrewarding but the patient is usually overweight and the presence of a goitre, cold dry skin or bradycardia should arouse suspicion. Loss of the outer third of the eyebrows is common in the elderly and is not a reliable sign of failing thyroid function. Scanty or absent axillary and pubic hair, on the other hand, is a feature of hypogonadism secondary to pituitary disease and other evidence of hypopituitarism should be sought.

In gross hypothyroidism, or myxoedema, the face is heavy and expressionless with a yellowish pallor and a malar flush. The eyes are puffy, the skin coarse and dry, the hair brittle and easily pulled out. The voice is deep and hoarse, and the slowness of speech and movement is only too apparent. It is in these patients that the characteristic slow relaxation of the tendon reflexes is most easily seen. Hypothermia is common but may not be recognised unless a low-reading rectal thermometer is used. Excessive salt and consequent water retention leads to oedema of the limbs, pericardial effusion, pleural effusions and occasionally ascites. This tendency to hang on to salt in this disorder may account for the high incidence of hypertension in the older patients. The gait is often unsteady and a severely-affected patient may be very confused and present in a semi-stuporose condition.

Investigations

The introduction of reliable radioimmunoassays for serum thyroxine (T_4) and thyroid-stimulating hormone (TSH) has greatly facilitated the diagnosis of both primary and secondary hypothyroidism. Needless to say, these tests should be carried out before any thyroid hormones are given to the patient. A low serum thyroxine will be found in both forms but an elevated TSH will be found only in those cases where the fault lies in the thyroid gland. Unfortunately there are exceptions to this general rule and some patients with primary hypothyroidism have total serum thyroxine levels which fall within the normal range.

The term *subclinical hypothyroidism* is often used to describe these patients who have suggestive symptoms or signs but apparently normal thyroxine levels and normal or slightly raised serum TSH levels. In this situation an exaggerated rise in the serum TSH levels following an intravenous injection of thyrotrophin-releasing hormone (TRH) will provide confirmatory evidence of a failing thyroid gland. This procedure is probably the most sensitive test available at present, but some doctors prefer to rely on low free thyroxine or triiodothyronine levels in the serum to confirm the diagnosis. These radioimmunoassays are more difficult to do and are not always available to the clinician.

The presence of thyroid microsomal antibodies in the blood will confirm the autoimmune nature of this disease, and an elevated ESR is sometimes found in Hashimoto's thyroiditis. A mild normochromic, normocytic anaemia is not uncommon and responds to replacement therapy alone. The megaloblastic anaemia which is sometimes found is probably due to vitamin B_{12} deficiency for parietal cell antibodies may also be present in hypothyroid patients with auto-immune thyroid disease; a low serum vitamin B_{12} level and an abnormal Schilling test will confirm the presence of pernicious anaemia in these cases. The fasting lipids and serum cholesterol are often elevated but normal levels do not rule out hypothyroidism.

In the more florid case the ECG will reveal the characteristic low voltage QRS complexes, with flat or inverted T waves in the standard chest leads.

A chest X-ray may show cardiac enlargement with pleural or pericardial effusions. In juvenile hypothyroidism X-rays of the hands, wrists and femoral heads may show the typical stippled appearance of epiphyseal dysplasia. A skull X-ray is only indicated if secondary hypothyroidism is suspected; enlargement of the sella turcica with erosion of the surrounding bone is indicative of a pituitary tumour.

Cushing's syndrome

Aetiology

This uncommon disorder is rare in childhood and old age and occurs most frequently in women during the reproductive period of life. It results from the prolonged excessive secretion of cortisol (hydrocortisone) by one or both adrenal glands; in some cases there is also evidence of androgen or mineralocorticoid excess. It may be due to the inappropriate secretion of corticotrophin (ACTH) by the pituitary gland, to the production of corticotrophin by an ectopic source such as a carcinoid tumour or oat cell carcinoma of the bronchus, or to an adrenal tumour.

Pituitary-dependent Cushing's syndrome accounts for about 75% of cases and some of these patients harbour a small ACTH-secreting pituitary tumour. Although these tumours may not be apparent on the initial skull X-rays they sometimes increase in size following bilateral adrenalectomy (Nelson's syndrome). In this form of the disease both adrenal glands will be moderately enlarged and, in long-standing cases, autonomous nodules develop in the hyperplastic glands.

Pseudo-Cushing's syndrome is seen occasionally in chronic alcoholics.

The clinical picture is identical to that of the naturally-occurring disorder but the increased adrenocortical activity subsides when the drinking stops; whether alcohol has a direct stimulatory effect on the adrenal cells or works indirectly via the hypothalamus or pituitary is still undecided.

In the ectopic ACTH syndrome gross hyperplasia of the adrenals is found at autopsy. This form of Cushing's syndrome is seen mainly in middle-aged or elderly male cigarette smokers with oat cell bronchial carcinomas, but it can occur with other polypeptide-secreting neoplasms. Adrenal tumours account for the remaining 10–20% of cases; about half of these are benign adenomas arising in one or other adrenal gland and appear to occur exclusively in females. Adrenal carcinomas, on the other hand, are found in both sexes and have usually spread to the liver or lungs by the time they present.

Clinical features
The onset of pituitary-dependent Cushing's syndrome is usually very insidious and it may be many years before the condition is even suspected. Obesity, often accompanied by irregular periods or amenorrhoea, may be traced back to a previous pregnancy. In children the onset is more rapid and always associated with stunting of growth; this is usually obvious from a height and weight chart. Impaired glucose tolerance is present in about half of these patients but thirst and polyuria are usually absent. Back pain from osteoporosis is not uncommon, depression is a prominent feature in many patients, and nocturnal sweating is complained of by a few.

In a severe case the diagnosis can be made on sight. The face is plethoric and rounded, the fat is more prominent on the trunk than on the limbs and characteristic broad red or purple striae will be found over the upper arms, thighs and lower abdomen. Hirsutism and acne will be present if there is excessive production of adrenal androgens and are seen in about half the female patients; they will not be accompanied by other signs of virilism unless the underlying lesion is an adrenal carcinoma. The blood pressure is often normal in the younger patients but hypertension is the rule over the age of 40. In milder cases the only evidence of increased adrenocortical activity may be generalised obesity and some rounding of the face.

A short history with florid signs is typical of an adrenal carcinoma and, depending on the mixture of steroids being produced by the tumour, there may be virilism in the female or feminisation in the male. In the ectopic ACTH syndrome loss of weight rather than obesity is one of the presenting features; these patients often complain of increasing pigmentation caused by the high levels of ACTH in the blood.

Investigations
The urine may contain glucose, especially after a meal, but ketones are usually absent. The fasting blood glucose level is often normal but a diabetic glucose tolerance curve is found in at least 20% of cases. Hypokalaemia, due to excess mineralocorticoids, may occur in pituitary-dependent disease but is more commonly associated with an adrenal carcinoma or the ectopic ACTH syndrome. In such cases a chest X-ray may

reveal a bronchial neoplasm or 'cannon-ball' secondaries. X-rays of the spine and skull will show generalised osteoporosis in a high proportion of cases but the characteristic 'cod-fish' vertebrae are seldom seen. A double contour to the floor of the pituitary fossa is the earliest radiological sign of a pituitary tumour, and its presence may be confirmed by computed tomography.

Although these preliminary investigations are often valuable pointers to the diagnosis and its probable aetiology, only reliable steroid assays will confirm the presence of increased adrenocortical activity. The simplest screening tests, which can be done as an outpatient, are the single-dose dexamethasone suppression test, the estimation of 11-hydroxycorticoids by fluorimetry in an overnight urine specimen, or a 24-hour urinary free cortisol level. None of these tests are infallible and patients should be referred to an endocrine clinic for assessment. Unfortunately morning plasma cortisol levels are often within the normal range in pituitary-dependent cases, but midnight levels are usually elevated, reflecting the absent or reduced circadian rhythm of pituitary-adrenal activity in Cushing's syndrome. Both plasma and urinary steroids will be grossly elevated in the ectopic ACTH syndrome and adrenal cancer.

Bilateral adrenal enlargement and solitary adrenal tumours may be visualised by computed tomography, but adrenal scans using radioactively-labelled cholesterol are more certain to differentiate between bilateral hyperplasia and tumour. Finally, plasma ACTH levels, estimated by radioimmunoassay, can be helpful in confirming the cause. The levels will be low if an autonomous adrenal tumour is present, normal or moderately increased in pituitary-dependent disease, and markedly elevated in the ectopic ACTH syndrome.

Stein–Leventhal syndrome

Aetiology
This combination of hirsutism, menstrual irregularities and bilateral poly-cystic ovaries was first recognised by Stein and Leventhal in 1934. It is also known as the *polycystic ovary syndrome*. In vitro studies have shown defec-tive conversion of androgens to oestrogens in these ovaries, with the result that excessive amounts of androgenic steroids are released into the blood. Whether this is due to congenital enzyme deficiencies in the ovaries or to some disturbance of gonadotrophin secretion from the pituitary gland is still unresolved.

The Stein–Leventhal syndrome is the commonest cause of postpubertal hirsutism in the female in Britain, and many of these patients will be infer-tile. Obesity is present in about 40% of cases which justifies its inclusion in this chapter.

Clinical features
This disorder usually presents in adolescence or early adult life with increasing body hair and irregular or absent periods. The hair growth is

often noticed soon after the onset of the menstrual periods, whilst the girl is still at school; primary amenorrhoea is uncommon but can occur. Acne is particularly troublesome in some patients and may precede or accompany the hirsutism. The latter varies from a mild excess of hair on the face to an extensive growth of coarse pigmented hair of masculine distribution, requiring frequent removal. In contrast to other more serious causes of postpubertal hirsutism there are no other signs of virilism and the clitoris is normal in size. The breasts develop normally but tend to be on the small side. The blood pressure is invariably normal, but when obesity is present the condition can be mistaken for normotensive Cushing's syndrome. Iliac fossa pain has occasionally led to a false diagnosis of acute appendicitis. Infertility is common in the older woman.

Investigations
Plasma and urinary cortisol concentrations will be normal, but the urinary 17-oxosteroids are moderately increased in about a quarter of the cases. Plasma testosterone levels are slightly elevated in the more hirsute females, but even when they fall within the normal range the free androgen index is often elevated; this is due to a reduction in the serum sex-hormone binding globulin and a consequent increase in the concentration of free testosterone in the tissues. Elevated serum LH levels are commonly found, but may fluctuate from day to day. The serum LH/FSH ratio usually exceeds 2.0.

A basal temperature chart will show anovulatory cycles as a rule but ovulation may occur from time to time. The enlarged ovaries are seldom palpable on pelvic examination, but computed tomography or ultrasound scanning may demonstrate enlargement and cystic changes.

At laparoscopy the ovaries will be moderately enlarged and have a characteristic, pearly-white appearance which is due to thickening of the capsule. Bilateral wedge resection of both ovaries will confirm their polycystic nature and reduces their androgen production proportionately. This operation often restores the periods to normal, increases fertility and cures the acne. The hirsutism rarely improves, although it may be prevented from getting worse. Similar results have been claimed for unilateral oophorectomy.

Hypopituitarism

Aetiology
This may result from infarction following a postpartum haemorrhage but is more commonly due to a pituitary tumour. Most of these growths are non-functioning chromophobe adenomas but partial or complete pituitary failure may eventually develop in acromegalics and patients harbouring prolactinomas. It is an unusual cause of obesity which may be present years before there is any clinical evidence of secondary hypothyroidism. Lack of the lipolytic hormones may contribute to this tendency to put on weight. Fröhlich's syndrome of obesity, hypogonadism and a pituitary tumour in

childhood must be incredibly rare; most fat children with delayed puberty have no endocrine disease and will respond to vigorous dieting.

Clinical features

Small neoplasms which are confined to the pituitary fossa may long remain undiscovered. Larger tumours often present with non-specific headaches or deteriorating vision from pressure on the optic chiasma. Acromegalic facies and large hands, persistent galactorrhea or prolonged amenorrhoea are obvious clues. Pituitary failure is usually insidious in onset and there is often a vague history of indifferent health for several years. Failure to grow and short stature in children may be due to growth hormone deficiency or secondary hypothyroidism.

Gonadotrophin deficiency in women will result in amenorrhoea, loss of libido and atrophy of the breasts; in men it will lead to diminished beard growth, atrophic testes and impotence. In both sexes there will be scanty pubic and axillary hair and the facial skin is characteristically thin, finely wrinkled and unusually pale from loss of skin pigment. The slow, delayed relaxation of the peripheral reflexes from hypothyroidism may be seen, and postural hypotension may be present if adrenocortical function is seriously impaired. Temporal field defects may be detected by confrontation and confirmed by perimetry.

Investigations

Depending upon the size of the tumour, lateral X-rays of the skull may show an enlarged fossa, erosion of the posterior clinoids or merely a double contour to its floor. Suprasellar calcification is indicative of a craniopharyngioma and this is the commonest lesion presenting in childhood or adolescence.

A mild normocytic, normochromic anaemia is common and severe hyponatraemia is often found in patients with adrenal insufficiency.

The diagnosis is usually confirmed by demonstrating secondary atrophy of the thyroid and adrenal glands. If hypothyroidism is present the serum thyroxine will be low and serum TSH levels will not rise normally after an intravenous injection of thyrotrophin-releasing hormone. Pituitary–adrenal insufficiency may be demonstrated by low plasma and urinary steroid levels, but an apparently normal adrenal response to corticotrophin does not necessarily rule this out. In doubtful cases it may be necessary to proceed to an insulin tolerance test, taking suitable precautions to avoid prolonged hypoglycaemia. Low gonadotrophin levels are not very helpful except in postmenopausal women when they would normally be high. Elevated serum prolactin levels exceeding 1000 mU/l are compatible with a prolactinoma but may be due to drugs such as phenothiazines, oestrogens or methyldopa.

Hypogonadism

In the male hypogonadism is often associated with moderate obesity which may diminish when androgens are given. It is either secondary to a pituitary lesion or results from primary gonadal failure, of which the commonest cause is undescended testicles. A history of infrequent shaving, impotence and lack of libido will be obtained. On examination smooth hairless skin, flabby paunch and small or absent testes will be found. The external genitalia will be infantile in appearance if puberty has not occurred.

Plasma testosterone levels will be low. Plasma FSH and LH estimations will enable a distinction to be made between primary and secondary hypogonadism, since elevated levels will only be found if the fault lies in the testes. In secondary hypogonadism further tests may be necessary to determine the cause. This may be a pituitary tumour or a selective deficiency of gonadotrophin secretion of congenital origin. Bone X-rays will show delayed fusion of the ephiphyses if the condition began in childhood before the onset of puberty.

CHAPTER 24
Fever

PHYSIOLOGY

The body temperature in health is controlled within narrow limits by the thermoregulatory centre in the hypothalamus. In most individuals, regardless of climate or race, it varies between 36 and 37.5°C, increasing by a degree or so in the evening and following exertion. It rises readily in children from minor causes, but in the elderly may show little response even to life-threatening infection. Measurements of temperature in the mouth or rectum are about half a degree below that of the blood, whilst axillary or groin readings are at least a degree lower.

Fever is said to be present when there is an episodic or persistent rise of body temperature above normal. Hyperthermia results from the stimulation of the thermoregulatory centre in the hypothalamus by a circulating endogenous pyrogen. This low molecular weight protein is synthesised by polymorphonuclear leukocytes, monocytes and tissue macrophages. Substances which cause its release into the circulation include bacterial toxins, breakdown products of tissue damage and immune complexes. This pyrogen is also produced by some neoplasms, notably lymphomas and renal carcinomas.

When the thermoregulatory centre is stimulated in this way it sends messages to the neighbouring vasomotor centre which raises the body temperature by increasing heat production and reducing heat loss. The neurotransmitters involved have not yet been identified, but may be prostaglandins. This could explain the antipyretic effect of aspirin and other prostaglandin inhibitors which do not appear to inhibit the production of the pyrogen itself.

Fever is usually accompanied by non-specific symptoms such as malaise, headache, aching muscles and a feeling of heat or coldness. In addition, the more specific symptoms and signs of the causal disease may be present. Fever is a feature of such diverse disorders as myocardial infarction, the connective tissue diseases and some neoplasms, but is most frequently due to bacterial or viral infection.

EPIDEMIOLOGY

Febrile illnesses are very common in the community, particularly in children, and are often viral in origin and self-limiting in nature. The prevalence of more serious infections in the UK has altered dramatically in recent decades as a consequence of various public health measures such as better housing, modern sanitation, clean food, pure water supplies, the isolation of infectious cases and preventive immunisation. The influence of other factors such as the introduction of antibiotics and changes in microbial virulence are more difficult to assess, but have obviously played a part.

There has followed in the UK the virtual disappearance of diphtheria and poliomyelitis and a greatly reduced incidence of scarlet fever, brucellosis and leptospirosis. The incidence of tuberculosis continues to fall slowly but the disease is still to be reckoned with, particularly in the immigrant population. Viruses have come to occupy a major role in febrile disorders, but food poisoning is on the increase and meningococcal meningitis is still a major hazard amongst children in some parts of the country.

This remarkable change in the prevalence of the infectious fevers is shown by a tabular comparison of notifications of selected infectious diseases in England and Wales between 1950 and 1986.

Disease	1950	1986
Whooping cough	157 752	36 841
Scarlet fever	65 878	6 877
Pulmonary tuberculosis	42 290	4 469
Poliomyelitis	5 557	3
Diphtheria	959	4
Enteric fever	506	250

The incidence of whooping cough fell to less than 10 000 cases annually in the 1970s, but has risen since then as a result of adverse publicity concerning the possible neurological complications of immunisation. The figures for enteric fever include all cases of typhoid and paratyphoid fever; about 70% of these infections are contracted abroad.

Air travel has, however, greatly increased the spread of microorganisms, so that there is no disease in any endemic area which cannot be carried elsewhere in the world in less time than its incubation period. At risk in this way are members of the armed forces, airline crews, business men, students, tourists and immigrants, particularly those returning from a holiday in their country of origin. As a consequence Britain, after decades of freedom from tropical diseases, has lost its sea-girt immunity, as indeed has the world as a whole.

In individuals arriving from abroad with fever the infection may of course be due to some common condition such as tonsillitis, upper respiratory tract infection, infectious mononucleosis, hepatitis or renal infection. If exotic disease remains a possibility it is essential to ask where they have been, and whether they stopped off somewhere on the way.

For the purposes of discussion this extensive subject is divided into the causes of acute and chronic fever. It must however be borne in mind that some diseases may manifest themselves in either way. Acute fever is pyrexia of short duration which rarely lasts more than a week or two before a diagnosis is made. Chronic fever, on the other hand, encompasses those conditions which give rise to intermittent or continuous pyrexia for weeks or even months without much indication of their aetiology; pyrexia of unknown origin (PUO) is a common diagnostic problem.

ACUTE FEVER

SYNOPSIS OF CAUSES*

GENERAL

Influenza; **Exanthemas**; Rheumatic fever; **Mumps**; **Infectious mononucleosis**; Leptospirosis; Brucellosis; Enteric fever; Malaria; Drugs; Blood disorders; **Septicaemia**; Toxic shock syndrome; Septic arthritis.

LOCAL

RESPIRATORY

Upper respiratory infections; **Tonsillitis**; Diphtheria; **Lower respiratory infections**; **Bronchitis**; **Bacterial pneumonias**; Legionnaires' disease; **Non-bacterial pneumonias**.

ABDOMINAL

Gastro-enteritis; **Hepatitis**; **Cholangitis**; **Pyelonephritis**.

* Bold type is used for causes more commonly found in Europe and North America.

DIAGNOSTIC APPROACH

In 1868 Carl Wunderlich published a treatise on fever which led Garrison to declare that he had 'found fever a disease and left it a symptom'. And therein lies our dilemma when faced with a febrile patient — so many conditions can produce a rise in body temperature.

Acute febrile illnesses are due in the great majority of cases to influenza, upper respiratory infections or one of the exanthemas which will declare themselves within a day or two of the onset. This is particularly true of children, and enquiry should be made about similar symptoms in other members of the family and contacts at school; the presence of a local epidemic of a particular disease will obviously have to be taken into account when reaching a decision. When taking a history a note should be made of any other illness suffered by the patient and whether drugs are being taken for this.

The presence of other symptoms and signs should be sought. Headache is common to many febrile illnesses but neck stiffness, photophobia or confusion may be due to encephalitis or meningitis and can only be excluded by a lumbar puncture. The skin should be examined carefully for the tell-tale rash of one of the exanthemas or the purpura associated with meningococcal infection. Cough, dyspnoea and chest pain may be due to bronchitis, pneumonia or, less commonly, pulmonary embolism, and the chest will be examined for the appropriate physical signs. Abdominal pain, vomiting and diarrhoea may be caused by gastroenteritis but appendicitis, cholecystitis, pancreatitis, salpingitis and hepatitis should be considered in the differential diagnosis. Acute pyelonephritis does not always present with much in the way of urinary symptoms, particularly in children, and the physical examination is incomplete without looking at a urine specimen.

The occupation of the patient may be relevant. Leptospirosis, psittacosis and Q fever, for example, are very uncommon in the UK but may occasionally be encountered in farmers, veterinary surgeons, miners, abbatoir workers and those who handle birds. If the patient appears ill and no cause can be found it is safer to admit him to hospital than to keep him at home. This particularly applies to the sick traveller from abroad. Because of the rapidity of air transport the general practitioner is often the first doctor to see such a person. It is essential in such cases to ask where such patients have been, what prophylactic immunisation they had before setting out, whether they took antimalarial drugs, drank untreated water, came into contact with any infectious disease or if any other member of their party has been taken ill. Enteric fever is not uncommon in Southern Europe and nearly 2000 cases of malaria are imported into the UK each year.

Investigations

If the diagnosis is not immediately apparent a throat swab, urine sample and sputum should be send for bacteriological examination. A full blood count may disclose a polymorph leukocytosis, suggesting a bacterial infection, or a relative lymphocytosis which is seen in many viral diseases. A chest X-ray should be done if respiratory symptoms or signs are present.

Where special investigations are called for they are mentioned in the text.

GENERAL CAUSES

Under the heading of general causes are included those viral and bacterial infections which are commonly seen in the UK, together with a few selected diseases which are important in other parts of the world and may occasionally be encountered in this country. Smallpox has been omitted, since the last known case was reported from Somalia in 1977; according to the World Health Organisation this disease has been totally eradicated and is very unlikely to return in endemic form.

Influenza

This highly infectious disease is due to a myxovirus having three distinct serotypes, A, B and C; type A is responsible for the worldwide epidemics which have occurred this century. The source of the markedly different strains of serotype which have caused these pandemics is unknown.

The virus gains entry to the respiratory tract by droplet infection and the incubation period is less than 2 days. Epidemics occur during the winter months and the infection is usually noticed first in schoolchildren, before spreading rapidly to the older members of the population.

Although the primary lesion is a necrosis of the ciliated epithelium of the respiratory tract, the symptoms are out of all proportion to the local damage and justify its inclusion in this section. The onset is abrupt with prostration, severe headache, sweating, myalgia, an unproductive cough and sometimes rigors. The temperature rises rapidly, falling to normal within 5 days at most in the uncomplicated case. During epidemics influenza itself may cause a primary pneumonia, but more often than not pneumonia is due to secondary infection by pneumococci or staphylococci. This complication is seen more frequently in those with pre-existing cardiac or pulmonary disease.

Other complications include sinusitis, otitis media and bronchitis. Influenza in children has been implicated as the cause of Reye's syndrome, a rare and often fatal encephalopathy which is associated with a fatty liver and hepatic failure. If fever persists beyond the fifth day complications should be looked for, particularly in the lungs. The diagnosis of influenza can be confirmed in retrospect by demonstrating a fourfold rise in complement-fixing antibody in the serum taken in the acute and convalescent stages.

EXANTHEMAS

The acute exanthemas of childhood all begin with fever, followed by a characteristic rash. The microorganisms responsible for these common diseases are conveyed by direct contact, droplet infection or airborne spread and enter the body via the upper respiratory tract.

With the exception of scarlet fever such diseases are caused by viruses.

Measles

This viral infection appears in epidemic form every 2 years, occurring mainly in the early winter and spring. The incubation period is about 12 days until the onset of fever and the child continues to shed the virus until the rash starts to fade.

The illness commences as a febrile cold with running eyes and nose, sore throat and cough. Conjunctivitis is marked and photophobia is often present. A minute white stippling on the inside of the cheek near the upper second molar is often seen before the rash appears and is only found in measles. These *Koplik's spots* may also be present on the mucous membrane of the gums.

The rash appears about the fourth day of the illness, beginning behind the ears and spreading rapidly to involve the face and trunk. It consists of a deep red macular eruption which in some areas coalesces to form blotchy patches. The rash fades within a week of its appearance, leaving a brownish staining and fine desquamation of the skin.

The fever increases until the rash is fully developed and then subsides. Cough is invariable and crepitations are often audible in the chest. A few patients go on to get a secondary bronchopneumonia but this is uncommon in the UK. Otitis media and tonsillitis are more common complications, and the mouth and eardrums should be inspected daily. Febrile convulsions are the most frequent neurological complication of this disease and may precede the onset of a post-measles encephalitis.

In the developing countries measles is a very serious illness, with a high mortality rate in malnourished children.

Rubella

This viral infection has an incubation period of about 18 days. The patient is infective for a week beforehand and remains so until the rash has been present for about 4 days.

Rubella is a mild disorder in childhood and may be misdiagnosed, as a number of other viruses produce a similar clinical picture. In adults the infection may have more serious consequences, particularly in women. Some develop a prolonged arthritis, mainly affecting the hands and feet, which can persist for months after the initial illness. When contracted during the first 4 months of pregnancy fetal abnormalities occur in about 20% of cases. Blindness, deafness and cardiac defects are the commonest complications of the congenital rubella syndrome. Prevention lies in immunising all seronegative schoolgirls with live attenuated virus vaccine.

The temperature, especially in children, is but slightly raised. It may be accompanied by a mild conjunctivitis and pharyngitis. The rash may be the first sign of the disease and is usually present within 4 days of the rise in temperature. It consists of pale red spots, smaller and less florid than those of measles, and appears first on the face before spreading to involve the trunk and limbs. Enlarged lymph nodes in the postauricular and suboccipital areas are characteristically found. Thrombocytopenia and postrubella encephalitis are rare complications but arthritis is common in women. During pregnancy the diagnosis should be confirmed by antibody studies.

Chickenpox

This widespread infectious disease is caused by the varicella-zoster virus. It may follow exposure to a case of herpes zoster and the causal organism is the same. The incubation period is about 15 days and the patient is infective for several days before the appearance of the rash and for about a week after the last vesicle is seen.

The illness commences with fever, malaise, sore throat and occasionally abdominal pain. Within 24 hours the typical rash appears on the trunk, face and, to a lesser extent, on the limbs. The lesions begin as small, red macules capped by vesicles containing clear fluid which rapidly progress to form pustules and finally scabs. Pruritus is invariable and scratching may result in secondary infection. The rash differs from that of smallpox in that it appears in successive crops so that all stages may be seen together. The crusts may persist for several weeks, depending upon the severity of the infection. The fever may continue as new lesions appear.

The disease is usually more severe in adults and smokers are particularly at risk from developing a viral pneumonia, which may prove fatal. In later years the fibrotic scars in the lungs calcify and their radiological appearance may be mistaken for that of miliary tuberculosis. Encephalitis is a rare complication and typically affects the cerebellum, causing ataxia and incoordination.

Erythema infectiosum

This mild exanthem is clinically indistinguishable from rubella for which it is often mistaken. It is caused by the human parvovirus which belongs to a group of small single-stranded DNA viruses of insects and vertebrates. In children it presents with a low-grade fever, general malaise and a rash. This usually starts on the face and is characteristically confluent and maculopapular in appearance, hence the alternative title of 'slapped-face syndrome'. On the trunk the rash is typically lacy or reticular in pattern, but it may take many forms and has a tendency to fade and then recur.

In adults the typical rash is uncommon but the illness is usually more severe. Arthralgia is a common presenting symptom, particularly in women. This starts in the hands and knees but rapidly spreads to involve the wrists, ankles, feet, elbows and shoulders. Occasionally the spinal joints are also involved, leading to severe backache. The arthralgia may persist for weeks or even months, and a few patients have gone on to develop classical rheumatoid arthritis. It is thought that this virus may be one of the environmental factors which triggers off rheumatoid arthritis in genetically susceptible individuals.

Human parvovirus infection has also been implicated in the aplastic crises of patients with sickle-cell anaemia and other haemoglobinopathies. Replication of this virus in the bone marrow apparently depresses normal erythropoiesis and exacerbates an existing anaemia. Recent parvovirus infection can be confirmed by demonstrating rising antibody titres to this organism in serial blood samples.

Scarlet fever

This is due to infection by a group-A haemolytic streptococcus that produces an erythrogenic toxin. It starts with a follicular tonsillitis and presents with high fever, malaise and sore throat. The rash usually appears within the next 2 days as a punctate erythema on the trunk and limbs which blanches on pressure; the face is spared. It fades with desquamation in a week or two. The tongue is coated with a thick white fur which eventually peels to leave a 'strawberry' tongue. Complications include sinusitis, otitis media and occasionally rheumatic fever or glomerulonephritis.

The disease is much less common and milder than it used to be 50 years ago, and the local suppurative complications can usually be avoided by the prompt administration of antibiotics.

Rheumatic fever

Aetiology
Acute rheumatic fever is probably an autoimmune disorder in which the tissue damage is produced by the patient's immunological response to a group-A beta-haemolytic streptococcal infection. The similarity of certain streptococcal and human antigens has been known for some time, and the autoimmune theory provides the most plausible explanation for the association of rheumatic fever with an antecedent streptococcal infection.

The pathological changes consist of inflammatory lesions in the connective tissues, particularly those of the heart and joints. Rheumatic fever chiefly affects children and adolescents and there is commonly a history of an upper respiratory tract infection a week or two prior to its onset. In the UK the incidence of rheumatic fever has declined dramatically during the past 50 years, but it is still the commonest cause of heart disease in the developing countries.

Clinical features
Rheumatic fever usually begins abruptly with severe pain and swelling of the knees, ankles, wrists and shoulders, characteristically flitting from joint to joint. A low-grade fever is apparent from the outset and is accompanied by sweating and tachycardia; the presence of erythema marginatum on the trunk or limbs is pathognomonic of this disease.

Cardiac failure may result from myocarditis or damage to the mitral and aortic valves. The heart is clinically enlarged and a transient pericardial rub may be heard. Mitral and aortic murmurs are often audible during the illness but may disappear on recovery.

The clinical course is very variable; some patients recover completely but others suffer from recurrent attacks, and many of the cases beginning in childhood are left with valvular damage. Painless subcutaneous nodules sometimes appear about the joints and over the occiput, spine and scapulae some weeks after the acute onset.

Investigations
A throat swab is unlikely to grow the streptococcus but the antistreptolysin-O-titre is elevated in the majority of cases. The ESR is often high and a mild leukocytosis may be present.

A chest X-ray may show an enlarged cardiac shadow due to dilatation of the heart or a pericardial effusion; echocardiography will differentiate between the two. A prolonged PR interval is often seen on the electrocardiogram.

Mumps

The causal agent of this common infectious disease is a paramyxovirus which is present in saliva and is spread by droplet infection. Like many other viruses it enters the body via the upper respiratory tract. Mumps has an incubation period of 16–18 days, and the period of infectivity starts several days before the onset of the illness and lasts until the swollen parotid glands subside. It commonly affects children of school age and occurs in epidemics in the winter or early spring.

Fever and general malaise usually precede the painful swelling of the parotid glands by a day or two. This may be followed by enlargement of the submandibular or sublingual salivary glands. In an uncomplicated case the swellings normally subside in about a week. A transient meningitis is not uncommon and should be suspected if the patient complains of neck stiffness, headache, nausea and vomiting; the CSF will show an excess of lymphocytes. Rare complications include encephalitis, myocarditis, nephritis, pancreatitis and unilateral nerve deafness. In adults it may cause orchitis, oöphoritis, mastitis and prostatitis.

Infectious mononucleosis

Aetiology

Glandular fever is caused by the Epstein–Barr virus, a member of the herpes group. It is common in childhood and early adult life and is particularly prevalent in such communities as nurses' homes and student hostels. The organism is excreted in the saliva and the salivary glands are probably the major site of virus production. For obvious reasons it is sometimes known as the 'kissing' disease. The incubation period is very variable, ranging from a few days in children to several weeks in the adult.

In tropical countries the Epstein–Barr virus has a more sinister role. It is almost certainly the cause of Burkitt's lymphoma of childhood, which is endemic in parts of Africa, and has been implicated in the development of nasopharyngeal carcinoma in adults in Africa and Asia. Infection by cytomegalovirus, another member of the herpes family, can produce a very similar clinical picture to infectious mononucleosis.

Clinical features

These include fever, sore throat, lymphadenopathy and splenic enlargement. The fever persists for a week or two and may be preceded by a few days of general malaise, headache and unusual tiredness. An exudative tonsillitis is seen in about half the cases and petechiae on the palate are found in about one-third by the end of the first week. A transient erythematous or maculopapular rash may appear on the trunk and is more likely to occur if the patient is given ampicillin.

The lymph nodes, particularly those in the neck, are enlarged and tender and may persist for several months. Hepatitis is common but jaundice is seen in only about 10% of cases. The spleen is palpable in at least half of patients. Encephalitis is a rare but serious complication.

Investigations

The white cell count is often elevated and atypical lymphocytes are usually seen by the fifth day of the illness; these abnormal cells account for at least 10% of the total.

The *monospot test* has replaced the classical Paul–Bunnell test in screening for heterophil antibodies; it usually becomes positive within a fortnight of the onset. A negative result after this period should make one think of other causes of a mononucleosis, such as cytomegalovirus infection or toxoplasmosis. Thrombocytopenia occurs occasionally. Liver function tests are frequently abnormal and may remain so for weeks after apparent recovery.

Leptospirosis

Aetiology

This infection has become rare in the UK. During 1986 only 28 cases of leptospirosis were confirmed by the Public Health Laboratory Service. Some of these infections were thought to have been contracted abroad.

The usual causes are *Leptospira icterohaemorrhagiae*, the hosts of which include rats, field mice, voles and hedgehogs, *Leptospira hebdomadis*, which is found in cattle, and *Leptospira canicola*, the host of which is the dog. All these animals harbour the organisms in their renal tubules and their urine contaminates the soil along the banks of streams or canals, sewers and other rodent-infested working places, and milking parlours. Those at risk include farm workers, veterinary surgeons, sewer and abattoir workers, miners and fish cleaners.

Infection in man takes place through abrasions and the mucous membranes of the conjunctiva, nose and mouth. Swimming or partial immersion in contaminated water accounts for some cases. The incubation period is 1–2 weeks.

In Malaysia and Indonesia leptospirosis is a common cause of a mild influenza-like illness; jaundice is seen in about 20%. It can range in severity, however, from a mild illness to death from renal failure. During the first week the organisms may invade the meninges, kidneys, liver or lungs.

Clinical features

In the severe form, more often seen in the UK in association with icterohaemorrhagiae infections, the onset is sudden with prostration, photophobia, conjunctivitis, severe headache, high fever and rigors. The muscles of the lower back and upper thighs are painful and may be tender on palpation. Subconjunctival haemorrhage, epistaxis, haemoptysis, spontaneous bruising and other forms of bleeding may be seen and are probably due to disseminated intravascular coagulation. Uncommon findings include jaundice, maculopapular or urticarial rashes on the trunk, erythema nodosum and enlargement of the liver or spleen.

It is not unusual for the fever and other symptoms to subside after the first week, only to reappear after a relatively asymptomatic period of a few days. This second phase of the illness coincides with the appearance of circulating antibodies to the leptospira, and examination of the CSF at this stage will often reveal an increase in protein and neutrophils or mononuclear cells, even in the absence of meningeal symptoms or signs. Rare complications include thrombocytopenia, a haemolytic anaemia, myocarditis, pancreatitis, optic neuritis, encephalitis, myelitis and a peripheral neuropathy.

Investigations
Anaemia and a polymorph leukocytosis may be present, particularly in jaundiced patients; the ESR is usually raised. Elevated serum creatinine levels and disturbed liver function tests will give some indication of renal and hepatic impairment. Protein, casts and cells may be found in the urine, even when there is no biochemical evidence of renal involvement. The CSF may show the changes described above.

The definitive diagnosis usually depends upon demonstrating a fourfold rise or greater in serum antibodies, using agglutination or complement fixation tests. Leptospira may be isolated from the urine and detected by dark field microscopy during the second phase of the illness.

Brucellosis

Aetiology
Human brucellosis is now a rare disease in the UK. This is entirely due to the success of the eradication scheme in dairy herds. In 1986 only 30 cases were reported, compared with over 600 cases in 1975, and some patients had acquired their infection abroad. Most infections in this country have been due to *Brucella abortus* in untreated milk or cream, or by direct contact with an infected animal. Farmers, veterinary surgeons and slaughter-house workers are most at risk.

Infection with *B. abortus* or *B. melitensis* is seen occasionally in travellers from the Middle East and Mediterranean countries, where this disease is still endemic in sheep and goats.

Clinical features
The disease may present acutely as a mild influenza-like illness or more dramatically with high fever, rigors, headache, sweating and intense depression. In the chronic stage of the illness, which may not necessarily be preceded by an acute episode, lassitude, backache, arthralgia and depression are the main symptoms; fever is slight and intermittent.

On examination there may be no abnormal signs, but in a minority the liver and spleen are enlarged and superficial lymph nodes are palpable. Complications include spondylitis, arthritis affecting the knees and ankles, and epididymo-orchitis.

Investigations

Leukopenia with a relative lymphocytosis is common; a raised white cell count makes this diagnosis unlikely. Blood cultures should be taken daily for a week, since a positive result is the only certain proof of active infection. Marrow culture is sometimes successful when the organism has not been found in the blood. A rising antibody titre in paired sera will confirm the diagnosis but the interpretation of serological data in chronic cases is often extremely difficult.

Enteric fever

Aetiology

This is due to *Salmonella typhi* and *S. paratyphi*, which differ from the other salmonellae in being confined to man and in causing a systemic illness. The organisms are excreted in the faeces and urine and thus infection is spread by sewage-contaminated food and water. Following their ingestion they invade Peyer's patches and the mesenteric lymph nodes, multiply there and, after an incubation period of 10–14 days, enter the bloodstream.

With increasing travel enteric fever may be expected to persist in Britain where, in 1986, typhoid was notified in 170 cases and paratyphoid fever in 80. The great majority of these infections were contracted on the Indian subcontinent, in Spain and, to a lesser extent, in the Middle East and West Africa.

Clinical features

The symptoms of typhoid fever are non-specific and somewhat insidious. In the first week headache and malaise are accompanied by a mild fever which rises daily; the pulse is proportionately slower. Cough is usually accompanied by bronchitis. The lassitude and relative bradycardia with soiled tongue, constipation and distended abdomen are characteristic.

During the second week the patient is languid, apathetic and obviously ill. The temperature is remittent and may reach 40°C (104°F). By this time the headache may have disappeared. In 10–20% of cases the typical 'rose' spots, scanty pink papules about 1–3 mm in diameter, are seen on the abdomen or chest. Hypotension is common and the spleen may be palpable.

In the third week improvement normally begins, but this is the time when complications such as intestinal haemorrhage, perforation, meteorism, pneumonia and thrombophlebitis occur.

Paratyphoid fever is clinically indistinguishable from typhoid but is commonly milder. While there is usually constipation at the onset, paratyphoid may otherwise take the form of typical food poisoning.

Investigations

A normocytic, normochromic anaemia is common, and is accompanied by leukopenia. Cultures should be positive in the blood in the first week, and in the stools in the second and third weeks of the illness. Agglutination tests become positive after the second week and a rising titre confirms the diagnosis. In immunised subjects interpretation of these tests may be difficult, if not impossible.

Malaria

Indigenous malaria has long ceased to occur in the UK, but the disease continues to be introduced in increasing numbers from endemic areas such as the Indian subcontinent and Africa. Air travel has greatly increased this risk and 1815 cases were notified in this country in 1986. *Plasmodium vivax* is responsible for the majority of the imported cases seen in Europe and has an incubation period of 2–3 weeks. *P. falciparum* has a shorter incubation period of about 12 days and is a more serious infection in non-immune people. The organism is spread by the bite of the female *Anopheles* mosquito and multiplies in the liver during the incubation period.

The clinical picture is very variable, but after a premonitory headache with malaise and nausea suggestive of influenza a feeling of cold or a rigor is followed by fever and sweating. Vomiting, abdominal pain and diarrhoea may occur, and may be mistaken for acute gastroenteritis. Initially, the fever is persistent but later it may become paroxysmal in character, recurring at intervals of 1–3 days. On examination the liver may be enlarged and the spleen is usually palpable.

Thick and thin blood films taken promptly should show the parasite and enable the species to be identified. Life-threatening complications are seen chiefly in *P. falciparum* or 'malignant' malaria and consist of coma, severe haemolytic anaemia, pulmonary oedema and acute renal failure. Cerebral malaria should always be suspected in a confused, febrile patient who has just returned from a holiday in Africa or Asia.

Drugs

Fever is an uncommon manifestation of hypersensitivity to drugs. It usually appears within a week or two of starting treatment, but not always. Cases have been reported of drug-induced fever developing months after the onset of therapy.

In the case of antibiotics such as the cephalosporins, penicillins, streptomycin and sulphonamides it is often impossible to be certain if the fever is due to the drugs, or to the underlying infection for which they are being given.

The *neuroleptic malignant syndrome* is an uncommon but potentially lethal reaction to neuroleptic drugs. A number of compounds which interact with the dopaminergic systems in the brain have been implicated, particularly chlorpromazine, haloperidol and flupenthixol. Hyperthermia is accompanied by pallor, sweating, tachycardia, a labile blood pressure, urinary incontinence and fluctuating levels of consciousness. Dystonia and other extrapyramidal signs may also be present. Recovery usually follows within a week or two of stopping oral therapy, but it takes much longer if the patient has been given depot preparations.

If drug fever is suspected a textbook of adverse reactions to drugs should be consulted. Other features which may draw attention to this possibility are an unexplained anaemia, leukopenia, rash or disturbed liver function tests.

Blood disorders

The acute forms of *leukaemia* often present with fever. The patient is obviously ill but there may be little else to find. Purpura and enlargement of lymph nodes, liver and spleen should be looked for.

Pancytopenia from bone marrow depression will also present acutely, with prostration, rigors and high fever. A full blood count and marrow biopsy will enable a diagnosis to be reached in both these disorders. Septicaemia is a common and very serious complication of the leukopenic state and blood cultures should always be taken when this is present.

In the *haemolytic anaemias* the onset of a haemolytic crisis may be heralded by fever and even rigors. Whether this is due to the haemolytic process itself or to intercurrent disease may be difficult to determine, for crises are often precipitated by bacterial or viral infection.

Septicaemia

Aetiology
Invasion of the bloodstream by Gram-positive or Gram-negative organisms is potentially lethal. Those most commonly involved are staphylococci, streptococci, *Esch. coli*, *Pseudomonas*, *Bacteroides* and occasionally the clostridial organisms which give rise to gas gangrene. The infection may gain entry from wounds or burns, a carbuncle or an intravenous injection site in drug addicts. A common route in hospital is via an indwelling intravenous needle or cannula, particularly when left in situ for several days.

Infection is more likely to occur in the very young or very old, in patients on corticosteroids and other immunosuppressive therapy, and after abdominal operations. In one series of 112 cases of *Bacteroides* septicaemia it followed appendicitis in 37%, hysterectomy in 13% and parturition or abortion in 10%. The focus may be in the middle ear, respiratory or urinary tract; thus it may follow middle-ear disease, suppuration in the lungs or urethral instrumentation.

Clinical features
The entry of the organisms into the bloodstream is signalled by prostration, fever and rigors, tachycardia, hypotension and often mental confusion. The patient's condition worsens rapidly and they may become delirious or unconscious. A loud and previously unheard heart murmur is very suggestive of acute bacterial endocarditis. Inflammation at a venepuncture site is usually due to *Staphylococcus aureus* or a Gram-positive enterococcus.

Investigations
Immediate blood cultures are called for and must be followed at once by appropriate antibiotic therapy. A polymorphonuclear leukocytosis is usual and the haemoglobin level may fall as a result of marrow suppression or intravascular haemolysis. If an indwelling needle or cannula is suspected as being the culprit it should be removed and sent to the laboratory for culture.

Toxic shock syndrome

Aetiology
Although this disease was first described in children in 1978 it primarily affects previously healthy women during or soon after a menstrual period. It is thought to be due to the vaginal absorption of a unique epidermal toxin secreted by a particular strain of *Staph. aureus*. Most individuals over the age of 20 have antibodies to this toxin, and it has been postulated that susceptible females have an isolated immunodeficiency which renders them vulnerable.

Over 2500 cases have been reported in the United States since 1979, but only a few isolated cases have appeared so far in the UK and other parts of the world. The mortality rate lies somewhere between 5 and 10% of cases. Women using vaginal tampons or contraceptive sponges seem to be particularly at risk, but a few non-menstrual cases have been described in association with childbirth or abortion, skin infection, osteomyelitis, pneumonia and even endocarditis.

Clinical features
Shortly after the onset of the menstrual period the woman becomes acutely ill with a high fever, rigors, sore throat, conjunctivitis, myalgia, vomiting, watery diarrhoea, vaginal discharge and a widespread erythematous rash which blanches on pressure. Headache and abdominal tenderness may also occur. Over the next few days the patient becomes lethargic, irritable and confused, with severe hypotension and peripheral vasoconstriction. Acute renal failure may develop and a petechial rash, due to thrombocytopenia or disseminated intravascular coagulation, may appear. Recovery usually takes place within 2 weeks of onset, with desquamation of the skin of the palms and soles of the feet. In some cases it takes longer and recurrences are not uncommon, usually occurring within two menstrual cycles of the initial attack.

The differential diagnosis depends to some extent on the predominant symptoms, but the rash can be mistaken for that of a drug eruption, erythema multiforme, scarlet fever, or toxic epidermal necrolysis. Vomiting and diarrhoea will suggest an acute gastroenteritis and the association with menstruation will inevitably raise the possibility of pelvic inflammatory disease.

Investigations
Staphylococcus aureus can usually be cultured from cervical or vaginal swabs

in the menstrual cases, but is rarely found in the blood. A polymorpho-nuclear leukocytosis and normochromic, normocytic anaemia are frequently found. Thrombocytopenia may be accompanied by prolonged prothrombin and partial thromboplastin times suggesting disseminated intravascular coagulation. Liver function tests are often abnormal but frank jaundice is rare. Hyponatraemia and hypokalaemia may develop if the diarrhoea is severe and prolonged. The blood urea and serum creatinine levels will be elevated in those who progress to renal failure.

Septic arthritis

Bacterial infection of one or more joints usually results from blood-borne spread of pathogenic organisms from infection elsewhere. It should be suspected in all cases of acute monoarthritis and in patients with established joint disease presenting with fever and a neutrophil leukocytosis. The diagnosis must be confirmed by aspirating the joint and sending the synovial fluid for culture.

In childhood it commonly affects the hip and, less frequently, the knee or elbow. Boys are more often affected than girls. *Haemophilus influenzae* from infection in the nasal passages or middle ear is most frequently found.

Gonococcal arthritis is not uncommon following venereal infection in young adults. The knees and wrists are usually involved and it is often accompanied by tenosinovitis of the hands or feet. Blood cultures may grow *Neisseria gonorrhoeae* when synovial cultures are negative.

Patients with pre-existing joint disease are particularly at risk. In someone with rheumatoid arthritis the sudden exacerbation of symptoms in a single joint, when accompanied by fever, should arouse suspicion.

LOCAL CAUSES

Pyrexia of sudden onset due to inflammation of a particular organ is usually accompanied by other symptoms or signs which help to identify its source. Severe headache, for example, is a much more prominent symptom than fever in meningitis and encephalitis, except in infancy. Similarly, the fever associated with myocardial infarction, pulmonary embolism or pericarditis is inevitably overshadowed by chest pain or dyspnoea. These conditions have all been described in earlier chapters and will not be considered further here.

RESPIRATORY CAUSES

Infection of the respiratory tract is responsible for many cases of acute fever in practice. It is most frequently due to one of the many viruses which infect humans and cause a range of disorders from the common cold to bronchitis and pneumonia. Viral infection is, however, an uncommon cause of pneumonia, which is more often due to bacteria or *Mycoplasma pneumoniae*.

UPPER RESPIRATORY INFECTIONS

Acute coryza, or the common cold, is caused by more than a hundred different viruses, of which the *rhinoviruses* constitute the largest single group. There is an increased incidence during the winter months and parents often contract infection from their children. The organisms are spread by droplets in the air and produce inflammation of the mucous membranes in the nasal passages. After an incubation period of 1–4 days the typical symptoms of headache, sneezing, sore throat, nasal congestion and mucopurulent discharge appear. These symptoms usually subside in about a week, but a dry cough may persist for some time afterwards. Fever is rarely evident unless there is secondary bacterial infection of the sinuses or middle ear. Otitis media may be missed in an irritable, febrile infant unless the ears are routinely examined for the characteristic red, bulging tympanic membranes.

Pharyngoconjunctival fever is another viral infection which is common amongst schoolchildren. It begins abruptly with conjunctivitis, sore throat, headache, malaise and fever. The fauces are inflamed and the cervical lymph nodes may be palpable and tender.

When the viruses spread further down the air passages the mucosa of the larynx and bronchial tree become inflamed. *Croup* is the name given to an illness which results from involvement of the larynx with consequent oedema and stridor. It occurs in young children and can be mistaken for whooping cough, which is very common in this age group. *Bronchitis* and *bronchiolitis* of viral origin cause fever and a variable degree of airways obstruction. The respiratory syncytial virus is often involved in these more serious respiratory infections and can cause epidemics of an influenza-like illness. A viral bronchopneumonia is sometimes seen in children under 5 years of age.

Tonsillitis

Tonsillitis is often attributed to *Streptococcus*, but is more often due to a virus. In adolescence the possibility of infectious mononucleosis should not be forgotten, while in an older person on drugs tonsillitis may be the first manifestation of agranulocytosis.

The onset is acute with severe sore throat and pain on swallowing, malaise and high fever. The tonsils are usually enlarged and obviously inflamed. The upper cervical lymph nodes are sometimes palpable and tender. Throat swabs, white cell count and monospot test are indicated if the condition does not subside within a few days.

Diphtheria

Corynebacterium diphtheriae may attack patients of any age, but young children are the most susceptible, or perhaps are more exposed to infection.

Owing to the success of preventive inoculation, diphtheria is rare in the UK. In 1986 only 4 cases were notified in England and Wales compared with 959 cases in 1950. Diphtheria is, however, still common in other parts of the world.

Faucial diphtheria begins in the same way as a sore throat or tonsillitis due to other causes. The wash-leather membrane referred to in the name of the disease (Greek *diphthera* = 'leather') is typical, but the possibility of the nasopharynx being the site and giving rise to a yellow or blood-stained nasal discharge, or of the larynx producing a croupy cough and stridor, should be borne in mind. A swab for culture must be taken if the possibility of diphtheria exists.

LOWER RESPIRATORY INFECTIONS

Bronchitis (see also Cough, p. 230)

Fever is a minor feature of acute bronchitis, which may complicate influenza, measles and other upper respiratory infections. Cough and purulent sputum are present, and scattered rhonchi will be heard on auscultation.

Bacterial pneumonias

Aetiology
Primary pneumonia is due to pathogenic organisms invading the lungs and causing patchy or lobar consolidation in a previously healthy individual. Secondary pneumonia, on the other hand, occurs in lungs which have already been damaged by bronchitis, bronchiectasis or tumours, or results from the inhalation of a foreign body, vomit or some other chemical irritant. Infected material may be inhaled during anaesthesia or coma from other causes, while regurgitated food may enter the bronchial tree in patients with oesophageal obstruction from achalasia or a pharyngeal diverticulum.

Streptococcus pneumoniae is responsible for most primary pneumonias of lobar or segmental distribution. As a secondary invader it is seen, along with *Staph. aureus*, in the pneumonias occurring in an influenza epidemic. Organisms which cause bronchopneumonia include *Klebsiella pneumoniae*, which has a high mortality rate and is found in patients with pre-existing lung disease, *Pseudomonas aeruginosa*, which is seen mainly in intensive care units, particularly in those on mechanical ventilation, and anaerobic organisms, which are inhaled into the lungs in debilitated patients with poor dental hygiene, repeated vomiting, strokes or other conditions where the normal protective mechanisms are impaired. *Legionella pneumophila* is considered separately in the next section.

Clinical features

Lobar pneumonia is uncommon in the UK today and this may be partly due to the widespread use of antibiotics in upper respiratory infections. In the majority of cases it is caused by *Streptococcus pneumoniae*. The onset is abrupt, with a dry and sometimes painful cough from an accompanying pleurisy. The temperature rises rapidly, often with rigors, and pulse and respiratory rate are increased. Mucopurulent sputum appears within a day or two and may be rusty in appearance or frankly bloodstained. Herpes of the lips is often present at the onset or may appear later. As a rule one of the lower lobes is involved and over this percussion is impaired. Pleural friction may be audible, along with crepitations, bronchial breathing and whispering pectoriloquy.

Pulmonary embolism should be considered in the differential diagnosis, but this is usually preceded or accompanied by thrombophlebitis in the legs, and fever is not a prominent symptom. In the absence of a pleural effusion, resolution begins within a few days of starting appropriate antibiotic therapy, and the fever should subside within a week or so.

Bronchopneumonia is much commoner than lobar pneumonia in patients in hospital and is often more insidious in onset. Temperature, pulse and respiratory rate are usually increased, but fever may be minimal or absent in the elderly. The sputum is usually purulent. It can be distinguished from bronchitis by the presence of patchy bronchial breathing and crepitations at the bases. Pleural involvement is very uncommon and a pleural rub is rarely heard.

Lung abscess is a complication of staphylococcal and *Klebsiella* pneumonia, but empyema is rarely seen in the UK nowadays.

Despite the introduction of antibiotics, bronchopneumonia is still a common cause of death in old age. In 1986 over 40 000 deaths from pneumonia were notified in England and Wales.

Investigations

Sputum should be sent for microscopy and culture without delay, and before any antibiotics have been given. A gram stain may reveal the presence of pneumococci, staphylococci or *Klebsiella pneumoniae*. Occasionally tuberculosis presents as an acute pneumonia; if suspicion exists the sputum should be sent for Löwenstein–Jensen cultures. In a severe pneumonia bacteraemia commonly occurs and a blood culture may grow the organism. The white cell count is usually elevated, with a marked increase in the number of neutrophils.

Chest X-rays should be taken as soon as possible. In lobar pneumonia any lobe may be involved but the lower lobes are more often affected; a homogeneous opacity will be seen on the film. Bilateral patchy shadows are characteristically seen in bronchopneumonia but a similar appearance results from a chemical pneumonitis or acute allergic alveolitis; a history of exposure to toxic fumes or a known allergen will enable these conditions to be excluded.

Legionnaires' disease

Aetiology

This title was first given to an outbreak of severe pneumonia affecting members attending an American Legion Convention in 1976. After much investigation a newly-recognised species of Gram-negative bacteria was identified and named *Legionella pneumophila*. Later, this was also shown to be the cause of *Pontiac fever* — a mild, self-limiting disorder without respiratory involvement.

Legionella pneumophila has been found in standing and running water, in hotel and hospital water supplies and in the cooling systems of air-conditioning plants. Infection is by aerosol inhalation. The incubation period is usually 2–10 days but may be longer. Males are more frequently affected than females, and most of the victims have been over 40.

In the UK a total of 181 cases were reported in 1986. In one large outbreak the organism was traced to the cooling tower of a newly-built district general hospital, and many patients were infected.

Clinical features

This disease usually presents acutely with fever, profuse sweats, anorexia, headache and myalgia. Over the next 2 or 3 days cough, dyspnoea and pleuritic pain appear. By this time the patient is obviously very ill and may be cyanosed and producing purulent sputum. Signs of consolidation may be minimal despite the severity of the respiratory symptoms.

Neurological manifestations include confusion, hallucinations, paraesthesiae, ataxia and dysarthria. In some patients, vomiting, abdominal pain and diarrhoea may obscure the issue.

There is a mortality rate of 10–15%, even in patients given appropriate antibiotic therapy.

Investigations

A chest X-ray will show segmental or lobar consolidation, usually affecting the lower lobes. There is a moderate neutrophil leukocytosis and a high ESR. Culture of the organism is very difficult and the diagnosis is usually established by demonstrating a rise in antibody titre to *L. pneumophila* in paired sera. During the acute illness the liver function tests are often abnormal and hyponatraemia is not uncommon.

Non-bacterial pneumonias

These differ in their mode of onset from the bacterial forms which have just been described. The systemic features of malaise, anorexia, headache, myalgia and fever tend to predominate over the respiratory symptoms. The sputum is often scanty and mucoid in appearance, and, apart from scattered crepitations, there may be little to find in the chest. The pulse is relatively slow, the spleen may be palpable and the white count is usually normal.

The patchy shadows seen on the chest X-ray are often out of all proportion to the scanty physical signs.

These forms of pneumonia are distinguishable from each other only by complement-fixation tests against antigens prepared from the appropriate organisms; a fourfold rise in titre in paired sera provides the answer. In practice serum will only rarely be obtained early in an undiagnosed febrile disorder. In consequence, the true incidence of such infections is unknown. A high titre at the end of a fortnight's illness is, however, significant.

Viruses rarely cause pneumonia in otherwise healthy individuals, but often do so in patients with impaired immunity. Pneumonias due to cyto-megalovirus, fungi and *Pneumocystis carinii* are a common cause of death in AIDS patients and others receiving immunosuppressive therapy for malignant disease. The commonest non-bacterial pneumonia in the UK is probably that due to *Mycoplasma pneumoniae.*

Mycoplasma pneumonia

Mycoplasma pneumoniae resembles the viruses in causing upper respiratory infections which, in a minority of cases, proceed to pneumonia. These usually occur in the autumn and winter months. In the UK 1702 cases were confirmed in 1986, but the true incidence is probably much higher than this. *Mycoplasma* pneumonia should be suspected in any previously healthy individual with an atypical bronchopneumonia.

Although *Mycoplasma pneumoniae* can be cultured with difficulty from the sputum, the diagnosis normally depends upon demonstrating a rising titre of antibodies in paired sera. Cold agglutinins are found in many patients and may be associated with an autoimmune haemolytic anaemia. Other complications include a variety of neurological disorders, which may be due to the production of antibodies to nervous tissue, and erythema multiforme (Stevens–Johnson syndrome).

Chlamydial pneumonia

This infection is due to psittacosis–ornithosis organisms and is endemic in parrots, budgerigars, pigeons and ducks. Human infection may occur from inhalation of dust from their excreta or feathers. Veterinary surgeons and workers in the duck processing industry appear to be particularly at risk.

The incubation period is 6–20 days and 309 cases were confirmed in the UK in 1986. Not all patients had signs of pneumonia — most presented with the non-specific symptoms of malaise, fever, cough, headache and undue fatigue. Again, the diagnosis is made on a rising titre to antibodies in paired sera.

Q fever

The organism responsible for Q fever was originally called *Rickettsia burneti* but was later renamed *Coxiella burneti* because it has certain features which separate it from the true rickettsiae. The principal reservoir of human infection in Britain is cattle and sheep and the organism is excreted in their faeces. Airborne spread and unpasteurised milk are thought to be the main routes of infection. In 1986 the disease was confirmed in 148 cases in the UK. Most of these occurred in rural areas.

Q fever usually begins abruptly with fever and rigors followed by headache, myalgia and sweating. Some patients have a cough and chest X-rays show the patchy shadowing of a bronchopneumonia.

Complications include myocarditis, epididymo-orchitis, uveitis, hepatitis and particularly endocarditis. Of 839 cases of confirmed Q fever in England and Wales between 1975 and 1981 no less than 11% had an endocarditis which mainly affected the aortic valve. The diagnosis is usually made on finding raised serum antibody titres to the two polysaccharide antigens produced by the organism.

ABDOMINAL CAUSES

In appendicitis, cholecystitis, pancreatitis and salpingitis any fever is likely to be overshadowed by abdominal pain and vomiting. When these are present attention should be directed to their possible causes.

Gastroenteritis (see also Diarrhoea, p. 130)

Fever is present in acute gastritis, particularly if it is due to a viral infection, but epigastric pain and vomiting are more evident. Enteritis can hardly exist without diarrhoea except in typhoid or paratyphoid fever. In infants, while the fever may be considerable, the pain may not be defined or localised.

Hepatitis (see also Jaundice, p. 149)

Epigastric pain or discomfort with fever are usually present at the onset of a viral or drug-induced hepatitis. Jaundice may or may not appear a few days later. Mild cases will escape detection unless liver function tests are carried out routinely in all patients with fever of uncertain origin.

Cholangitis

Acute inflammation in the biliary tract is usually the result of partial obstruction of the common bile duct by gallstones or stricture following cholecystectomy. At times it may be due to the spread of a low-grade infection from a chronically inflamed gall-bladder. Fever, rigors, hypotension and mental confusion may precede any jaundice and overshadow any complaint of right upper quandrant pain. Tenderness under the right costal margin can be minimal or absent. A history of other episodes of unexplained fever over the previous weeks or months may be elicited.

The passage of dark urine containing urobilin and disturbed liver function tests will direct attention to the biliary tract. Blood cultures should be taken before starting antibiotics. A raised leukocyte count and a high ESR are commonly found. The presence of gallstones in the biliary tract may be detected by ultrasonography or computerised tomography.

Pyelonephritis

Aetiology

Acute pyelonephritis is commonly associated with obstruction in the urinary tract. In infants and young children this may be a congenital malformation or be due to ureteric reflux. In adults it is seen more frequently in women, especially during pregnancy, and it is often preceded by cystitis. When it occurs in men it is likely to be associated with prostatic enlargement or pre-existing renal disease.

Clinical features

A high fever, sometimes with rigors, marks the beginning of an attack. Loin pain is characteristic but not always complained of by the patient. On questioning they will usually admit to some dysuria or increased frequency of micturition. The inflamed kidney may be tender but is rarely palpable. Vomiting may occur and jaundice is sometimes seen in infants.

Investigations

The urine has a fishy odour and is opalescent or cloudy in appearance. Microscopy will show innumerable pus cells and possibly motile bacilli. Culture of a midstream urine specimen with a dip slide should be made before starting treatment; in infants and in pregnancy percutaneous suprapubic aspiration of the bladder may be necessary to avoid contamination. The infection is frequently caused by a coliform organism and a count of over 100 000 organisms per millilitre is diagnostic. A polymorph leukocytosis is usually present.

CHRONIC FEVER

SYNOPSIS OF CAUSES*

GENERAL CAUSES

Tuberculosis; Ankylosing spondylitis; **Systemic lupus erythematosus**; Polyarteritis nodosa; **Polymyalgia rheumatica; Cranial arteritis.**

LOCAL CAUSES

Infective endocarditis; Thyroid disorders; **Pulmonary embolism**; Hepatic disease; **Cholangitis**; Subphrenic abscess; **Renal infection**; Pelvic abscess; **Neoplasia.**

* Bold type is used for causes more common found in Europe and North America.

DIAGNOSTIC APPROACH

Chronic fever is arbitrarily defined as fever persisting for more than a fort-night. Only when the history, examination and preliminary investigations have failed to produce a diagnosis does it qualify to be called a pyrexia of unknown origin (PUO). This proves in most cases to be due to a familiar condition presenting in an unusual way. Infection is by far the most frequent cause and was found in 69% of one series of 494 cases.

The presence of non-specific symptoms such as malaise, anorexia, head-ache and aching muscles, sweating and loss of weight will help to determine its duration. Other symptoms may not be volunteered and should be enquired for. They include cough, chest pain, shortness of breath, pains in the joints, dysuria and frequency of micturition. A history of chest disease in the family, rheumatic fever, recent abdominal operation, change of bowel habit or of jaundice in the past may be significant. The patient should be asked if he has ever been abroad and where. Hepatic amoebiasis may not present for some time after their return, and relapses of malaria due to *Plasmodium vivax* and *P. malariae* emerging from their hiding places in the liver may occur months or even years after the initial attack.

Prolonged fever in a child is a particularly worrying problem. It may precede the joint changes of juvenile rheumatoid arthritis (Still's disease) by many months or be due to such unusual infections as brucellosis, toxocariasis, toxoplasmosis or a low-grade osteitis. More commonly it is due to urinary tract infection. Malignant disease is rare in childhood, with the exception of leukaemia, but fever can occur in the reticuloses and Wilm's tumour.

The patient's occupation and hobbies may be relevant. Dairy farmers, veterinary surgeons, bird fanciers and workers in poultry and meat processing plants may become chronically infected with brucellosis or psit-tacosis. Parrots are not the only birds to harbour *Chlamydia* and the owners of pigeon-infested buildings, pet shops and sick budgerigars are equally at risk.

No history is complete without a full record of any medication being taken. Drug-induced fever is relatively uncommon but can be caused by several antibiotics; fever due to an earlier infection may be prolonged or replaced by one due to hypersensitivity to the chemotherapy. Oppor-tunistic infection is the most likely cause in patients being given steroids or cytotoxic drugs.

Examination will include a search for enlarged lymph nodes, liver or spleen. The presence of any cardiac enlargement or murmurs should arouse suspicion of infective endocarditis, particularly if there is any history of rheumatic fever, recent dental treatment or cardiac surgery; other signs such as splinter haemorrhages or tender nodules in the fingers may be present. The optic fundi should be examined for haemorrhages or exudates.

Investigations

Over-investigation is often unproductive and unpleasant for the patient. The scope and order of the tests should be determined by any lead obtained from the history and physical signs. Preliminary investigations will include an examination of the urine, full blood count and chest X-ray. Blood cultures should be taken early on if infection is likely. The ESR may be grossly elevated in infection, malignant disease, drug allergy or one of the connective tissue disorders and is therefore of little help in differentiating between them. Nevertheless, it is of some value as an indicator of the activity of the underlying disease and should always be estimated. A normal blood count and ESR are so unusual with a prolonged fever that these findings should make one suspect malingering, particularly if the patient happens to be a nurse.

Further investigations will depend upon the most probable causes and may include a battery of serological tests for specific antibodies to known organisms, liver function tests, serum electrophoresis and a search for LE cells, antinuclear factor and DNA antibodies. Bone marrow examination or lymph node biopsy and special radiological procedures may be required in individual cases; these include ultrasonography and computed tomography. Laparotomy should not be delayed for too long if the cause is thought to lie in the abdomen and the results of these other tests are inconclusive.

GENERAL CAUSES

Infections are responsible for the majority of fevers. Many of these present acutely and have already been considered earlier in this chapter. Some however smoulder on for a considerable time in a subacute or chronic form without revealing their identity. *Tuberculosis* is the classical example of this and is discussed below. *Brucellosis* and *psittacosis* sometimes behave in this way and the diagnosis of these infections is made by carrying out the appropriate serological tests; they will not be discussed further. *Malaria* usually presents acutely but episodic fever may occur in individuals infected with *P. vivax* or *P. malariae* years after they have returned from the tropics; the organism is readily found on thick blood films provided that this possibility is borne in mind.

Connective tissue disorders are another cause of prolonged or intermittent fever which may precede other signs and symptoms for many months. This is certainly true of ankylosing spondylitis, polyarteritis nodosa, systemic lupus erythematosus and rheumatoid arthritis which has already been considered in the chapter on loss of weight. It now seems likely that most of these conditions are due to the deposition of immune complexes and consequent inflammation in blood vessels and synovial membranes, although the nature of the allergens which provoke this immunological response is still unknown. They are notoriously difficult to diagnose in the early stages and even at autopsy histological evidence of their presence may be scanty.

Drug-induced fever is usually of short duration and has been dealt with already.

Tuberculosis

Whilst its incidence in Britain has fallen dramatically from 42 290 reported cases in 1950 to 4469 in 1986 tuberculosis still remains an important cause of prolonged fever, particularly among the immigrant population from Africa, Asia and the West Indies. In tropical countries all the factors for its spread such as overcrowding, poverty and malnutrition still exist. *Mycobacterium tuberculosis* is inhaled or ingested in contaminated milk and the infection may be localised to the lungs or intestines or be carried in the blood to all parts of the body.

Pulmonary tuberculosis

This is still the commonest form of the disease in this country. The onset is often insidious with mild malaise, intermittent fever, night sweats and loss of weight. Cough, mucoid sputum and occasional haemoptysis may draw attention to its presence. Dyspnoea on exertion appears later. A pleural effusion in a young person should always be assumed to be tuberculous in origin until proved otherwise. There may be a family history of chest disease or of contact with a known case. The diagnosis is usually made on X-rays of the chest which show ill-defined opacities in the apices of the lungs; cavities may appear later. The tubercle bacillus should be sought in sputum or, in its absence, in a laryngeal swab or early morning specimen of gastric juice. Samples must be sent for Löwenstein–Jensen culture but it will be several weeks before the results are known. When an effusion is present a pleural biopsy may provide the answer. The tuberculin test is usually positive.

Non-pulmonary tuberculosis

Pulmonary tuberculosis should offer no difficulty in diagnosis provided that a chest X-ray is taken. This is not so however with the disseminated form which may present acutely or as a chronic illness. Acute miliary tuberculosis is sometimes seen in young adults presenting with high fever and marked prostration. The initial chest X-ray is often passed as normal and the characteristic miliary shadowing in the lung fields may not appear for several weeks. Hepatosplenomegaly may be present and choroid tubercles should be looked for repeatedly in the fundi.

Chronic miliary tuberculosis may affect any organ and presents in many guises. Its presence may be masked by the administration of corticosteroids for other diseases and there is some evidence to suggest that latent infection may be lit up by these drugs. Persistent headache, however bizarre, must be taken seriously for it may be the only manifestation of tuberculous meningitis in these patients; it can only be excluded by a lumbar puncture.

Intestinal tuberculosis is sometimes mistaken for Crohn's disease, even at laparotomy, but it can also appear insidiously with vague abdominal pain or discomfort, anorexia and loss of weight. On examination there may be ascites or the characteristic doughy feel of the tuberculous mesentery.

A tuberculous kidney may present with frequency of micturition and a sterile pyuria, whilst chronic inflammation of the pelvic organs may cause amenorrhoea and lower abdominal pain. Bone and joint tuberculosis are now rare in the UK but swelling of a single joint without much sign of inflammation should remind one of its existence.

Unusual manifestations of miliary tuberculosis include multiple ganglia at the wrists, 'cervical' spondylosis, epididymo-orchitis, pericarditis, 'cold' abscesses, granulomata on the skin, pancytopenia and Addison's disease. In elderly patients there may be only mild fever, slight loss of weight or painless enlarged lymph nodes in the neck.

Tuberculin testing is of little value in chronic miliary tuberculosis — many of these patients are tuberculin negative. Lung involvement is rare but X-rays may show calcification in the pericardium, kidneys, spleen or adrenal areas. The liver is infected in the majority and the characteristic granulomata may be found on liver biopsy, even when the liver function tests are normal. If renal tuberculosis is suspected the urine should be cultured on Löwenstein–Jensen media and an intravenous pyelogram organised. If all else fails the diagnosis of this treatable disorder may eventually depend upon a laparotomy.

Ankylosing spondylitis

This disorder has a high familial incidence and is much commoner in men. Although its cause is unknown it is linked to other disorders such as psoriatic arthritis, Reiter's syndrome and ulcerative colitis by the presence of the tissue antigen HLA-B27 in a high proportion of cases.

The first symptom is usually low back pain but it may present with loss of weight and intermittent fever in a young man. The backache is often worse at night and accompanied by stiffness after immobility. The peripheral joints are involved in some patients and occasionally this precedes the spinal symptoms.

In the early stages of the disease there may be little to find apart from some tenderness over the sacro-iliac joints and decreased mobility of the spine. Complications include iritis, myocarditis and rarely spinal cord compression.

A normal ESR does not exclude this diagnosis, and it may be years before the characteristic X-ray appearances of fusion of the sacro-iliac joints and 'squaring' of the vertebral bodies appear.

Systemic lupus erythematosus

Aetiology

This autoimmune disorder is characterised by the production of a variety of non-organ-specific antibodies. Deposition of circulating immune complexes with consequent complement fixation is thought to be responsible for the widespread inflammatory lesions that appear in the skin, heart, kidneys, serous membranes and central nervous system. The disease is much commoner in females and may run in families; there is a high incidence of the HLA antigens B8 and DRw3 in affected individuals.

Lupus erythematosus is seen predominantly in young women but can present in childhood and after the menopause. It usually follows an indolent course with acute exacerbations triggered off by exposure to strong sunlight, viral infections or drugs. Photosensitivity may help to explain why it is such a common illness in the West Indies and parts of South East Asia. Many drugs have been implicated in its causation; they include antibiotics, anticonvulsants, hypotensive agents and oral contraceptives.

Clinical features

The typical patient is a young woman with premenstrual fever, migraine, transient joint pains, recurrent skin rashes and falling hair. There may be a history of 'rheumatic' fever in childhood or unexplained psychiatric illness. The central nervous system is frequently involved and accounts for the high incidence of neuro-psychiatric manifestations which range from mild depression to epilepsy and psychotic behaviour. Minor forms of this disorder often go unrecognised for years.

The classical 'butterfly' rash on the face is seen in less than half the cases, but there may be ulcers on the finger tips and a characteristic periungual erythema with telangiectasia. Raynaud's phenomenon is common.

Dyspnoea and chest pain may be due to pleurisy, pericarditis or an allergic pneumonitis. Fluffy white exudates in the fundi may be the only objective evidence of damage to the central nervous system. Occasionally, the disease presents with acute glomerulonephritis or the nephrotic syndrome.

Arthralgia is common but destructive joint changes are rarely seen. Recurrent venous and arterial thromboses are not uncommon. The term 'mixed connective tissue disease' has been given to a group of patients with the overlapping features of systemic lupus erythematosus, scleroderma and polymyositis.

Investigations

Most cases have a normocytic, normochromic anaemia with a raised ESR. Leukopenia or thrombocytopenia may be present. The Coombs test is sometimes positive and false-positive tests for syphilis are seen in about 15% of cases. LE cells and antinuclear antibodies are found in a high proportion of cases but may also occur in other rheumatic disorders and in chronic active hepatitis. Antibodies to double-stranded DNA are present in high titre during periods of clinical activity and this has proved to be the most reliable test in practice.

Polyarteritis nodosa

Aetiology

The deposition of immune complexes in the walls of small arteries is thought to be responsible for the clinical manifestations of this disease. The nature of the allergens which trigger off this process is unknown. In some patients it appears to be associated with a persisting hepatitis B infection. Polyarteritis nodosa is a multisystem disorder which is commoner in males; it can occur at any age but its peak incidence is in the fifth and sixth decades of life.

The widespread distribution of the arterial lesions may impair the blood supply to many organs. Thus it can present with myocardial infarction, asthma, pneumonitis, glomerulonephritis, mononeuritis multiplex, gastrointestinal haemorrhage, ischaemia legs, tender muscles, painful joints and vasculitic rashes or nodules in the skin.

Clinical features

Prolonged fever, tachycardia, weight loss and evidence of multisystem involvement should bring this disease to mind, particularly in a middle-aged man. It may prove fatal within a matter of weeks or smoulder on for months or even a year or two. The kidneys are commonly involved and there may be hypertension or haematuria; in the variant known as Wegener's granulomatosis the renal lesions are usually preceded by granulomas in the nasal passages or lungs. Infarcts in the intestines present with rapid loss of weight, malabsorption and bloody diarrhoea. Death may result from heart failure, uraemia or pulmonary complications.

Investigations

A normocytic, normochromic anaemia is usually accompanied by a neutrophil leucocytosis; eosinophilia is sometimes present. The ESR is usually grossly elevated and tests for antinuclear factor are often positive. The urine will contain protein, red cells and casts if the kidneys are involved, and the blood urea and serum creatinine will rise with decreasing renal function. Histological proof of the diagnosis is often very difficult to obtain but a biopsy of muscle, kidney or occasionally a skin lesion may provide the answer. In some patients the diagnosis is only confirmed at autopsy.

Polymyalgia rheumatica

Polymyalgia rheumatica is not uncommon in the elderly and is seen most frequently in women. The aetiology is unknown but at least a third of patients have been shown to have an accompanying cranial arteritis, confirmed by biopsy of a temporal artery. It may be abrupt or insidious in onset and presents with pain and stiffness in the shoulder and pelvic girdles. The stiffness is particularly prominent on waking but may wear off during the day. These symptoms are often accompanied by a low-grade fever, anorexia and loss of weight and are characteristically relieved by small doses of corticosteroids. The ESR is usually elevated but antibodies to IgG (rheumatoid factor) are found in less than 10% of cases.

Cranial arteritis (see also Head pain, p. 15)

Like polymyalgia rheumatica this disorder appears to be confined to the elderly of both sexes. It is due to a giant-cell arteritis affecting the larger arteries and may involve the aorta as well as its branches to the head and neck. Systemic manifestations include fever, anaemia, loss of weight and, in a significant proportion of cases, the symptoms of polymyalgia rheumatica.

Severe headache, mental confusion and presenile dementia are caused by inflammation of the cerebral and temporal arteries. Transient diplopia from ischaemia of the extra-ocular muscles may precede the sudden onset of blindness from occlusion of the terminal branches of the ophthalmic artery. Involvement of the facial artery leads to pain on chewing. Disappearance of the peripheral pulses in the upper limbs is due to inflammation of the vessels arising from the arch of the aorta.

Anaemia is usually mild but the ESR is often very high. Early treatment with corticosteroids is essential if the sight is to be preserved. Biopsy of a temporal artery will often confirm the diagnosis.

LOCAL CAUSES

Local sepsis in the mouth and ears will have been excluded by the initial examination. The search for pus elsewhere may be long and difficult. The temptation to treat blindly with antibiotics should be resisted for this will only make the task even harder.

Infective endocarditis

Aetiology

This potentially fatal disease is due to the colonisation of the valves of the heart by pathogenic microorganisms which have entered the circulation as a result of a transient bacteraemia or septicaemia. This leads to damage to the valves themselves with consequent cardiac failure, the release of septic emboli which may lodge in any tissue but have particularly grave consequences in the brain, and the production of circulating immune complexes causing a widespread vasculitis which is particularly evident in the skin, nails and glomeruli of the kidneys.

Streptococcus viridans is still the main causative organism in patients with chronic rheumatic heart disease, but the declining incidence of rheumatic fever in the developed countries has markedly reduced the numbers at risk. In these patients the infection usually reaches the heart as a result of a transient bacteraemia produced by dental treatment without adequate antibiotic cover.

In the UK nearly half the cases seen today arise in patients without any obvious pre-existing cardiac lesions, and are not due to *Streptococcus viridans* infection. *Staphylococcus aureus* is responsible for about 20%. Other infecting agents include *Strep. faecalis, Staph. epidermidis, Esch. coli, Pseudomonas aeruginosa*, fungi in immune-suppressed subjects and Coxiella burneti. Q fever endocarditis is commoner in men and only one third of the reported cases in Britain had a pre-existing cardiac abnormality.

Predisposing causes include the increasing age of the population and the development of atherosclerosis of the aortic valve, mitral valve prolapse, cardiac surgery, renal dialysis, urinary instrumentation in elderly men, nasotracheal intubation, gall-bladder disease and the increased use of intravenous cannulae which provide a ready portal of entry for microorganisms into the circulation. Endocarditis is a tragic consequence of intravenous narcotic abuse and of opportunistic infections in debilitated patients on high doses of immunosuppressive drugs.

Clinical features
These are very variable and are due to valvular damage, septicaemia, systemic embolism or immune complex disease. In the elderly there may be little to suggest this diagnosis but unexplained cardiac failure, changing heart murmurs, fever and loss of weight should arouse suspicion. A history of rheumatic fever in childhood, cardiac surgery, dental treatment or prolonged intravenous infusions are obviously important.

Embolism may result in hemiplegia, sudden blindness, ischaemic limbs, splenic infarcts and prolonged angina or myocardial infarction from coronary artery occlusion. It is unusual to see cachexia or marked anaemia but the spleen may be palpable. The patient should be carefully examined for conjunctival haemorrhages, vasculitic rashes, petechiae, splinter haemorrhages and tender nodules on the tips of the fingers (Osler's nodes). Finger clubbing is sometimes seen. In a suspected drug addict a search should be made for puncture marks.

Investigations
A mild normocytic, normochromic anaemia is usual with a high ESR. The white count is often normal but there may be a polymorph leukocytosis. At least three and preferably six separate specimens should be taken for blood culture as soon as possible and before commencing therapy. The bacteriologist should be asked to advise on the most appropriate antibiotics to use. Unfortunately, cultures are often sterile, even in patients with convincing physical signs and symptoms; this may be due to previous antibiotic therapy or an unusual organism such as *Candida* or *Coxiella burneti*.

Microscopic haematuria should be looked for as evidence of diffuse glomerulonephritis and urine should be sent for culture. The serum immunoglobulins may be raised and about half have positive auto-antibodies to IgG (rheumatoid factor).

Chest X-rays may show enlargement of the heart.

Echocardiography, if available, will demonstrate vegetations on the aortic or mitral valve in about 30% of cases.

Thyroid disorders

Fever is sometimes seen in hyperthyroidism but the diagnosis is usually obvious from the presence of a goitre and other physical signs of thyroid overactivity. Autoimmune thyroiditis occasionally presents with malaise, fever and an enlarged tender thyroid gland. High titres of thyroid antibodies will be found.

Pulmonary embolism

Recurrent small pulmonary emboli can cause unexplained fever and increasing dyspnoea on exertion, particularly in the elderly. There may be no clinical or ECG evidence of pulmonary hypertension, or of thrombophlebitis in the legs. Some cardiac enlargement may be evident on a chest X-ray but lung scans are useless for the lesions are too small to demonstrate. It is impossible to confirm this diagnosis except at autopsy, but a rapid improvement in the patient's condition after a week or so on a continuous intravenous heparin infusion is strong supporting evidence. A search should be made for an underlying cause; in a recent case a man was found to have hypothyroidism due to autoimmune disease and systemic lupus erythematosus. Occult malignancy, particularly in the pancreas or large bowel, is also associated with an increased risk of thromboembolism.

Hepatic disease

A low-grade fever is sometimes seen in chronic active hepatitis which is usually due to autoimmune disease in young women or a sequel to viral hepatitis B infection in others. There is often a history of malaise, anorexia and fluctuating jaundice. The liver function tests will be disturbed and liver biopsy will show the characteristic pathology.

Occasionally patients with hepatic cirrhosis suffer from episodic febrile illnesses due to *Esch. coli* bacteraemia. These come out of the blue with little warning. On examination spider naevi and liver palms may be found. Blood cultures should reveal the causative organism.

Hepatitis commonly accompanies amoebic dysentery but responds promptly to therapy. Sometimes, however, abscess formation takes place over the years with little or no evidence of its presence. This diagnosis should always be thought of in patients with a PUO who have lived in the tropics. The liver may be enlarged and tender and there will be a neutrophil leukocytosis. Filling defects in the liver will be found by ultrasound scanning or computerised tomography. The complement fixation test for amoebiasis is positive in about 90% of cases.

Finally, pyogenic abscesses of the liver may present with high fever and rigors following penetrating abdominal wounds, an attack of cholangitis or infection spreading from a pelvic abscess. Blood cultures may grow the organism and a liver scan, using ultrasound or computed tomography, may show multiple small filling defects. Laparotomy is essential to confirm the diagnosis and to establish drainage.

Cholangitis

This has already been mentioned as a cause of acute fever but it can present in a much more insidious way with loss of weight, malaise and intermittent fever. There may be nothing in the history or examination to implicate the biliary tract. The ESR is often grossly elevated but the white cell count may be normal. Gallstones may be visible on a plain X-ray of the abdomen or be demonstrated by ultrasound scanning or computerised tomography. Jaundice is present only if there is obstruction to the bile ducts, but the liver function tests are likely to be abnormal even when this is absent.

Subphrenic abscess

The aphorism 'pus somewhere, pus nowhere, pus below the diaphragm' remains a useful reminder of a puzzling cause of fever. Subphrenic abscess is a complication of penetrating abdominal injuries, perforation of a duodenal ulcer, acute pancreatitis or operations on the gastrointestinal tract. It has an insidious onset and a paucity of physical signs which may be masked by the administration of antibiotics or steroids. Early recognition and prompt surgical treatment is important for there is a very high mortality rate in the untreated patient.

The white count is raised with a neutrophil leukocytosis. Plain X-rays of chest and abdomen may show a sympathetic pleural effusion and gas below the diaphragm on the affected side. Ultrasonography or computed tomography provides the answer in over 90% of cases. The place of isotope scanning with technetium-99 or gallium-67 citrate to localise inflammatory foci in the abdomen is still uncertain and few centres have the necessary facilities.

Renal infection

Pyelonephritis is a common cause of prolonged fever in young children. There may be no accompanying urinary symptoms or loin pain but a urine specimen will usually contain pus cells and organisms. Perinephric abscess is a rare cause of a PUO and is usually associated with long-standing obstruction of the renal tract by calculi; there is often a history of recurrent urinary infections but the urine at the time may appear normal. An intravenous pyelogram will usually demonstrate some abnormality in both these disorders and a perinephric abscess should show up on computerised tomography.

Pelvic abscess

Pelvic peritonitis may be due to perforation of an inflamed appendix or colonic diverticulum, Crohn's disease or tubo–ovarian abscess. It presents with fever which is usually accompanied by hypogastric pain, frequency, dysuria, tenesmus or diarrhoea. There may be tenderness over the lower abdomen and on rectal or vaginal examination, and a mass may be palpable. Laparotomy is usually necessary to establish the diagnosis.

Prostatitis may present with an intermittent fever but local symptoms are more prominent. They include deep-seated pain and heaviness felt in the perineum which is increased by sitting and during micturition. A rectal examination is painful and induration is felt.

Neoplasia

Fever is not uncommon in malignant disease and may result from secondary infection of the tumour mass or the release of endogenous pyrogen from the neoplastic cells. The fever is often mild and intermittent so that it may be weeks or even months before the patient seeks medical advice. Some accompanying loss of weight is usual.

A prolonged fever is a well-recognised feature of the leukaemias and lymphomas. The diagnosis is usually confirmed by the blood picture, marrow examination or lymph node biopsy.

The association of fever with renal carcinoma has been well-documented, but the tumour may not show up on an intravenous pyelogram and symptoms pointing to the urinary tract may be absent. Carcinoma of the stomach and pancreas occasionally present as a PUO without any other symptoms, and pyrexia is not uncommon when a malignant melanoma has spread to the liver.

Radiological examination of the chest, alimentary tract and skeleton may provide some evidence to suspect neoplasia. Ultrasound scanning or computed tomography may demonstrate the presence of hepatic secondaries, renal tumour or enlarged lymph nodes in the abdomen or mediastinum. Surgical exploration is usually necessary to obtain histological proof.

CHAPTER 25

Coma

G. H. Hall

SYNOPSIS OF CAUSES*

CEREBRAL

TRAUMATIC
Concussion; Extradural and subdural haematoma.

CEREBROVASCULAR
Thrombosis; Embolism; Intracerebral haemorrhage; Subarachnoid haemorrhage;
Hypertensive encephalopathy; Eclampsia.

INFLAMMATORY
Meningitis; Encephalitis and encephalomyelitis; Abscess.

IDIOPATHIC
Epilepsy; Narcolepsy.

NEOPLASTIC
Primary and metastatic tumours.

GENERAL

CARDIOVASCULAR
Bradycardia; Tachycardia; Myocardial infarction; Pulmonary embolism; **Valvular stenosis**;
Dissecting aortic aneurysm.

TOXIC AND INFECTIVE
Drugs and poisons (incl. alcohol); Severe infections.

METABOLIC
Renal failure; Cholaemia; Hyperthermia; Hypothermia; Hypercapnia; Hypoxia;
Hyponatraemia.

ENDOCRINE
Diabetes mellitus; Hypoglycaemia; Adrenal failure; Hypothyroidism; Hypoparathyroidism.

PSYCHOGENIC
Hysteria.

---

* Bold type is used for causes more commonly found in Europe and North America.

PHYSIOLOGY

In coma, motor activity and sensory responsiveness are markedly reduced and the patient cannot be awakened. Because sensible communication with the patient is impossible, it is best to avoid such terms as 'levels of consciousness'. No conclusion can be drawn about the state of mind of a comatose patient. There is no recollection of a period of coma.

Coma is always due to a disturbance of brain-functioning as a whole. Physical factors which may produce such a global disturbance include head injury, electric shock, epilepsy, raised intracranial pressure and alterations of body temperature. Chemical factors include anoxia, hypoglycaemia and endogenous or exogenous intoxication.

Of all organs, the brain is the most dependent on the continuous provision of arterial blood at normal pressure and of normal composition for its function and survival. Cessation of cerebral circulation is followed by coma in less than a minute, and by irreversible brain damage after 5 minutes. Focal brain damage (e.g. by infarction or tumour) does not cause coma unless secondary effects develop (e.g. elevation of intracranial pressure).

A normal state of wakefulness and the ability to respond appropriately to environmental stimulation depend on proper functioning of the reticular formation in the brain stem and its connexions to the cerebrum. The universal ramifications of these extralemniscal systems ensure that only those conditions which affect the brain as a whole will produce coma, apart from those damaging the brain stem where it passes through the tentorium cerebelli.

The electrical activity of the brain, as recorded by the electroencephalogram, shows synchronous slow waves in sleep and coma, in contrast to the desynchronised patterns seen in the waking state. Occasional exceptions are seen, e.g. in the paradoxical association of consciousness and synchronous waves in atropine poisoning, and sleep with desynchronised waves in reserpine poisoning and lesions of the pons and tegmentum. It is important to remember that awareness may be preserved even though a patient may not be able to move or speak. An EEG is valuable in determining what residual brain function exists in deeply comatose patients.

Coma is not, of course, an all-or-nothing phenomenon. A continuous spectrum of clinical states ranges from mild confusion to total inanition, where 'life' can be maintained only by artificial and extraordinary means. From a practical point of view, five levels may be defined (modified after Symonds).

1. Responsive to verbal commands, but drowsy
2. Responsive to painful stimuli
3. Corneal reflexes preserved
4. Pupils unresponsive to light
5. Respiration ceases

The chief merit of this classification is to facilitate recognition of changes of depth of coma.

DIAGNOSTIC APPROACH

Coma is one of the few conditions (like arterial haemorrhage) where action must precede analysis. The patient cannot help himself, and the first step is to ensure that ventilation is adequate and that the airway is clear. It is best to lay the patient on his side while a rapid assessment and measurements of pulse, blood pressure, respiration and temperature are made. In case of shock, an immediate intravenous infusion may be necessary.

History
Of necessity, this must be second-hand. All available attendants, relatives, friends and medical advisers must be interviewed and the following questions included:

1. How was he found and by whom? Circumstances may point clearly to head injury, self-poisoning, asphyxia or exposure.
2. How rapid was the onset of coma? An abrupt onset suggests a local or general vascular cause, epilepsy or cardiac dysrhythmia. Coma developing over several hours may be due to drugs, virulent infections or extradural haematoma. More slowly developing coma is likely to be due to elevation of intracranial pressure by neoplasm or metabolic disturbance as in diabetes, uraemia, liver failure or myxoedema.
3. Was a convulsion observed, and if so, what was its type?
4. Have there been any previous episodes of this kind? Recurrent syncope is found in epilepsy, vasovagal attacks, spontaneous hypoglycaemia, Stokes–Adams attacks, diabetes and drug addicts.
5. Is the patient a known diabetic receiving insulin, or taking drugs of any kind? Hypoglycaemic attacks are the commonest cause of coma in diabetes. By the nature of their complaint, patients receiving antidepressants and tranquillisers are likely to take an overdose.
6. Fuller routine enquiry must be made about other past illnesses and familial disorders. Concealed haemorrhage, as in peptic ulceration and ectopic pregnancy, may present as coma.

Examination
The age, sex and general appearance of the patient will often afford valuable clues as to the cause. In the middle-aged and elderly cardiovascular accidents are by far the commonest causes of coma. In the young, head injury and drug overdosage predominate.

The following diagnostic signs must be sought:

Pallor:	haemorrhage or cardiogenic shock
Cyanosis:	hypoxia, hypoventilation, pulmonary embolism, polycythaemia and stroke
Jaundice:	cholaemia
Odorous breath:	diabetic ketosis, cholaemia, uraemia, alcohol

Cold skin:	shock, hypothermia
Shallow respiration:	drug overdose, raised intracranial pressure
Deep respiration:	diabetic ketosis, acidosis, pulmonary embolism, cerebral haemorrhage, aspirin poisoning, hypotension, shock
Slow pulse:	heart block, Stokes–Adams attack, raised intracranial pressure; tricyclic antidepressants
High temperature:	local and general infection, aspirin poisoning, pontine haemorrhage
Low temperature:	myxoedema, exposure, pituitary or hypothalamic insufficiency
Hypertension:	malignant hypertension, uraemia, raised intracranial pressure
Hypotension:	haemorrhage, shock, pulmonary embolism, coronary thrombosis, pituitary/adrenal insufficiency, poisoning, fulminant infections
Neck stiffness:	meningitis, subarachnoid haemorrhage
Optic fundi:	papilloedema, exudates and haemorrhage in malignant hypertension, expanding intracerebral lesions and uraemia
Dilated pupils:	midbrain damage, atropine poisoning
Constricted pupils:	morphine poisoning
Unequal pupils:	lateralising intracranial lesion, Horner's syndrome, neurosyphilis
Ophthalmoplegia:	'false localising sign' of intracranial lesion, berry aneurysm, neurosyphilis
Cardiac murmurs:	cerebral embolism, mycotic aneurysm, uraemic pericarditis
Hemiparesis or hemianaesthesia:	cerebrovascular accident. Todd's palsy (postepileptic)
Urinalysis:	glycosuria and ketonuria in diabetes, proteinuria in uraemia, ferric chloride test positive in aspirin poisoning
Skin:	petechiae in meningitis, bullae in barbiturate poisoning, coarse and dry in myxoedema

The physical examination should then be completed thoroughly including a pelvic examination.

Investigations
It is probable that the history and examination will reveal the diagnosis in most cases of coma. Confirmation may require certain other tests:

X-ray:	*Chest* — heart, bronchial neoplasm
	Skull — for fracture or signs of intracranial neoplasm.
	Computed tomography — non-invasive, safe and capable of detecting and distinguishing between most types of intracranial mass lesion
	Angiography
	Ventriculography
Biochemical:	Blood sugar, urea, electrolytes, calcium and drug levels
	CSF protein
	Urine — for drug detection
Haematological:	Full blood count
	Blood culture
Lumbar puncture:	Not to be undertaken in the presence of papilloedema without neurosurgical advice because of the risk of tentorial herniation
	Pressure
	Red and white cells
	Organisms; Culture
Electro encephalography:	For detection of epileptogenic foci
Electrocardiogram:	Cardiac dysrhythmia, coronary thrombosis, pulmonary embolism

As is the case with other symptom complexes, diagnosis of the causes of coma requires the matching of the observed clinical pattern with previously defined criteria identifying a 'disease state'. Of course, this is not always possible because one is not able to carry out the 'clinching' investigation, or because of gaps in the anamnesis. There can, however, be no excuse for failing to make a complete physical examination. It may be a platitude to remind the reader that 'common things occur commonly'; but an obscure clinical picture is more likely to be an atypical presentation of a banal disease, rather than a rare condition.

CEREBRAL CAUSES
TRAUMATIC

Concussion (see also Head pain, p. 17)

Sudden acceleration or deceleration of the head may suspend cerebral activity by mechanical distortion of the neurones and their intracellular contents. The interruption of purposive activity is usually momentary but it is often associated with pretraumatic (retrograde) and post-traumatic (anterograde) amnesia. The duration in these gaps in memory is a valuable guide to the severity of the injury. When coma is prolonged cerebral contusion or haemorrhage may be suspected, particularly when fits and palsies are observed.

Extradural and subdural haematoma

These have been considered in the chapter on Head pain.

CEREBROVASCULAR CAUSES

Cerebral thrombosis

Arterial thrombosis seldom results in coma unless the occlusion is in the basilar artery. When this occurs examination shows small fixed pupils, paralysis of deglutition, loss of the cough reflex, with an immediate threat to the airways, and spastic or flaccid quadriplegia. Death is an inevitable sequel, though it may be delayed by skilled nursing care.

Venous thrombosis is now most commonly observed in women about the time of childbirth or when taking sex hormones for contraception or control of menstruation. When the thrombosis is extensive coma may develop but it is often preceded by fits and hemiparesis.

Lumbar puncture generally yields a clear CSF under normal pressure. Diagnosis may be confirmed by angiography with special attention to the late phase as the veins fill with the dye.

Cerebral embolism

The embolus is most commonly a thrombus but it may occasionally be an air bubble from surgical procedures, a nitrogen bubble in decompression sickness or fat from a fracture site. It causes abrupt cessation of function in the area of brain supplied by the occluded vessel. A brief convulsion may be observed followed by a short period of coma and a neurological deficit appropriate to the area affected.

The condition must be suspected in patients with atrial fibrillation, because thrombi may develop in the left atrium. These may be released at any time but particularly with a return to normal atrial contraction, or as a result of electrical or chemical defibrillation. Cerebral emboli may be seen in subacute bacterial endocarditis.

Intracerebral haemorrhage

The patient, commonly elderly and hypertensive, is felled by severe headache, vomiting, coma and hemiplegia. The coma is deep and may persist for several days. The CSF is usually bloodstained and under raised pressure.

Subarachnoid haemorrhage (see also Head pain, p. 18)

There may be a sudden onset of intense headache with vomiting and loss of consciousness.

Hypertensive encephalopathy (see also Head pain, p. 25)

In hypertension an acute episode of increased blood pressure may occur abruptly or evolve within minutes or hours along with headache, dizziness, vomiting, convulsions and coma. If the pressure remains unrelieved death ensues.

Eclampsia

Toxaemia of pregnancy occurs during the last trimester, usually in primi-parae in the thirties. Hypertension is an early sign along with proteinuria and oedema. Convulsions and coma may develop even after delivery if the condition is severe.

INFLAMMATORY CAUSES

Meningitis, encephalitis and encephalomyelitis (see also Head pain, p. 11)

Direct infection occurs in bacterial meningitis and may do so in certain viral infections, or symptoms may result from an auto-allergic process engendered by the virus. Similar clinical effects are seen in generalised vascular diseases such as polyarteritis nodosa and systemic lupus erythematosus, or from infiltration by malignant cells, especially in leukaemia.

Encephalitis as a complication of a specific infection may be suspected when exceptional drowsiness and coma supervene after a period of delirium, and when neurological abnormalities of irregular pattern appear, such as cranial nerve palsies, in association with mild meningism and papilloedema. The appearance of a typical rash such as that of herpes zoster or the purpura of meningococcal meningitis may reveal the aetiology. Enquiries should be made about recent vaccination.

Disturbances of sleep rhythm and personality are frequent sequelae and Parkinsonism has been traced in some cases to past infection with a neurotropic virus, as in epidemic encephalitis lethargica.

The CSF generally, but not invariably, shows a lymphocytosis with a normal glucose concentration. The virus may be isolated from the CSF and from the body secretions.

Cerebral abscess

This has been discussed in the chapter on Head pain.

IDIOPATHIC CAUSES

Epilepsy

An epileptic attack is most commonly of the idiopathic kind due to an inherently unstable nervous system. The possibility of an underlying cause must be borne in mind, especially when the attack occurs for the first time in middle or old age; in the young, metabolic abnormalities like hypoglycaemia or hypocalcaemia must be considered.

In minor epilepsy (petit mal) ordinary activities are interrupted very briefly and are hardly noticed by the patient or those around him. Major epilepsy (grand mal) is characterised by an initial tonic phase with body and limbs in extension, and apnoea; this is succeeded rapidly by a clonic phase with repeated convulsive movements of the limbs and head.

The attack usually subsides in a matter of minutes. Incontinence of urine or faeces may occur, and occasionally the tongue is bitten. Sometimes the convulsions are succeeded by longer periods of stupor, automatic behaviour of which the patient has no recollection and paralysis of one or more parts of the body (Todd's palsy). Rarely the clonic phase is prolonged, as in status epilepticus.

Focal (Jacksonian) epilepsy is manifested by twitching which gradually extends over the limb, face or half of the body (the 'march') and may indicate the area of the brain in which the lesion is situated.

Eye-witness accounts of the attack usually suffice to suggest the diagnosis of epilepsy, as does the brevity of the coma. There is often a history of previous attacks in the patient, perhaps as convulsions in infancy, or in the other members of the family. Physical examination may reveal possible precipitating causes; e.g. malignant hypertension with severe retinopathy; cerebral tumour, with papilloedema; hypoglycaemia with sweating, tachycardia and irrational behaviour.

Investigations should normally include an X-ray of the skull and chest, an EEG and, in appropriate cases, biochemical tests to exclude hypocalcaemia, hypoglycaemia and uraemia.

Narcolepsy

This seldom requires urgent consideration, for the patient can be easily awakened. A history of such attacks should be obtainable from attendants or the family.

NEOPLASTIC CAUSES

Coma is an unusual presenting sign of intracranial neoplasm, whether benign or malignant (primary or secondary). It may occur suddenly, taking the form of status epilepticus, or it may be brought on by coning.

Coning may result from midbrain compression by herniation of the uncus through the tentorium cerebelli or herniation of the cerebellar tonsil through the foramen magnum. It is especially liable to occur after lumbar puncture when the supratentorial pressure is unduly high. Lumbar puncture should therefore be avoided when such a pressure may exist — as in the presence of papilloedema.

Persistent drowsiness after a fit or a stroke may indicate the presence of an intracranial space-occupying lesion, either in the brain or pituitary gland.

Preliminary investigations must include an X-ray of the chest to exclude bronchogenic carcinoma, which is a common source of secondary cerebral tumour.

GENERAL CAUSES

CARDIOVASCULAR

Inadequate perfusion of the brain may result in coma because of an abrupt fall of blood pressure. This may be caused by a sudden internal or external haemorrhage, the circulatory collapse from severe infection or poisoning, or reduced cardiac stroke volume in massive pulmonary embolism or myocardial infarction.

Bradycardia

Vasovagal attacks are seen in some subjects from a simultaneous fall in blood pressure and slowing of the heart rate. The period of unconsciousness in this common form of fainting is brief.

Disease of the conducting mechanism of the heart affecting as a rule the atrioventricular node is due usually to arteriosclerotic ischaemia. It may also result from degenerative conditions or from a toxic cause such as digitalis overdosage. It is seen characteristically in Stokes–Adams attacks, in which an elderly subject falls abruptly and without warning; loss of consciousness is momentary. A history of such attacks should be obtainable.

In heart block an ECG is necessary for proper characterisation and localisation of the abnormality of conduction.

Tachycardia

The cause of tachycardia have been discussed elsewhere. When the heart rate is too great to permit adequate systole to occur (over 150/min) perfusion of the brain may be inadequate and loss of consciousness may result.

Cardiac infarction (see also Thoracic pain, p. 34)

Unconsciousness, commonly leading to a fatal termination, occurs in a severe attack.

Pulmonary embolism (see also Thoracic pain, p. 30)

Obstruction to the flow of blood through the great pulmonary vessels, and consequently through the heart, may result in loss of consciousness when a major embolism has occurred.

Valvular stenosis

Brief syncopal attacks are common in pulmonary and aortic stenosis. They are less often seen in myxoma and ball-valve thrombus of the left atrium. When the obstruction to blood flow is severe enough to cause cerebral symptoms, however, congestive manifestations in the lungs and jugular engorgement are predominant. In such cases extreme pallor and sweating occur. Whilst the characteristic murmurs should be audible they may disappear during periods of extremely low cardiac output.

Dissecting aortic aneurysm

Aneurysm of the aorta is discussed in the chapter on Thoracic pain.

TOXIC AND INFECTIVE CAUSES

Drugs and poisons

Inadvertent or deliberate administration of overdoses of analgesic, sedative or psychotropic drugs are possibly the commonest causes of coma nowadays among patients admitted to hospital. The diagnosis is often made clear by information obtained by the attendant concerning the subject's personal life; despair or disappointment makes a temporary escape into oblivion imperative; suicide is seldom intended. There may be a history of anxiety or depression or of previous attempts at suicide.

Insulin overdose

While it is strictly a drug cause, insulin overdose has been put with diabetic coma in the Endocrine section of causes of coma.

Digitalis poisoning

Overdose may induce heart block and unconsciousness. There should be a history of digitalis therapy for heart disease and preceding nausea and vomiting.

Barbiturate poisoning

In barbiturate poisoning, life appears to be at a low ebb with failure to reply to questions, to respond to commands or to respond to painful stimuli. The patient appears to be deeply asleep. The temperature, pulse rate and blood pressure are all depressed and corneal reflexes may disappear. Respiration may have to be maintained artificially if ventilation is poor, as judged clinically and by analysis of the arterial blood gases. There must be no delay in removing the poison from the body by gastric lavage, purging and forced diuresis when these measures are appropriate.

Psychotropic drug poisoning

The tranquillisers, antidepressant and euphoriant drugs may induce initial excitement, convulsions and cranial nerve dysfunction (e.g. oculogyric spasms) and these may precede coma.

Alcoholic poisoning

Familiarity with this condition should not breed contempt for its dangers. The circumstances and the appearance of the patient may be suggestive and the odour of the breath characteristic. The patient must be examined for other conditions such as cirrhosis or head injury.

Hypotensive drugs

These are a common cause of postural hypotension, which is seen typically on rising in the morning.

Aspirin poisoning

Of the drugs used for self-poisoning this is often the most lethal. Inhibition of aerobic glycolysis leads to severe acidosis and marked hyperpnoea. The body temperature fluctuates widely and ultimately respiratory and cardiac failure supervene unless treatment is begun early enough. The urine will show a positive ferric chloride test but a negative Rothera's test.

Carbon monoxide poisoning

The advent of natural (alkane) gas has reduced the hazard of poisoning by coal gas, in which carbon monoxide is present. The carbon monoxide displaces oxygen from haemoglobin even when present in small amounts. There is likely to be a history of exposure. The patient, though in coma from a state of severe tissue anoxia, may be pink in colour. The diagnosis may be confirmed by spectroscopic identification of carboxyhaemoglobin.

Poisoning in children

Children in the exploratory years (2–5) are at a risk from the taking not only of tablets from the drug cupboard but also of common household substances.

Severe infections

Fulminating infections and septicaemia may depress brain function to the point of coma. Prominent among the causes are meningococcal, strepto-coccal and staphylococcal infections of brain or lungs, typhoid and, in the tropics, cerebral malaria and trypanosomiasis.

The onset is usually rapid, coming within hours of onset of the illness the specific features of which may be apparent. Fever and hypotension are likely to be present. A blood film and culture and CSF examination may be necessary to establish diagnosis.

METABOLIC CAUSES

Renal failure

Coma is a late event in renal failure and death is near unless resuscitation by dialysis is possible. The diagnosis may be clear from the nature of the preceding illness but occasionally the possibility has not been considered or the patient is seen by the medical attendant for the first time and without a history.

The complexion is muddy and the mucous membranes are pale. Breathing is deep and rapid because of the state of acidosis and the breath is foul and ammoniacal in odour. The degree of hydration is variable and often the upper part of the body is dehydrated, while oedema is present in the dependent parts. Generalised twitching and occasional convulsions may be seen. Hypertension and retinopathy are always present and a pericardial friction rub can usually be heard.

The urine is scanty and contains protein. The blood urea is high, perhaps 50 mmol/l (300 mg/100 ml) or more, and there is usually a normochromic anaemia. Hyperkalaemia (over 7 mmol/l) is a common cause of death.

Cholaemia

Coma from cerebral complications in acute liver failure is thought to be due to the inability to detoxicate nitrogenous substances such as ammonia and glutamine absorbed from the bowel. In acute liver failure, although blood passes through the liver the cells are unable to perform their function of detoxication.

In cirrhosis these nitrogenous substances may enter the systemic circulation through the portal–systemic anastomoses which develop when drainage of the portal vein is impeded by cirrhosis. In either event, the brain is progressively affected. The patient will pass through phases of disordered thought and behaviour, delirium, stupor and finally coma. Foetor hepatis is pathognomonic and is thought to be due to volatile mercaptans. The flapping tremor is not, as was once believed, confined to liver failure, but is seen also in uraemia and hypercapnia. Spider naevi and red palms are useful indications of severe liver dysfunction, jaundice is usually present and the liver and spleen may be enlarged.

Tests of liver function will be grossly disturbed and the EEG will show characteristic abnormalities.

Hyperthermia

Oral temperatures of over 41.0°C (106°F) are rare in man and lead to impairment of consciousness and convulsions. Hyperpyrexia, or heat stroke, may occur in the healthy in hot weather with high humidity and a cessation of sweating. Hyperthermia may occur in cerebral lesions, including strokes and in severe infections.

Hypothermia

This condition is easily overlooked if an ordinary clinical thermometer is used. It is seen most commonly in the elderly who, through poverty and neglect, inhabit cold rooms. Such patients are often admitted to hospital with the diagnosis of 'a stroke'. The possibility of primary or secondary hypothyroidism must be borne in mind. The circumstance and history are important and the examiner's hand is the best guide to the state of hypothermia. A low registering thermometer may give a reading as low as 33°C (91°F) or less. At this level there is loss of consciousness.

Hypercapnia

Carbon dioxide retention may be due to inadequate elimination by the alveoli and is seen chiefly in chronic lung disease and particularly in emphysema complicated by bronchitis. It leads to narcosis, muscular twitching, flapping tremor and unconsciousness and may be aggravated by the giving of oxygen. Breathing is laboured or depressed and there is venous dilatation of the extremities; papilloedema may be present.

The onset may be insidious or precipitated by secondary lung infection. The arterial blood will show a raised Pco_2 and HCO_3 content. The pH may be normal or low depending upon the degree of renal compensation of the respiratory acidosis.

Hypoxia

Deficient intake of oxygen may occur in the asphyxia of drowning, in acute pulmonary oedema, from the inhalation of non-oxygen containing gases or carbon monoxide (referred to above under Poisons), in severe anaemia and in congestive cardiac failure. If acute, hypoxia will cause immediate coma.

Chronic hypoxia with slow adaptation is characterised by cyanosis. However, coma itself, arising from other causes, may precipitate hypoxia by depression of the respiratory centre or by allowing airway obstruction to occur uncorrected by the normal reflexes of coughing and swallowing.

If assisted respiration is applied the gases given must be checked regularly, especially in the presence of cyanosis. Measurement of the arterial blood oxygen saturation and Po_2 will confirm the presence of significant hypoxia.

Hyponatraemia

Stupor or even coma may occur when the serum sodium level falls below

120 mmol/l. This happens after excessive diuretic administration and in certain forms of acute and chronic chest disease, especially oat-cell carcinoma of the bronchus (syndrome of inappropriate secretion of antidiuretic hormone).

ENDOCRINE CAUSES

Diabetes mellitus (see also Loss of weight, p. 280)

Happily, the symptoms of diabetes are sufficiently troublesome to stimulate the sufferer to obtain medical help before coma develops. In an established diabetic who is insulin-dependent, omission of the usual dose leads to a rise in the blood sugar and ketosis. This omission may be because of anorexia from an infective process which will itself accentuate the hyperglycaemia and ketosis. In occasional cases coma may develop with extreme hyperglycaemia in the absence of ketosis.

This condition is thought to be due to extreme hyperosmolality of the blood, leading to cerebral dehydration. It may be contrasted with the 'dysequilibrium syndrome' which often produces coma and may appear after rapid dialysis; the brain becomes oedematous because of hypoosmolality of the blood.

In diabetic coma the patient is flushed and dehydrated, there is dyspnoea and the blood pressure is low. The smell of exhaled ketones may be apparent on approaching the bed.

The urine contains large amounts of sugar and ketones and the blood sugar is much raised, often over 25 mmol/l (500 mg/100 ml). The serum bicarbonate may be less than 10 mmol/l.

Hypoglycaemia

Even well-controlled insulin-dependent diabetics may suffer from occasional attacks of hypoglycaemia. These may be precipitated by actual overdose or by accidental intravenous injection, by omission of a meal or by untoward exertion.

The onset of coma may be abrupt or it may be preceded by irrational or violent behaviour. It differs in this way from diabetic coma, which usually takes several hours or days to develop. In insulin coma the patient is usually pale, sweating and restless; tachycardia and a low blood pressure are present, the pupils are dilated and there may be convulsions.

Because of the time lag, examination of the urine may be misleading because of the presence of sugar secreted earlier. Acetone is absent. The blood sugar is invariably less than 2.0 mmol/l (38 mg/100 ml) and recovery is prompt following the intravenous injection of 20–40 g of glucose. This is a useful therapeutic trial in the absence of biochemical facilities.

A blood sugar level persisting below 1.5 mmol/l (27 mg/100 ml) for an hour or two may result in hypoglycaemic encephalopathy. Coma is profound with convulsions and irreversible cerebral damage may occur.

Coma may result from an excessive secretion of insulin by an islet-cell tumour of the pancreas. Retroperitoneal sarcomas may also produce hypoglycaemia.

Adrenal failure (see also Loss of weight, p. 283)

A crisis of acute adrenal insufficiency may arise in Addison's disease, taking the form of vomiting, abdominal pain and often fever, along with collapse and even coma.

Hypothyroidism (see also Obesity, p. 291)

In this chronic and commonly unrecognised disorder a sudden stress such as infection, trauma or anaesthesia may precipitate a crisis. Hypothermia, hypoglycaemia and arterial hypotension are likely to be present. A thyroidectomy scar should be looked for. Secondary hypothyroidism may result from pituitary ablation by tumour or following postpartum shock (Sheehan's syndrome).

Hypoparathyroidism

In this condition tetany and fits may precede actual coma. Diarrhoea may be an important premonitory symptom. The presence of a thyroidectomy scar should arouse suspicion. The symptoms are due to a low serum calcium level and may also be seen in steatorrhoea, rickets and uraemia. The serum calcium is usually below 1.5 mmol/l (6 mg/100 ml).

PSYCHOGENIC CAUSES

Hysteria

Classical hysteria is very rare in men. A history of instability commonly goes back to adolescence and a full account of the subject's reaction to illnesses and to difficulties at home, at school and later should be obtained.

Almost any physiological system may be involved and the patient may be brought to hospital with amnesia or simulated loss of consciousness. Whilst the usual careful examination must not be omitted a vigorous test of the corneal reflex rapidly determines the issue.

Appendix
Normal values

The international system of units (SI units) has been adopted in many countries including the UK, but the more traditional units are still widely employed elsewhere. It is therefore necessary to list normal values in both SI and traditional units in the tables which follow. In some instances, however, particularly in biochemistry, it is not possible to give an SI value as the precise molecular structure of the substance being estimated is unknown.

Results in SI units can be converted to other units by multiplying them by the conversion factors shown in the tables; conversely, results in other units can be changed to SI units by dividing them by the appropriate conversion factor.

Normal ranges vary from one laboratory to another depending upon the methods used and the age and sex of the patient. The figures given here are those in use at the Royal Devon and Exeter Hospital and apply to adults; where sex differences are known to exist these are indicated in the tables.

Consultation between clinician and pathologist is essential when special investigations are requested or when there is doubt about the correct procedure for obtaining specimens. This should be the rule rather than, as it tends to be at present, the exception. Polypeptide hormone assays, in particular, can produce misleading results if the samples are collected at the wrong time of day and are not kept on ice until they reach the endocrine laboratory.

It is important that all specimens reach the laboratory without delay and are properly labelled with the patient's name, time of sampling and the date. The accompanying form should contain such relevant information as the full name, age and sex of the patient. In hospital the consultant's name, ward or department and patient's index number must be supplied if the results of the tests are to reach their proper destination. In general practice the name of the doctor requesting the test should be given.

If pathologists are to help in the interpretation of the results they must be provided with sufficient clinical details to understand the problem. Details of any drugs currently or recently taken should be recorded on the form in all cases of blood disorders, jaundice or suspected endocrine disease. Whilst they may not necessarily be responsible for the patient's condition they may, by interfering with the assay, produce spurious results.

HAEMATOLOGY

Estimation		SI units	Factor	Other units
Haemoglobin	— men	14–18 g/dl	1	14–18 g/100 ml
	— women	12–16 g/dl	1	12–16 g/100 ml
RBC	— men	$4.5–6.5 \times 10^{12}/l$	1	$4.5–6.5$ M/mm^3
	— women	$3.9–5.6 \times 10^{12}/l$	1	$3.9–5.6$ M/mm^3
PCV	— men	0.40–0.54	100	40–54%
	— women	0.36–0.47	100	36–47%
MCV		75–95 fl	1	75–95 cμ
MCH		27–32 pg	1	27–32 pg
MCHC		30–35 g/dl	1	30–35%
WBC		$4–11 \times 10^9/l$	1000	4000–11 000/mm^3
Polymorphs		$2.5–7.5 \times 10^9/l$	1000	2500–7500/mm^3
Lymphocytes		$1.5–3.5 \times 10^9/l$	1000	1500–3500/mm^3
Monocytes		$0.2–0.8 \times 10^9/l$	1000	200–800/mm^3
Eosinophils		$0.04–0.44 \times 10^9/l$	1000	40–440/mm^3
Basophils		$0.02–0.10 \times 10^9/l$	1000	20–100/mm^3
Platelets		$150–400 \times 10^9/l$	1000	150 000–400 000/mm^3
Reticulocytes		—	—	0.2–2.0%
ESR (Westergren)		—	—	< 15 mm/h
Serum iron		14–29 μmol/l	5.7	80–165 μg/dl
Total iron-binding capacity (TIBC)		45–72 μmol/l	5.7	256–410 μg/dl
Serum ferritin		15–300 μg/l	—	—
Serum B$_{12}$		160–950 ng/l	1	160–950 pg/ml
Serum folate		3–20 μg/l	1	3–20 ng/ml
Plasma fibrinogen		1.5–4.0 g/l	100	150–400 mg/dl
Prothrombin time		—	—	10–14 s
Partial thromboplastin time (Eastham)		—	—	34–42 s

BLOOD BIOCHEMISTRY

Estimation	SI units	Factor	Other units
Carbon dioxide (P$_a$co$_2$)	4.5–6.1 kPa	7.5	34–46 mmHg
Glucose (fasting)	3.3–5.8 mmol/l	18	59–104 mg/dl
Glycosylated haemoglobin			5.4–7.8%
Lead	0.5–2.0 μmol/l	20	10–40 μg/dl
Oxygen, arterial (P$_a$o$_2$)	12–15 kPA	7.5	90–110 mmHg
Pyruvate	41–67 μmol/l	0.009	0.4–0.6 mg/dl

SERUM BIOCHEMISTRY

Estimation	SI units	Factor	Other units
Acid phosphatase	—	—	0–3 IU/l
Albumin	32–50 g/l	0.1	3.2–5.0 g/dl
Alanine aminotransferase	—	—	5–50 IU/l
Alkaline phosphatase	—	—	25–85 IU/l
Amylase	—	—	70–300 U/l
Aspartate aminotransferase	—	—	0–25 IU/l
Bicarbonate	22–30 mmol/l	1	22–30 mEq/l
Bilirubin	3–17 μmol/l	0.06	0.2–1.0 mg/dl
Calcium (total)	2.2–2.62 mmol/l	4	8.8–10.5 mg/dl
Calcium (ionised)	1.07–1.27 mmol/l	4	4.3–5.1 mg/dl
Carotene	0.9–3.6 μmol/l	56	50–200 μg/dl
Chloride	96–106 mmol/l	1	96–106 mEq/l
Cholesterol	3.7–6.9 mmol/l	39	145–270 mg/dl
Copper	13–24 μmol/l	6.2	80–150 μg/dl
Creatine kinase (CK)			
— male	—	—	0–182 IU/l
— female	—	—	0–130 IU/l
Creatinine	44–124 μmol/l	0.011	0.5–1.4 mg/dl
Fibrinogen (plasma)	1.5–4.0 g/l	100	150–400 mg/dl
Gammaglutamyl transferase	—	—	0–60 IU/l
Glucose, plasma (fasting)	4.2–6.5 mmol/l	18	76–117 mg/dl
Iron	14–29 μmol/l	5.7	80–165 μg/dl
Immunoglobulins — IgA	1.3–4.3 g/l	—	—
— IgG	5.0–16.0 g/l	—	—
— IgM	0.5–1.7 g/l	—	—
Lactate dehydrogenase	—	—	160–480 IU/l
Magnesium	0.7–1.0 mmol/l	2.4	1.7–2.4 mg/dl
Phosphate	0.8–1.45 mmol/l	3.1	2.5–4.5 mg/dl
Potassium	3.5–5.5 mmol/l	1	3.5–5.5 mEq/l
Protein (total)	61–80 g/l	0.1	6.1–8.0 g/dl
Sodium	132–144 mmol/l	1	132–144 mEq/l
Triglycerides (fasting)	0.82–1.93 mmol/l	89	73–172 mg/dl
Urate — male	0.21–0.43 mmol/l	17	3.6–7.3 mg/dl
— female	0.16–0.36 mmol/l	17	2.7–6.1 mg/dl
Urea	2.5–6.6 mmol/l	6	15–40 mg/dl
Zinc	11.5–25.0 μmol/l	6.4	74–160 μg/dl

URINE BIOCHEMISTRY

Estimation	SI units	Factor	Other units
Adrenaline	0–0.1 μmol/24 h	183	0–18 μg/24 h
Calcium	2.5–7.5 mmol/24 h	40	100–300 mg/24 h
Catecholamines (total)	0.04–0.55 μmol/24 h	170	7–94 μg/24 h
Creatinine	9–17 mmol/24 h	0.115	1.0–2.0 g/24 h
Hydroxyindole-acetic acid	4.6–36.2 μmol/24 h	0.2	0.9–7.2 mg/24 h
Hydroxymethoxy-mandelic acid (HMMA)	10–35 μmol/24 h	0.2	2–7 mg/24 h
Hydroxyproline	3–31 μmol/mmol creatinine	1.16	3–36 mg/g creatinine
Noradrenaline	0–0.45 μmol/24 h	169	0–76 μg/24 h
Porphobilinogen	0.9–8.8 μmol/24 h	0.225	0.2–2.0 mg/24 h
Potassium	30–90 mmol/24 h	1	30–90 mEq/24 h
Protein	< 0.06 g/24 h	1000	< 60 mg/24 h
Uric acid	1.4–4.4 mmol/24 h	0.17	0.2–0.8 g/24 h

CEREBROSPINAL FLUID

Estimation	SI units	Factor	Other units
White cell count	< 0.005 × 10⁹/l	1000	< 5/mm³
Protein	0.15–0.50 g/l	100	15–50 mg/dl
Glucose	2.5–5.5 mmol/l	18	45–99 mg/dl

FAECES

Estimation	SI units	Factor	Other units
Fat★	11–25 mmol/24 h	0.28	3–7 g/24 h
Coproporphyrin	0–31 nmol/g dry weight	0.66	0–20 μg/g dry weight
Protoporphyrin	0–53 nmol/g dry weight	0.57	0–30 μg/g dry weight

★ Average over at least four consecutive 24-hour periods: fat intake > 100 g/day

SERUM HORMONE ASSAYS

Estimation	SI units	Factors	Other units
Aldosterone — morning	0.28–0.84 nmol/l	36	10–30 ng/dl
ACTH — 0900 h	10–80 ng/l	—	—
Cortisol — 0900 h	160–725 nmol/l	0.036	6–26 µg/dl
— midnight	< 185 nmol/l	0.036	< 7 µg/dl
FSH — men	—	—	1.0–10.0 IU/l
— women			
Follicular phase	—	—	2.0–10.6 IU/l
Midcycle	—	—	9.0–31.0 IU/l
Luteal phase	—	—	2.0–9.0 IU/l
Growth hormone (fasting)	< 20 mU/l	0.5	< 10 ng/ml
11-Hydroxycorticoids — 0900 h	140–666 nmol/l	0.036	5–24 µg/100 ml
— midnight	< 220 nmol/l	0.036	< 8 µg/100 ml
25-Hydroxycholecalciferol	8–80 nmol/l	0.38	3–30 µg/ml
17-Hydroxyprogesterone — newborn infant	< 5 nmol/l	33	< 165 ng/100ml
— adults	0.9–18 nmol/l	33	30–600 ng/100 ml
LH — men	—	—	2.2–12.0 IU/l
— women			
Follicular phase	—	—	3.0–13.0 IU/l
Midcycle	—	—	20–70 IU/l
Luteal phase	—	—	3.0–13.0 IU/l
Oestradiol — men	55–165 pmol/l	0.0272	1.5–4.5 ng/dl
— women			
Early follicular phase	110–183 pmol/l	0.0272	3–5 ng/dl
Pre-ovulatory peak	550–1650 pmol/l	0.0272	15–45 ng/dl
Luteal phase	550–845 pmol/l	0.0272	15–23 ng/dl
Parathyroid hormone	0–60 pmol/l	—	—
Progesterone — women			
Follicular phase	1.1–5.2 nmol/l	31	34–161 ng/dl
Luteal phase	13.7–72.4 nmol/l	31	425–2244 ng/dl
Mid-luteal phase	25.3–74.3 nmol/l	31	784–2300 ng/dl
Prolactin — men	—	—	0–380 mIU/l
— women			
Premenopausal	—	—	0–624 mIU/l
Postmenopausal	—	—	0–416 mIU/l
Testosterone — men	10.4–34.6 nmol/l	28.9	300–1000 ng/dl
— women	0.7–2.8 nmol/l	28.9	20–81 ng/dl
Thyroxine (T_4)	58–170 nmol/l	0.08	4.6–13.6 µg/dl
Triiodothyronine (T_3)	1.2–2.8 nmol/l	65	78–182 ng/dl
Thyroxine-binding globulin (TBG)	6–16 mg/l	—	—
TSH	0.15–3.5 mu/l	—	—

URINE HORMONE ASSAYS

Estimation	SI units	Factor	Other units
Adrenaline	0–0.1 μmol/24 h	183	0–18 μg/24 h
Aldosterone (18-conjugate)	14–56 nmol/24 h	0.36	5–20 μg/24 h
Catecholamines (total)	0.04–0.55 μmol/24 h	170	7–94 μg/24 h
Cortisol	160–462 nmol/24 h	0.36	58–166 μg/24 h
11-Hydroxycorticoids	220–880 nmol/24 h	0.36	80–320 μg/24 h
Overnight urine	< 280 nmol/8 h	0.36	< 100 μg/8 h
HMMA	10–35 μmol/24 h	0.2	2–7 mg/24 h
Noradrenaline	0–0.45 μmol/24 h	169	0–76 μg/24 h

Index

Main references are in bold type